Innovations in Stroke Recovery and Rehabilitation

Editors

JOAN STILLING
JOEL STEIN

PHYSICAL MEDICINE AND REHABILITATION CLINICS OF NORTH AMERICA

www.pmr.theclinics.com

Consulting Editor
BLESSEN C. EAPEN

May 2024 • Volume 35 • Number 2

ELSEVIER

1600 John F. Kennedy Boulevard • Suite 1800 • Philadelphia, Pennsylvania, 19103-2899

http://www.theclinics.com

PHYSICAL MEDICINE AND REHABILITATION CLINICS OF NORTH AMERICA Volume 35, Number 2 May 2024 ISSN 1047-9651, 978-0-443-13117-2

Editor: Megan Ashdown
Developmental Editor: Nitesh Barthwal

Reprints. For copies of 100 or more of articles in this publication, please contact the Commercial Reprints Department, Elsevier Inc., 360 Park Avenue South, New York, NY 10010-1710. Tel.: 212-633-3874; Fax: 212-633-3820; E-mail: reprints@elsevier.com.

Physical Medicine and Rehabilitation Clinics of North America (ISSN 1047-9651) is published quarterly by Elsevier Inc., 360 Park Avenue South, New York, NY 10010-1710. Months of issue are February, May, August, and November. Business and Editorial Offices: 1600 John F. Kennedy Blvd., Suite 1800, Philadelphia, PA 19103-2899. Customer Service Office: 3251 Riverport Lane, Maryland Heights, MO 63043. Periodicals postage paid at New York, NY and additional mailing offices. Subscription price per year is $352.00 (US individuals), $100.00 (US students), $400.00 (Canadian individuals), $100.00 (Canadian students), $506.00 (foreign individuals), and $210.00 (foreign students). For institutional access pricing please contact Customer Service via the contact information below. Foreign air speed delivery is included in all *Clinics* subscription prices. All prices are subject to change without notice. **POSTMASTER:** Send address changes to *Physical Medicine and Rehabilitation Clinics of North America*, Customer Service Office: Elsevier Health Sciences Division, Subscription Customer Service, 3251 Riverport Lane, Maryland Heights, MO 63043. **Customer Service: 1-800-654-2452 (US). From outside of the United States, call 314-447-8871. Fax: 314-447-8029. E-mail: JournalsCustomerService-usa@elsevier.com (for print support); JournalsOnlineSupport-usa@elsevier.com (for online support).**

Physical Medicine and Rehabilitation Clinics of North America is indexed in *Excerpta Medica, MEDLINE/ PubMed (Index Medicus), Cinahl, and Cumulative Index to Nursing and Allied Health Literature.*

Contributors

CONSULTING EDITOR

BLESSEN C. EAPEN, MD
Chief, VA Greater Los Angeles Health Care System, Associate Clinical Professor Division of Physical Medicine and Rehabilitation, Department of Medicine David Geffen School of Medicine at UCLA Los Angeles, California, USA

EDITORS

JOAN STILLING, MD, MS, FRCPC
Assistant Professor, Department of Rehabilitation Medicine, Weill Cornell Medicine, NewYork-Presbyterian Hospital; Adjunct Assistant Professor, Department of Rehabilitation and Regenerative Medicine, Columbia University Vagelos College of Physicians and Surgeons, New York, New York, USA

JOEL STEIN, MD
Physiatrist-in-Chief, NewYork-Presbyterian Hospital; Simon Baruch Professor, Department of Rehabilitation and Regenerative Medicine, Columbia University Vagelos College of Physicians and Surgeons; Professor, Department of Rehabilitation Medicine, Weill Cornell Medicine, New York, New York, USA

AUTHORS

SUZANNE ACKERLEY, PhD
Senior Research Fellow, School of Sport and Health Sciences, University of Central Lancashire, Preston, United Kingdom

JODI ARATA, MS, CCC-SLP
Speech Language Pathologist, Rehabilitation Research Lab, University of Maryland Rehabilitation and Orthopedic Institute, Baltimore, Maryland, USA

ALEXA BOYER, MASc
Masters Student, Department of Clinical Neurosciences, Cumming School of Medicine; Department of Biomedical Engineering, Schulich School of Engineering, University of Calgary, Calgary, Alberta, Canada

ROBYNNE G. BRAUN, MD, PhD
Assistant Professor, Department of Neurology, University of Maryland School of Medicine; Director, Brain Rehab and Recovery Lab, University of Maryland, Baltimore, Maryland, USA

JOHN CHAE, MD
Professor, MetroHealth Rehabilitation Institute, MetroHealth System, Case Western Reserve University, Cleveland, Ohio, USA

TRACY Y. CHANG, MD
Neurologist, Department of Neurology, UCLA, California Rehabilitation Institute, Los Angeles, California, USA

AUDRIE A. CHAVEZ, MD, MPH
Brain Injury Medicine Fellow, Spaulding Rehabilitation, Harvard University, Cambridge, Massachusetts, USA

CHIH-HAO CHEN, MD, PhD
Clinical Assistant Professor, Department of Clinical Neurosciences, University of Calgary, Calgary, Alberta, Canada; Department of Neurology, National Taiwan University Hospital, Taipei, Taiwan

STEVEN C. CRAMER, MD
Stroke Neurologist, Department of Neurology, UCLA, California Rehabilitation Institute, Los Angeles, California, USA

SARA J. CUCCURULLO, MD
Physiatrist, Department of Physical Medicine and Rehabilitation, JFK Johnson Rehabilitation Institute at Hackensack Meridian Health, Edison, New Jersey, USA

DAVID A. CUNNINGHAM, PhD
Cleveland FES Center; Assistant Professor, Department of Physical Medicine and Rehabilitation, MetroHealth System, MetroHealth Center for Rehabilitation Research, Case Western Reserve University, Cleveland, Ohio, USA

SEAN P. DUKELOW, PhD, MD, FRCPC
Professor, Division of Physical Medicine and Rehabilitation, Department of Clinical Neurosciences, Cumming School of Medicine, University of Calgary; Hotchkiss Brain Institute, Calgary, Alberta, Canada

JAMIE L. FLEET, MD, FRCPC
Physiatrist, Parkwood Institute Research, Parkwood Institute, St. Joseph's Health Care London; Department of Physical Medicine and Rehabilitation, Schulich School of Medicine and Dentistry, University of Western Ontario, London, Ontario, Canada

TALYA K. FLEMING, MD
Physiatrist, Department of Physical Medicine and Rehabilitation, JFK Johnson Rehabilitation Institute at Hackensack Meridian Health, Edison, New Jersey, USA

ARAVIND GANESH, MD, DPhil(Oxon) FRCPC
Assistant Professor, Department of Clinical Neurosciences, University of Calgary, Calgary, Alberta, Canada

MARLIS GONZALEZ-FERNANDEZ, MD, PhD
Associate Professor of PM&R and Orthopedic Surgery, Vice Chair of Clinical Affairs, Department of PM&R, Johns Hopkins University School of Medicine, Baltimore, Maryland, USA

AMBER HARNETT, RN, MSc
Parkwood Institute Research, Parkwood Institute, London, Ontario, Canada

ARGYE E. HILLIS, MD, MA
Neurologist, Department of Neurology, Johns Hopkins School of Medicine, Baltimore, Maryland, USA

NNEKA L. IFEJIKA, MD, MPH
Section Chief of Stroke Rehabilitation and Professor, Departments of Physical Medicine and Rehabilitation, and Neurology, UT Southwestern Medical Center, Dallas, Texas, USA

ABHISHEK JAYWANT, PhD
Psychologist, Departments of Psychiatry and Rehabilitation Medicine, Weill Cornell Medicine, NewYork-Presbyterian Hospital, Weill Cornell Medical Center, New York, New York, USA

HARRY JORDAN, PhD
Research Fellow, Department of Medicine, University of Auckland, Auckland, New Zealand

ALEXANDRA KEENAN, BA
Department of Rehabilitation Medicine, Weill Cornell Medicine, New York, New York, USA

JAYME S. KNUTSON, PhD
Director of Research, Department of Physical Medicine and Rehabilitation, MetroHealth Center for Rehabilitation Research, Cleveland FES Center, Case Western Reserve University, Cleveland, Ohio, USA

KELLY A. LARKIN-KAISER, PhD
Assistant Research Professor, Department of Clinical Neurosciences, Cumming School of Medicine, Hotchkiss Brain Institute, Ablerta Children's Hospital Research Institute, University of Calgary, Calgary, Alberta, Canada

SHENG LI, MD, PhD
Professor, Department of Physical Medicine and Rehabilitation, McGovern Medical School, University of Texas Health Science Center – Houston, TIRR Memorial Herman, Houston Texas, USA

NATHAN S. MAKOWSKI, PhD
Instructor, Department of Physical Medicine and Rehabilitation, MetroHealth Center for Rehabilitation Research, Cleveland FES Center, Case Western Reserve University, Cleveland, Ohio, USA

MANUEL F. MAS, MD
Physiatrist, Department of Physical Medicine and Rehabilitation, School of Medicine, University of Puerto Rico, San Juan, Puerto Rico

DAWN M. NILSEN, EdD, OTR/L, FAOTA
Director, Programs in Occupational Therapy, Vice Chair, Professor, Department of Rehabilitation and Regenerative Medicine; Assistant Dean, Vagelos College of Physicians and Surgeons, Columbia University; Honorary Adjunct Professor of Movement Sciences and Education, Department of Biobehavioral Sciences, Teachers College, Columbia University, New York, New York, USA

HALA OSMAN, PhD
Postdoctoral Fellow, MetroHealth Center for Rehabilitation Research, Cleveland FES Center, Cleveland, Ohio, USA

HAYK PETROSYAN, PhD
Director of Resident and Fellow Research, Department of Physical Medicine and Rehabilitation, JFK Johnson Rehabilitation Institute at Hackensack Meridian Health, Edison, New Jersey, USA

PREETI RAGHAVAN, MD
Associate Professor, Departments of Physical Medicine and Rehabilitation and Neurology, Johns Hopkins University School of Medicine, Baltimore, Maryland, USA

DEEPTHI RAJASHEKAR, PhD
Post Doctoral Fellow, Department of Clinical Neurosciences, Cumming School of Medicine, University of Calgary, Calgary, Alberta, Canada

ANNE SCHWARZ, PT, PhD
Postdoctoral Researcher, Department of Neurology, California Rehabilitation Institute, UCLA, Los Angeles, California, USA

KENT P. SIMMONDS, DO, PhD, MPH
Resident, Department of Physical Medicine and Rehabilitation, UT Southwestern Medical Center, Dallas, Texas, USA

RICARDO SIU, PhD
Postdoctoral Scholar, MetroHealth Center for Rehabilitation Research, Cleveland FES Center, Cleveland, Ohio, USA

MARIE-CLAIRE SMITH, PhD
Senior Lecturer, Department of Exercise Sciences, University of Auckland, Auckland, New Zealand

CATHY M. STINEAR, PhD
Professor, Department of Medicine, University of Auckland, Auckland, New Zealand

MICHAEL SU, MD
Associate Medical Director, Department of Neurology, UCLA, California Rehabilitation Institute, Los Angeles, California, USA

ROBERT TEASELL, MD, FRCPC
Physiatrist, Parkwood Institute Research, Parkwood Institute, St. Joseph's Health Care London; Physical Medicine and Rehabilitation, Schulich School of Medicine and Dentistry, University of Western Ontario, London, Ontario, Canada

VICTORIA E. TILTON-BOLOWSKY, PhD
Postdoctoral Research Fellow, Department of Neurology, Johns Hopkins School of Medicine, Baltimore, Maryland, USA

AARDHRA M. VENKATACHALAM, MPH, CCRC (MS2)
Ross University School of Medicine, Miramar, Florida, USA

RICHARD D. WILSON, MD
Professor, MetroHealth Rehabilitation Institute, MetroHealth System, Case Western Reserve University, Cleveland, Ohio, USA

PAUL WINSTON, MD
Division of Physical Medicine and Rehabilitation, University of British Columbia, Canadian Advances in Neuro-Orthopedics for Spasticity Consortium, Victoria, British Columbia, Canada

LAUREN WINTERBOTTOM, MS, MM, OTR/L
Research Occupational Therapist and Instructor in Clinical Rehabilitation and Regenerative Medicine (Occupational Therapy), Department of Rehabilitation and Regenerative Medicine, Columbia University, EdD Candidate in Movement Sciences and Education, Department of Biobehavioral Sciences, Teachers College, Columbia University, New York, New York, USA

BRITTANY M. YOUNG, MD, PhD
Neurologist, Department of Neurology, UCLA, California Rehabilitation Institute, Los Angeles, California, USA

JULIET ZAKEL, MD
Assistant Professor, MetroHealth Rehabilitation Institute, MetroHealth System, Case Western Reserve University, Cleveland, Ohio, USA

Contents

> Stroke remains a leading cause of disability. Motor recovery requires the interaction of top-down and bottom-up mechanisms, which reinforce each other. Injury to the brain initiates a biphasic neuroimmune process, which opens a window for spontaneous recovery during which the brain is particularly sensitive to activity. Physical activity during this sensitive period can lead to rapid recovery by potentiating anti-inflammatory and neuroplastic processes. On the other hand, lack of physical activity can lead to early closure of the sensitive period and downstream changes in muscles, such as sarcopenia, muscle stiffness, and reduced cardiovascular capacity, and blood flow that impede recovery.

> Predicting motor outcomes after stroke based on clinical judgment alone is often inaccurate and can lead to inefficient and inequitable allocation of rehabilitation resources. Prediction tools are being developed so that clinicians can make evidence-based, accurate, and reproducible prognoses for individual patients. Biomarkers of corticospinal tract structure and function can improve prediction tool performance, particularly for patients with initially moderate to severe motor impairment. Being able to make accurate predictions for individual patients supports rehabilitation planning and communication with patients and families.

> Sensorimotor impairments are common after stroke requiring stroke survivors to relearn lost motor skills or acquire new ones in order to engage in daily activities. Thus, motor skill learning is a cornerstone of stroke rehabilitation. This article provides an overview of motor control and learning theories that inform stroke rehabilitation interventions, discusses principles of neuroplasticity, and provides a summary of practice conditions and techniques that can be used to augment motor learning and neuroplasticity in stroke rehabilitation.

Stroke remains a top contributor to long-term disability in the United States and substantially limits a person's physical activity. Decreased cardiovascular capacity is a major contributing factor to activity limitations and is a significant health concern. Addressing the cardiovascular capacity of stroke survivors as part of poststroke management results in significant improvements in their endurance, functional recovery, and medical outcomes such as all-cause rehospitalization and mortality. Incorporation of a structured approach similar to the cardiac rehabilitation program, including aerobic exercise and risk factor education, can lead to improved cardiovascular function, health benefits, and quality of life in stroke survivors.

Neural stimulation technology aids stroke survivors in regaining lost motor functions. This article explores its applications in upper and lower limb stroke rehabilitation. The authors review various methods to target the corticomotor system, including transcranial direct current stimulation, repetitive transcranial magnetic stimulation, and vagus nerve stimulation. In addition, the authors review the use of peripheral neuromuscular electrical stimulation for therapeutic and assistive purposes, including transcutaneous electrical nerve stimulation, neuromuscular electrical stimulation, and functional electrical stimulation. For each, the authors examine the potential benefits, limitations, safety considerations, and FDA status.

Robotic technology and virtual reality (VR) have been widely studied technologies in stroke rehabilitation over the last few decades. Both technologies have typically been considered as ways to enhance recovery through promoting intensive, repetitive, and engaging therapies. In this review, we present the current evidence from interventional clinical trials that employ either robotics, VR, or a combination of both modalities to facilitate poststroke recovery. Broadly speaking, both technologies have demonstrated some success in improving post-stroke outcomes and complementing conventional therapy. However, more high-quality, randomized, multicenter trials are required to confirm our current understanding of their role in precision stroke recovery.

Botulinum toxin (BonT) is the mainstream treatment option for post-stroke spasticity. BoNT therapy may not be adequate in those with severe spasticity. There are a number of emerging treatment options for spasticity management. In this paper, we focus on innovative and revived treatment options that can be alternative or complementary to BoNT therapy, including phenol neurolysis, cryoneurolysis, and extracorporeal shock wave therapy.

Poststroke aphasia, which impacts expressive and receptive communication, can have detrimental effects on the psychosocial well-being and the quality of life of those affected. Aphasia recovery is multidimensional and can be influenced by several baseline, stroke-related, and treatment-related factors, including preexisting cerebrovascular conditions, stroke size and location, and amount of therapy received. Importantly, aphasia recovery can continue for many years after aphasia onset. Behavioral speech and language therapy with a speech–language pathologist is the most common form of aphasia therapy. In this review, the authors also discuss augmentative treatment methodologies, collaborative goal setting frameworks, and recommendations for future research.

Physiatrists play a vital role in post-stroke dysphagia management not only by providing guidance on the risks, benefits, and efficacy of various treatment options but also as advocates for patients' independence and quality of life. While swallow study results are often discussed broadly by acute stroke clinicians as "pass/fail" findings, physiatrists need a more nuanced working knowledge of dysphagia diagnosis and treatment that encompasses swallow pathophysiology, targeted treatment strategies, and prognosis for recovery. To that end, this review summarizes current clinical practice guidelines on dysphagia, nutrition and oral care, risks and benefits of differing enteral access routes, prognostic factors, and approaches to rehabilitation.

Pain can be a significant barrier to a stroke survivors' functional recovery and can also lead to a decreased quality of life. Common pain conditions after stroke include headache, musculoskeletal pain, spasticity-related pain, complex regional pain syndrome, and central poststroke pain. This review investigates the evidence of diagnostic and management guidelines for various pain syndromes after stroke and identifies opportunities for future research to advance the field of poststroke pain.

Post-stroke cognitive impairment, depression, and fatigue are common, persistent, and disabling. This review summarizes current knowledge on the pathophysiology, assessment, and management of these debilitating neuropsychiatric sequelae of stroke. We briefly review evolving knowledge on the neural mechanisms and risk factors for each condition. We describe patient-reported outcome measures and clinician rating techniques that can be used to assist in screening and comprehensive assessment. We then discuss behavioral and pharmacologic management strategies. Heterogeneity of stroke remains a challenge in management and new research is still needed to optimize and personalize treatments for stroke survivors.

PHYSICAL MEDICINE AND REHABILITATION CLINICS OF NORTH AMERICA

SERIES OF RELATED INTEREST

Orthopedic Clinics
https://www.orthopedic.theclinics.com/
Neurologic Clinics
https://www.neurologic.theclinics.com/
Clinics in Sports Medicine
https://www.sportsmed.theclinics.com/

VISIT THE CLINICS ONLINE!
Access your subscription at:
www.theclinics.com

Stroke Recovery, Rehabilitation, and Innovation

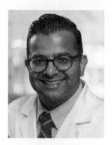

Blessen C. Eapen, MD
Consulting Editor

Stroke is a leading cause of death and disability worldwide with an annual incidence of over 1.5 million cases. In the United States, the Centers for Disease Control and Prevention estimates approximately eight hundred thousand strokes occur annually with an expected increase in incidence due to the aging "baby-boomer" population. Over the last decade, there have been significant advancements in both the medical and surgical management of acute stroke, leading to increased survival rates. Consequently, in the United States, there are over 4 million stroke survivors, with persistent physical, cognitive, and emotional symptoms requiring interdisciplinary stroke rehabilitation care.

The stroke rehabilitation team is typically led by a *physiatrist*, and the team often comprises physical therapists, occupational therapists, speech and language therapists, rehabilitation nurses, recreational therapists, and psychologists depending on the individualized needs of the stroke survivor. The goal of stroke rehabilitation is to help patients regain independence, promote functional abilities, and enhance quality of life.

Stroke rehabilitation is typically an ongoing and individualized process that continues after discharge from the hospital. It may take weeks, months, or even years to achieve optimal recovery, and the rehabilitation plan may be adjusted based on progress and changing needs. Family support and involvement play a crucial role in the rehabilitation process, and caregivers may be educated on how to assist and support the stroke survivor.

We hope this timely special issue provides comprehensive guidance on the management of stroke rehabilitation and provides insight into current rehabilitation programming and innovations in stroke care. We want to thank Dr. Stein and Dr. Stilling for

Phys Med Rehabil Clin N Am 35 (2024) xv–xvi
https://doi.org/10.1016/j.pmr.2024.01.001
1047-9651/24/© 2024 Elsevier Inc. All rights reserved.

leading this special issue and our esteemed colleagues for sharing their valuable experience and expertise with the physical medicine and rehabilitation community!

Blessen C. Eapen, MD
Division of Physical Medicine and Rehabilitation
David Geffen School of Medicine at UCLA
VA Greater Los Angeles Health Care System
11301 Wilshire Boulevard
Los Angeles, CA 90073, USA

E-mail addresses:
beapen@ucla.mednet.edu; blessen.eapen2@va.gov

Preface

Innovations in Stroke Recovery and Rehabilitation

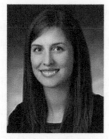 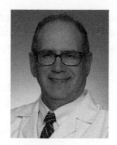

Joan Stilling, MD, MS, FRCPC   Joel Stein, MD
Editors

Despite improvements in acute stroke management, many stroke survivors remain with substantial disability. Efforts to more effectively harness the brain's plasticity and capacity for recovery have been gradually providing a more robust array of evidence to help guide practitioners. At the same time, new treatments, such as cryoneurolysis, are being incorporated into the management of long-term sequelae of stroke. In this special issue focusing on stroke rehabilitation, contributors review our current understanding of mechanisms involved in motor recovery and motor learning following stroke. Techniques to impact and augment motor control and motor learning are discussed. Biomarkers of functional outcomes following stroke are presented with regards to prognostication of both upper and lower limb recovery, with the expectation that these predictive models will ultimately be used to guide individualized treatment.

Next, the delivery of stroke rehabilitation is explored, outlining how health care disparities may play a role in treatment prescription, level of rehabilitation care, and functional outcomes across the continuum of care. Innovative methods of treatment through telerehabilitation are presented, and a novel example of a telerehabilitation program is discussed in detail as an example of how this can be implemented effectively.

Motor rehabilitation therapies, which can be delivered across the acute, subacute, and chronic poststroke stages, are discussed, including remote ischemic conditioning, exercise (ie, dosing, intensity, timing, utilization of a modified cardiac rehabilitation program), neurostimulation (ie, transcranial magnetic, direct current, and vagus nerve stimulation, peripheral neuromuscular electrical stimulation), virtual reality, and robotics.

Finally, treatments to manage the secondary sequalae of stroke associated with impaired functional outcomes are outlined. Spasticity treatment beyond botulinum

Phys Med Rehabil Clin N Am 35 (2024) xvii–xviii
https://doi.org/10.1016/j.pmr.2023.07.003
1047-9651/24/© 2023 Published by Elsevier Inc.

pmr.theclinics.com

toxins, including phenol injection, cryoneurolysis, and extracorporeal shockwave therapy, is described. The complexities of recovery and treatment of aphasia (ie, behavioral speech and language therapy, brain stimulation, medications, computer practice) and current clinical practice guidelines on management of dysphagia, nutrition, oral care, enteral feeding, and delivery of rehabilitative approaches are all considered. The spectrum of poststroke pain (ie, headache, musculoskeletal, shoulder, complex regional pain syndrome, central pain), mood, cognition, and fatigue are also discussed.

We hope that readers will find the content in this special review on innovations in stroke recovery and rehabilitation both stimulating and useful, as we come to understand the complexities and future opportunities for stroke rehabilitation techniques and delivery of care.

Joan Stilling, MD, MS, FRCPC
Department of Rehabilitation Medicine
Weill Cornell Medicine
New York Presbyterian Hospital
525 East 68th Street, Baker Pavilion, F-1602
New York, NY 10065, USA

Joel Stein, MD
Department of Rehabilitation and Regenerative Medicine
Columbia University Vagelos College of Physicians and Surgeons
180 Ft. Washington Avenue, Harkness Pavilion Room 1-165
New York, NY 10032, USA

E-mail addresses:
qsi9001@med.cornell.edu (J. Stilling)
js1165@cumc.columbia.edu (J. Stein)

Top-Down and Bottom-Up Mechanisms of Motor Recovery Poststroke

Preeti Raghavan, MD[a,b,*]

KEYWORDS

- Stroke • Rehabilitation • Muscle • Neuroplasticity • Cardiovascular

KEY POINTS

- Brain injury triggers neuroimmune mechanisms that open a window for spontaneous motor recovery.
- Aligning rehabilitation interventions, including high-frequency physical activity, with the window for spontaneous recovery reinforces top-down neural mechanisms.
- Physical activity has anti-inflammatory effects, can prevent poststroke sarcopenia, preserves muscle mechanical properties, and builds cardiovascular capacity after stroke.
- Understanding top-down and bottom-up mechanisms of recovery can assist in optimizing the timing, dosing, and specificity of rehabilitation interventions.

INTRODUCTION

The annual number of strokes continues to increase particularly among people younger than 70 years, making it a leading cause of disability.[1,2] Ischemia from occlusion or severe stenosis of cerebral arteries is the leading cause of stroke. Reperfusion therapies for ischemic stroke, such as intravenous thrombolysis and endovascular therapy, are only used in 5% to 10% of cases.[3] Intracerebral hemorrhage is the second most common and the most devastating type of stroke, as only 20% of survivors of intracerebral hemorrhage are functionally independent 6 months after stroke with high rates of disability.[4,5] The disability after stroke is characterized by a sudden loss in bodily function, activities, and participation in societal roles.[6] Although disability may be due to impairment in motor, sensory, language, swallowing, and/or cognitive abilities, and the mechanisms of recovery across these domains overlap and interact,

[a] Department of Physical Medicine and Rehabilitation, Johns Hopkins University School of Medicine, 600 North Wolfe Street, Baltimore, MD 21287, USA; [b] Department of Neurology, Johns Hopkins University School of Medicine, 600 North Wolfe Street, Baltimore, MD 21287, USA
* Department of Physical Medicine and Rehabilitation and Neurology, Johns Hopkins University School of Medicine, 600 North Wolfe Street, Baltimore, MD 21287, USA.
E-mail address: praghavan@jhmi.edu

Phys Med Rehabil Clin N Am 35 (2024) 235–257
https://doi.org/10.1016/j.pmr.2023.07.006
1047-9651/24/© 2023 Elsevier Inc. All rights reserved.

motor recovery often receives the most attention. This is partly because hemiparesis, or loss of control on one side of the body, causes significant disability. However, recent literature points to the need to expand the idea of motor disability beyond hemiparesis to include changes in body composition, or sarcopenia, which occurs throughout the body.[7-9] Thus, although stroke is caused by a focal neurologic deficit, its consequences are systemic, and indeed even societal. The mechanisms of recovery after stroke also involve multiple levels. From the perspective of recovery of disability, recovery must occur across the levels of body or body part function (impairment at the tissue or organ level), whole person function (restoration of activity), and whole person and environment level (restoration of participation in societal roles) as per the international classification of disability and function framework.[10] Because the key impairment in stroke occurs from injury to the brain, the mechanisms of recovery were also thought to be top-down, stemming entirely from neuroplastic processes. Recent data suggest that although top-down mechanisms are important, there are changes downstream from the brain and the nervous system that greatly influence recovery. These bottom-up mechanisms in the musculoskeletal system must also be addressed to facilitate top-down processes (**Fig. 1**). It is critical that we understand these mechanisms to develop comprehensive systems of care to facilitate recovery and mitigate disability to the greatest extent possible.

WHAT IS MOTOR RECOVERY?

Motor recovery has been defined as the restitution of "normal" motor performance or skill that existed before the neural injury.[11,12] In contrast, compensatory motor behavior is defined as the appearance of new motor patterns resulting from the adaptation of remaining motor elements or substitution, that is, functions are taken over, replaced, or substituted by different body segments. It is important to keep in mind that "true" recovery of motor performance may not involve the same neural networks as before the injury. A natural question that follows is: is "true" motor recovery possible? The answer at this time depends on the extent of initial motor impairment.[13,14] A recent case report of a patient with complete right hemiplegia who was

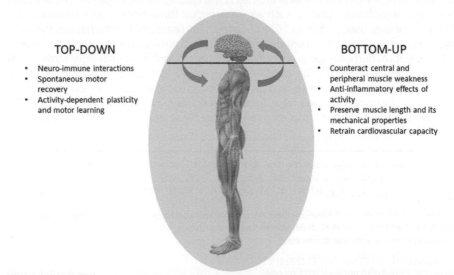

TOP-DOWN

- Neuro-immune interactions
- Spontaneous motor recovery
- Activity-dependent plasticity and motor learning

BOTTOM-UP

- Counteract central and peripheral muscle weakness
- Anti-inflammatory effects of activity
- Preserve muscle length and its mechanical properties
- Retrain cardiovascular capacity

Fig. 1. Top-down and bottom-up mechanisms of motor recovery after stroke.

examined longitudinally over 12 years showed complete recovery of dexterous finger movements that only began after the first 5 years;[15] imaging at 12 years after the stroke revealed partially intact motor pathways on the lesioned side. Practitioners of rehabilitation also often witness recovery of motor functions long after the injury, suggesting that the window for "true" motor recovery may be longer than currently thought, should the right conditions exist. What are these conditions, and how can we reproduce them systematically? This review attempts to summarize recent developments in understanding the mechanisms underlying motor recovery.

TOP-DOWN MECHANISMS
Neuroimmune Interactions

Cerebral ischemia, neuronal cell death, and disruption of the blood-brain barrier activate resident and infiltrating immune cells, which trigger sterile neuroinflammatory processes.[16] The inflammatory response is biphasic: it initially exacerbates ischemic neuronal injury and impairs neurologic function and then triggers and accelerates neural repair and recovery mechanisms.[17] Microglia are the first immune cells to be activated to produce inflammatory neurotoxic molecules; they also engulf dying and surviving neurons. The molecules released from injured brain cells activate neutrophils and macrophages, which produce inflammatory cytokines and activate T lymphocytes to exacerbate the sterile inflammatory process leading to further neuronal loss. However, approximately 1 week after stroke onset, the immune cells adopt anti-inflammatory phenotypes to facilitate neural repair. Macrophages produce trophic factors necessary for angiogenesis and survival of peri-infarct neurons, and microglia produce trophic factors to promote synaptogenesis, remyelination, and tissue repair, which are necessary for neuronal circuit reorganization both locally and remotely in regions connected to the injured region; this change in the phenotype of immune cells to a reparative state facilitates spontaneous motor recovery (**Fig. 2**).[18]

After hemorrhagic stroke, extravascular blood causes more prolonged inflammation that peaks within the first 72 hours but may last for weeks at both local and distant sites.[19,20] The time course and regions showing chronic inflammation are variable across individuals and may depend on biological variables, such as sex and comorbid conditions.[21] Anti-inflammatory and reparative pathways become more dominant after 72 hours, although the acute and subacute stages cannot be cleanly divided into inflammatory and reparative stages as after ischemic stroke.[22–25] Blood components at the site of the hemorrhage also trigger inflammation. Iron increases local inflammation by activating astrocytes, and free heme, bilirubin, and hemoglobin activate microglia and other immune cells.[26–30] The protective activity of macrophages and microglia is linked to their ability to phagocytose red blood cells, clear iron from the brain, and inhibit cell death.

Given the biphasic response of the immune cells in both producing injury and stimulating repair, it is not surprising that suppressing the acute inflammatory process after stroke using systemic anti-inflammatory agents, such as steroids and hypothermia, is not beneficial in the long term. They may temporarily reduce edema, but result in rebound swelling and damage 1 week later.[17] Clinical trials of immunomodulators have also failed to show a significant benefit after stroke.[31,32] Furthermore, ablation of proliferating microglia in a mouse model of ischemic stroke led to a significant increase in the size of the cerebral infarct associated with a decrease in neurotrophic growth factor levels, whereas stimulation of microglial proliferation after cerebral ischemia had the opposite effect, suggesting that proliferating microglia may serve as an endogenous pool of neurotrophic molecules that have a neuroprotective

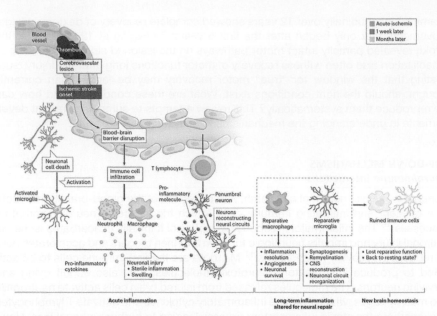

Fig. 2. Timeline of neuroimmune interactions after ischemic stroke. CNS, central nervous system. (*From* Shichita T, Ooboshi H, Yoshimura A. Neuroimmune mechanisms and therapies mediating post-ischaemic brain injury and repair. Nat Rev Neurosci. 2023;24(5):299-312.)

effect.[33] Treatment strategies that accelerate the resolution of the acute inflammatory state and promote transition to the reparative neuroimmune state could potentially reduce neural damage and facilitate early recovery after stroke. For example, vagus nerve stimulation is a novel, recently Food and Drug Administration–approved, adjunctive treatment option, which may release neuroimmune modulators to enhance synaptic plasticity and facilitate poststroke recovery, although the mechanisms are still unclear.[34–38] Several other techniques, including noninvasive brain stimulation, manipulation of gut microbiota, and cellular and molecular interventions, are also being actively investigated as immune-modulators.[39–42]

Spontaneous Motor Recovery

Spontaneous recovery occurs when the brain injury leads to a time-limited window of enhanced synaptic plasticity, which includes changes in gene expression, dendritic spine proliferation, sprouting of new axons, and the formation of new synapses in the peri-infarct cortex associated with motor recovery and sensory-motor reorganization (**Fig. 3**).[43–45] The brain injury also disrupts the perineural extracellular matrix (ECM) or perineural nets, which normally create an inhibitory environment for activity-dependent plasticity; their disruption opens up a critical period during which the cortex is particularly sensitive to experience.[46] The opening of the plasticity window coincides with the change of the neuroimmune cells to an anti-inflammatory phenotype, and its closure coincides with the gradual disappearance of immune cells. Activated microglia, in particular, participate in poststroke plasticity, with effects on neurogenesis, axonal regeneration, reorganization of neural network and circuits, and interhemispheric connections.[47] Increased extrasynaptic GABA signaling ends the sensitive period.[48] A recent study in a mouse model showed that the spontaneously recovered perilesional cortex showed highly correlated patterns of activity with the homologous

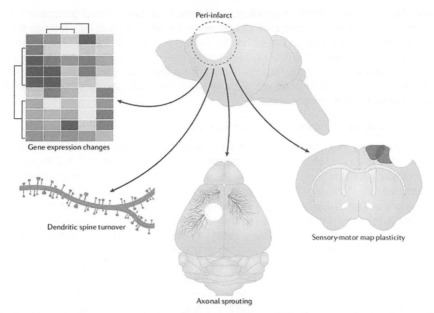

Fig. 3. Neuroplastic processes during spontaneous recovery in the mouse brain after stroke. (*From* Joy MT, Carmichael ST. Encouraging an excitable brain state: mechanisms of brain repair in stroke. Nat Rev Neurosci. 2021;22(1):38-53.)

areas in the contralesional hemisphere. However, chronic stimulation of the contralesional hemisphere inhibited the newly established functional connections via callosal connections.[49] These data suggest that although the contralesional hemisphere facilitates spontaneous recovery naturally, chronic stimulation, for example, with exclusive use or compensation using the contralateral arm, may result in early closure of the sensitive period.

Most studies on the mechanisms of spontaneous recovery have been done in animal models of stroke, as cortical plasticity is difficult to measure directly in humans. Recently, continuous theta burst (cTBS) transcranial magnetic stimulation was used to assess whether there is an early period of enhanced synaptic plasticity at a neural level in humans after stroke.[50] cTBS repetitively inhibits synaptic connections in the motor cortex by a long-term depression-like process. The investigators surmised that if there was increased synaptic plasticity in the early weeks after stroke, cTBS would reduce excitability to a greater extent soon after stroke, and the magnitude of the response would decrease over a 12-month period. Depression of cortical excitability by cTBS was most prominent shortly after stroke in the contralesional hemisphere and diminished over subsequent sessions. However, contrary to what was expected, the cTBS response did not differ across the 12-month follow-up period in the ipsilesional hemisphere. It is possible that these results were due to already reduced baseline excitability in the ipsilesional cortex.[51] Nevertheless, these data provide the first neurophysiologic evidence consistent with a period of enhanced synaptic plasticity bilaterally in the human brain early after stroke.

Furthermore, most studies that examined spontaneous recovery have used an ischemic stroke model. A recent study in rats compared the mechanisms of recovery in intracerebral hemorrhage and ischemia, focusing on synapses, glial cells, and dopamine expression, which are considered fundamental for neural recovery after stroke. Although there were no significant differences between the 2 groups in terms of lesion volume in the striatum, motor recovery in the intracerebral hemorrhage group occurred more rapidly than in the ischemia group, and the intracerebral hemorrhage group exhibited higher protein expression in the motor cortex associated with changes in astrocytes in brain regions remote from the injury site.[52] These data suggest that it is important to separate patients with ischemic and hemorrhagic stroke when examining rates of recovery.

Activity-dependent plasticity and motor learning

Synaptic plasticity that occurs during spontaneous recovery is enhanced in an activity-dependent manner and shares similar processes with motor learning.[53] Activity induces synchronous neuronal firing, which enhances excitability and long-term potentiation, and reduces tonic inhibitory GABAergic signaling to promote learning and motor recovery. The population of neurons engaged in synchronized neural firing determines the activity that is reinforced or the behavior that is learned. Defining this neural population involves 3 processes: active searching, neuronal selection, and refinement.[54–57] In the active searching phase, neurons within a motor network demonstrate loosely correlated spatiotemporal activity patterns associated with the activity. Repetitive activity or closely spaced practice then leads to the selection of a neuronal circuit that shows little variability. Further practice leads to a period of refinement in which spatial and temporal activation patterns become highly efficient and sparse.[58,59] This sparse neuronal circuit is then strengthened structurally by the formation of new dendritic spines and axons in local and distant sites and the release of neurotrophic factors that support a state of enhanced plasticity.[60–62] It is thus critically important to select the neural circuits that result in the desired motor behavior.[63,64]

How does one select the desirable circuits to be reinforced through practice? Selecting the right circuits to facilitate "true" motor recovery is particularly challenging after stroke due to loss of neural substrate. Animal models suggest that the spatial and temporal processing of sensory information is critical for sensorimotor remapping after stroke and occurs in the peri-infarct zone as well as at more distant sites.[65,66] Somatosensory stimuli from a specific body part are preferentially routed through the thalamus to the primary sensory areas that are dedicated to that body part, but can also exhibit widely divergent activation patterns.[67] Sensory information is critical for motor control in both the presence and absence of sensory impairment.[68–70] When sensory stimulation is temporally and spatially specific, sensorimotor maps are more accurate.[71] However, when sensory stimuli are processed in divergent networks, The sensorimotor maps may be less precise. In fact, human imaging studies show that individuals with severe somatosensory impairment after stroke show reduced interhemispheric and ipsilesional intrahemispheric somatosensory network connectivity involving bilateral primary sensorimotor cortices, supplementary motor area, insula, cerebellum, and inferior and superior parietal regions compared with individuals with mild to moderate somatosensory impairment at approximately 6 days after stroke.[72] In addition, chronic poststroke sensorimotor impairment is associated with smaller ipsilesional hippocampal volume that is not lesion related.[73] In individuals with chronic stroke, functional MRI during unilateral tactile stimulation showed increased activation in the postcentral gyrus, and structural MRI showed increased cortical thickness in the same area, demonstrating that structural plasticity is colocalized with areas exhibiting functional plasticity in the human brain after stroke.[74] These results suggest that sensorimotor plasticity can occur even in individuals in the chronic stage after stroke. Although the role of sensory information in enhancing motor recovery is still under study,[75–77] the relative ease of providing more accurate sensory information to elicit specific motor behaviors is a potential area that can enhance the selectivity of functional neural networks for motor recovery in more severely impaired individuals who need to use more distributed neural resources.[78–82] For example, a new study shows that exposure to sensory information from the nonparetic side of the body can lead to an immediate transient change in functionally relevant sensori-motor integration on the paretic side in individuals with chronic stroke.[83]

Retrospective resting-state functional MRI studies in individuals with subacute stroke showed that cognition-related networks were also correlated with motor recovery of the upper limb.[84] Specifically, cognition-related networks were associated with motor recovery in patients with a lower strength of motor-related networks; that is, the greater the damage to the motor network, the more important the cognition-related networks are in motor recovery.

Damage to the corticospinal tract has repeatedly been linked to the severity of motor impairment, whereas the role of the extrapyramidal pathways, specifically the rubrospinal and reticulospinal tracts, is controversial in humans—some studies suggest that their recruitment results in spasticity and abnormal motor synergies, whereas others suggest it promotes recovery.[85–87] A new study that examined compartment-wise anisotropy of the corticospinal and extrapyramidal tracts showed that, as expected, degeneration of the descending ipsilesional corticospinal tract is associated with upper and lower limb motor impairment. In addition, anisotropy of bihemispheric rubrospinal and reticulospinal tracts was linked to lower limb deficits, whereas anisotropy of two-directional contralesional rubrospinal tracts explained gross motor performance of the affected hand. The extrapyramidal tracts also contained fibers crossing the midline that appear to compensate for impaired gross arm and leg movements resulting from loss of ipsilesional corticospinal tract integrity.[88] These results, along with others, suggest that the integrity of the extrapyramidal pathways is important in motor recovery.[89,90]

Clinical observations also suggest that arousal and motivation are critical to learning and recovery. Cholinergic innervation mediates arousal through the basal forebrain and has been shown to be critical in skill learning.[91–94] Endogenous dopamine is also required for recovery of motor skill after stroke, and blockade of dopamine receptors in rats decreases motivation and impedes motor learning.[95] Hence it is thought that reward feedback may augment motivation through stimulation of midbrain dopaminergic pathways. A recent human study that directly tested whether reward feedback would augment poststroke motor learning showed that the rewarded group had significantly greater improvements from baseline in clinical measures of motor impairment and function, although measures of reaching did not show a significant difference.[96] Longitudinal resting state functional MRI has been used to determine whether brain network connectivity patterns after stroke can predict longitudinal behavioral outcomes. The findings suggest that functional coupling between the dorsal attention and limbic networks after stroke predicts subsequent clinical motor recovery.[97] Indeed, interventions using music that is known to stimulate arousal and motivation have shown measurable changes in motivation, self-efficacy, mood, motor impairment, function, and participation mediated via increases in levels of brain-derived neurotrophic factor.[98,99]

A better understanding of the neural circuitry for motor function has led to the development of brain-machine interfaces that capitalize on available circuits and strengthen them more precisely.[100,101] However, changes in the musculoskeletal system often act as barriers to recovery and must also be addressed to reap the full benefits of neuroplastic mechanisms.

BOTTOM-UP MECHANISMS
Counteract Central and Peripheral Muscle Weakness

Neural activity serves as the conductor of an orchestra, coordinating activity of more than 600 muscles that serve as the players or effectors that produce the movements. The bottom-up changes in muscle structure and function may determine why patients with stroke show heterogeneous responses to treatment. A defining consequence of a stroke is focal weakness or paresis of muscles, making them the chief organ of disability. The descending motor pathways provide input to the spinal cord neuronal network that activates the motor neurons to stimulate motor units in the muscles. A motor unit consists of a motor neuron and all the muscle fibers it innervates. Motor units generate force: small motor units generate low forces, and larger motor units are recruited to generate higher forces. A stroke leads to loss of motor units in the skeletal muscles, which produces focal weakness. The decrease in motor units starts within 4 to 30 hours after an infarction, when T1-weighted MR images of the brain involved are still normal and is correlated with the degree of clinical weakness.[102] In individuals with chronic stroke, the motor units become saturated, and they are not able to be recruited progressively to generate the required forces in the paretic limb.[103,104] However, grip strength is reduced in both the paretic and the nonparetic limbs after stroke, and the grip strength on the paretic side predicts the gains in rehabilitation.[105] Although a stroke can produce central deficits in strength in both hands owing to involvement of ipsilesional descending tracts,[106] the loss in grip strength may also be due to peripheral causes of weakness.

In addition to central focal paresis, individuals with stroke may have varying degrees of generalized peripheral age-related loss of muscle mass, muscle strength, or function, also known as sarcopenia.[107,108] There is a higher prevalence of sarcopenia among individuals with stroke compared with healthy individuals after controlling for age, sex, and race.[9,109-111] Stroke-related muscle wasting is multifactorial and depends on impaired neurovegetative control, loss of motor neurons, degeneration of neuromuscular junctions, systemic catabolic-anabolic imbalance, and local muscle metabolic alterations.[112] Poststroke sarcopenia is more evident in the upper than in the lower limbs; spasticity and walking may be protective for sarcopenia in the lower limb muscles.[8]

It is not routine or easy to differentiate between central (eg, stroke-related reduction in motor units) and peripheral (eg, disuse muscle atrophy) causes of poststroke weakness.[113] In contrast to age-related sarcopenia whereby there is a shift from fast-twitch type IIa/b to slow-twitch type I fibers, which is mainly attributed to disuse of fast fibers, stroke survivors show a shift from slow-twitch to fast-twitch muscle fibers.[114] In addition, the atrophy after central lesions is thought to be due to increased proteolysis rather than to reduced muscle protein synthesis, which is more common with aging.[115-117] Physical activity can however prevent and treat sarcopenia.[118-120] Specifically, muscle strength training along with appropriate nutritional supplementation has a significant effect on muscle mass, muscle strength, and physical performance.[121-124]

Anti-inflammatory Effects of Physical Activity

Individuals with stroke show an early and sustained peripheral inflammatory response with or without evidence of infection.[125] Inflammatory cytokines may access the systemic circulation through the disrupted blood-brain barrier or the venous and lymphatic outflows of cerebrospinal fluid circulation.[126] The ensuing systemic inflammatory response is followed by systemic immunodepression, which predisposes to infections, as well as poststroke fatigue.[127,128] Poststroke fatigue, in turn, leads to further inactivity and impedes rehabilitation.[129] Thus, inflammation impacts the muscle, but muscle activity also impacts inflammation.[130]

Muscle strengthening exercises have strong anti-inflammatory effects that counteract the chronic low-grade inflammatory profile associated with many chronic diseases.[131–136] Contracting skeletal muscles produce molecules called myokines, for example interleukin-6 (IL-6) is a prototypical myokine, that mediate the anti-inflammatory effects of exercise.[137] IL-6 works as an energy sensor and exerts both local and endocrine metabolic effects. When the endocrine function of the largest organ in the body, the skeletal muscles, is not stimulated through contractions, it causes malfunction of several organs and tissues.[138] Muscle-induced myokines enable direct cross talk between muscle and brain function. Muscles secretes myokines that contribute to the regulation of hippocampal function, production of BDNF, neurogenesis, learning and memory, suppression of feeding, and antidepressant effects.[139] In contrast, ongoing inflammation impairs recovery of muscle strength and fatigability, as well as muscle gain after strength training.[140–142]

Preserve Muscle Length and its Mechanical Properties

In addition to being the effectors that produce movement, muscles also contain the receptors that sense muscle length and tension both at rest and during movement. The muscle sensory receptors, known as muscle spindles lie in the extracellular space of the muscle, specifically, in the perimysium, and are innervated by primary and secondary nerve endings that fire in response to passive stretch and shortening of the muscle.[143]

Immobility leads to muscle unloading, which results in changes in muscle composition and in its mechanical properties. A recent study examined the effect of stroke versus immobilization within 14 days in a rat model with 4 groups that underwent the following: (1) immobilization of one forelimb without stroke, (2) stroke without immobilization, or (3) stroke with immobilization of the paretic forelimb, and also (4) a control group. The investigators found that immobilization rather than stroke was responsible for muscle atrophy, connective tissue thickening, and alteration of passive mechanical muscle properties.[144] Immobilization has also been shown to increase the content of glycosaminoglycans, specifically hyaluronic acid (HA), in the ECM of the muscle, which precedes the thickening and disorganization of collagen fibrils.[145] In human muscle, HA is especially abundant in the perivascular and perineural connective tissue of the perimysium where the muscle spindles are located. The muscle spindle capsule consists of 2 distinct portions, the inner and the outer capsule.[146] The inner capsule encloses the intrafusal fibers within an innermost axial space, whereas the outer capsule is multilayered and encloses a fluid-filled space in the equatorial region of the spindle called the periaxial space (**Fig. 4**A). HA is abundant in the axial and periaxial spaces of the muscle spindles, in all layers of the spindle capsule, as well as in the endoneurium and in the space in between individual axons in the perimysium (**Fig. 4**B).[147] The presence of HA in the periaxial fluid has been shown to be responsible for the transcapsular potential, which increases the sensitivity of the sensory endings to mechanical stimuli.[148] Alteration in the viscosity of the HA solution in the muscle spindle can thus increase the sensitivity of the muscle spindle to stretch based on models of mechanosensation.[149] Furthermore, a muscle that is in a shortened position shows increased sensitivity to stretch.[150] Taken together, paresis and immobility can lead to HA accumulation in the ECM of muscle, which may increase the stretch-sensitivity of the muscle spindle in shortened paretic muscles. This along with the

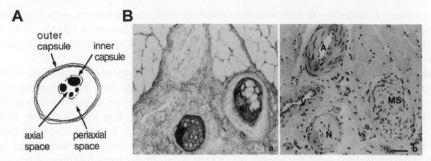

outer
capsule   inner
           capsule

axial   periaxial
space   space

Fig. 4. Muscle spindle structure, location, and HA content. (*A*) The structure of the muscle spindle in the equatorial region. The intrafusal fibers are shown in the axial spaces within the inner capsule. (*B*) Serial cross-sections of human lumbrical muscle stained with brown staining biotinylated HA binding protein (HABP) (a) and toluidine blue (b) showing a neurovascular bundle (A artery; V vein; N nerve) and a muscle spindle (MS). Notice the strong HABP staining filling the capsular space of the muscle spindle and surrounding the nerve fibers. Bar, 50 μm. (*Modified from* Pedrosa-Domellof F, Hellstrom S, Thornell LE. Hyaluronan in human and rat muscle spindles. Histochem Cell Biol. 1998;110(2):179-182.)

excitatory-inhibitory imbalance in the spinal cord interneuronal network after upper motor neuron lesions may further potentiate stretch reflex hyperexcitability that is characteristic of spastic muscles.

The hyaluronan hypothesis of muscle stiffness postulated that the deposition of HA in the ECM of muscle contributes to the development of muscle stiffness by dramatically altering its viscosity.[151,152] Immobility-induced hyperviscous HA in the ECM can increase passive stiffness of the ECM and cause the myofibers to stick to each other. Exercise, on the other hand, mobilizes HA and increases serum HA concentration, which rapidly returns to resting levels by 30 minutes after exercise.[153] Short-term exercise for 10 weeks reduces HA levels in previously less active individuals as measured using relaxation times with T1rho MRI.[154] However, when immobility and overuse coexist, for example, in patients with spastic paresis, the homeostasis of HA is disrupted, leading to excessive accumulation of HA and the ensuing changes in the mechanical properties of the muscle. Treatment with the enzyme hyaluronidase, which hydrolyzes high-molecular-weight HA into smaller fragments, has been shown to lead to a reduction in resistance to passive motion measured using the Modified Ashworth Scale, and consequently increased passive and active range of motion.[151] In addition, T1rho muscle MRI, which images intramuscular GAG content, showed increased signal in patients with poststroke muscle stiffness, and a reduction in signal to more normal levels after treatment with hyaluronidase.[155]

Retrain Cardiovascular Capacity

Abnormal movement patterns in the lower limb, which are likely caused by a combination of neural and nonneural changes, alter the mechanics of walking, which in turn increase the metabolic cost of walking, and result in reduced walking speed.[156] Reduction in mobility and walking speed is associated with high fall risk, increased comorbidities, reduced quality of life, and increased risk of hospitalizations, leading to a downward spiral.[157–161] Furthermore, individuals with stroke spend ~80% of their time in sedentary activities and engage in less than half the physical activity of their age-matched peers without stroke.[162,163] Recent guidelines for secondary prevention after stroke recommend moderate-intensity aerobic activity for a minimum of

10 minutes 4 times a week or vigorous-intensity aerobic activity for a minimum of 20 minutes twice a week[164] and suggest that individuals after stroke should aim to achieve population-based recommendations of 20 to 60 minutes of moderate-intensity aerobic exercise performed 3 to 5 times a week.[165] However, poststroke fatigue is common, and many individuals reach their maximum aerobic capacity by simply performing their daily activities because of decreased endurance, reduced oxygen uptake, and a decline in cardiovascular capacity.[166–168]

Studies in animal models show that moderate forced exercise (10 m/min, 5–7 days per week for about 30 minutes), initiated early after injury (24–48 hours after stroke), reduced lesion volume and protected perilesional tissue against oxidative damage and inflammation for at least 4 weeks by increasing neurotrophic factors and synaptogenesis in multiple brain regions.[169,170] Furthermore, sustained aerobic physical exercise promotes adult hippocampal neurogenesis even in animals who are not genetically predisposed to training effects.[171] Vascular restoration is critical for the enhancement of neurogenesis and neuroplasticity.[172] A recent meta-analysis shows that although individuals may have attenuated cerebrovascular hemodynamics during acute moderate-intensity exercise after stroke, exercise training increases cerebral blood flow and cerebrovascular reactivity to carbon dioxide.[173] However, neuroplastic effects tend to be more robust with moderate- to high-intensity exercise training.[174,175] Exercise training induces skeletal muscle myofibers to express vascular endothelial growth factor, which can maintain hippocampal cerebral blood flow necessary for neurogenesis.[176,177] The optimal time to deliver aerobic exercise to amplify the biological recovery processes is during the acute and subacute stages of recovery after stroke, which is both feasible and safe.[178–180] Exercise training delivered during this optimal time window has been shown to significantly improve cardiovascular function as well as physical and cognitive function and decrease 1-year all-cause hospital readmission by 22%,[181–183] thus mitigating disability and controlling health care costs.

SUMMARY

Motor recovery after stroke depends on top-down neuroimmune processes that likely limit neuronal damage and trigger open the window for spontaneous motor recovery, during which the brain is particularly sensitive to sensory, motor, cognitive, and social stimuli. These stimuli produce synchronous distributed firing in local and remote regions, which become selected and reinforced to shape recovery. The selection and shaping of neural circuitry are influenced by activity, which is highly dependent on bottom-up mechanisms. Both central and peripheral muscle weakness limit activity-dependent plasticity. Poststroke immobility potentiates mechanical changes in muscles, which potentiates spasticity, muscle stiffness, and abnormal movement patterns. These in turn lead to further reduced mobility, limit cardiovascular capacity, and reduce cerebral blood flow. In contrast, physical activity has anti-inflammatory effects that facilitate positive neuroimmune interactions.

CLINICS CARE POINTS

Translating the top-down and bottom-up mechanisms into clinical practice requires the following:

- Alignment of the timing of rehabilitation interventions with the window for spontaneous recovery. This means ensuring that stroke survivors are provided the opportunity to receive high-frequency interventions continuously rather than episodically in the first 3 months regardless of the severity of their deficits as demonstrated by the critical period after stroke study.[184]

- Facilitating high-frequency physical activity to promote its anti-inflammatory effects on neuroimmune interactions, prevent poststroke sarcopenia, and prevent changes in muscle mechanical properties. This may be achieved by enabling early mobility starting in the stroke unit.[185,186]

- Preventing muscle mechanical changes by incorporating early and frequent joint mobilization.[187,188]

- Supporting "true" motor recovery, while minimizing the use of compensatory strategies that may impede recovery over the long term; this requires assessment of impairment, function, and participation across the care continuum.[189]

- Retraining cardiovascular capacity as soon as feasible after stroke, ideally within the first 3 months, which has been shown to be possible.[181,183]

FUTURE DIRECTIONS

The future is optimistic for motor recovery after stroke. On the one hand, there has been exciting progress in understanding neuroimmune and neuroplastic mechanisms and their interactions with physical activity, exercise-mimetics, and technology.[39,100,190] On the other hand, there have been advances in the organization of systems of care and treatments to translate mechanistic understanding into clinical practice.[191–194] The rubber will meet the road when these 2 directions converge toward data-driven mechanistic precision rehabilitation that is accessible to individuals after stroke. We need to hasten progress toward this goal.

AUTHOR DISCLOSURES

The author declares no disclosures specific to this work. This work is partly funded by the Johns Hopkins Sheikh Khalifa Stroke Institute and NIH R61AT012279.

REFERENCES

1. Collaborators GBDS. Global, regional, and national burden of stroke and its risk factors, 1990-2019: a systematic analysis for the Global Burden of Disease Study 2019. Lancet Neurol 2021;20(10):795–820.
2. Tsao CW, Aday AW, Almarzooq ZI, et al. Heart Disease and Stroke Statistics-2022 Update: A Report From the American Heart Association. Circulation 2022;145(8):e153–639.
3. Akbik F, Xu H, Xian Y, et al. Trends in Reperfusion Therapy for In-Hospital Ischemic Stroke in the Endovascular Therapy Era. JAMA Neurol 2020;77(12): 1486–95.
4. Broderick JP, Grotta JC, Naidech AM, et al. The Story of Intracerebral Hemorrhage: From Recalcitrant to Treatable Disease. Stroke 2021;52(5):1905–14.
5. Toyoda K, Yoshimura S, Nakai M, et al. Twenty-Year Change in Severity and Outcome of Ischemic and Hemorrhagic Strokes. JAMA Neurol 2022;79(1):61–9.
6. Martins Dos Santos H, Pereira GS, de Oliveira LC, et al. Biopsychosocial factors associated with the state of disability after hemiparesis in the chronic phase of stroke: exploratory analysis based on the International Classification of Functioning, Disability and Health. Disabil Rehabil 2023;1–8.

7. Chang KV, Wu WT, Huang KC, et al. Segmental body composition transitions in stroke patients: Trunks are different from extremities and strokes are as important as hemiparesis. Clin Nutr 2020;39(6):1968–73.
8. Li S, Gonzalez-Buonomo J, Ghuman J, et al. Aging after stroke: how to define post-stroke sarcopenia and what are its risk factors? Eur J Phys Rehabil Med 2022;58(5):683–92.
9. Mas MF, Gonzalez J, Frontera WR. Stroke and sarcopenia. Curr Phys Med Rehabil Rep 2020;8(4):452–60.
10. World Health Organization International Classification of Functioning, Disability and Health. World Health Organization; 2001. Available at: https://www.who.int/standards/classifications/international-classification-of-functioning-disability-and-health.
11. Levin MF, Kleim JA, Wolf SL. What do motor "recovery" and "compensation" mean in patients following stroke? Neurorehabil Neural Repair 2009;23(4): 313–9.
12. Raghavan P. Upper Limb Motor Impairment After Stroke. Phys Med Rehabil Clin N Am 2015;26(4):599–610.
13. Stinear CM, Byblow WD, Ackerley SJ, et al. Predicting Recovery Potential for Individual Stroke Patients Increases Rehabilitation Efficiency. Stroke 2017;48(4): 1011–9.
14. Prabhakaran S, Zarahn E, Riley C, et al. Inter-individual variability in the capacity for motor recovery after ischemic stroke. Neurorehabil Neural Repair 2008; 22(1):64–71.
15. Ciceron C, Sappey-Marinier D, Riffo P, et al. Case Report: True Motor Recovery of Upper Limb Beyond 5 Years Post-stroke. Front Neurol 2022;13:804528.
16. Kono H, Rock KL. How dying cells alert the immune system to danger. Nat Rev Immunol 2008;8(4):279–89.
17. Buckley CD, Gilroy DW, Serhan CN, et al. The resolution of inflammation. Nat Rev Immunol 2013;13(1):59–66.
18. Shichita T, Ooboshi H, Yoshimura A. Neuroimmune mechanisms and therapies mediating post-ischaemic brain injury and repair. Nat Rev Neurosci 2023;24(5): 299–312.
19. Xue M, Del Bigio MR. Intracerebral injection of autologous whole blood in rats: time course of inflammation and cell death. Neurosci Lett 2000;283(3):230–2.
20. Shi E, Shi K, Qiu S, et al. Chronic inflammation, cognitive impairment, and distal brain region alteration following intracerebral hemorrhage. FASEB J 2019;33(8): 9616–26.
21. Puy L, Leboullenger C, Auger F, et al. Intracerebral Hemorrhage-Induced Cognitive Impairment in Rats Is Associated With Brain Atrophy, Hypometabolism, and Network Dysconnectivity. Front Neurosci 2022;16:882996.
22. Ohashi SN, DeLong JH, Kozberg MG, et al. Role of Inflammatory Processes in Hemorrhagic Stroke. Stroke 2023;54(2):605–19.
23. Yang Z, Liu B, Zhong L, et al. Toll-like receptor-4-mediated autophagy contributes to microglial activation and inflammatory injury in mouse models of intracerebral haemorrhage. Neuropathol Appl Neurobiol 2015;41(4):e95–106.
24. Liu B, Hu B, Shao S, et al. CD163/Hemoglobin Oxygenase-1 Pathway Regulates Inflammation in Hematoma Surrounding Tissues after Intracerebral Hemorrhage. J Stroke Cerebrovasc Dis 2015;24(12):2800–9.
25. Lei C, Lin S, Zhang C, et al. Effects of high-mobility group box1 on cerebral angiogenesis and neurogenesis after intracerebral hemorrhage. Neuroscience 2013;229:12–9.

26. Wang YC, Zhou Y, Fang H, et al. Toll-like receptor 2/4 heterodimer mediates inflammatory injury in intracerebral hemorrhage. Ann Neurol 2014;75(6):876–89.

27. Su X, Wang H, Zhu L, et al. Ethyl pyruvate ameliorates intracerebral hemorrhage-induced brain injury through anti-cell death and anti-inflammatory mechanisms. Neuroscience 2013;245:99–108.

28. Lin S, Yin Q, Zhong Q, et al. Heme activates TLR4-mediated inflammatory injury via MyD88/TRIF signaling pathway in intracerebral hemorrhage. J Neuroinflammation 2012;9:46.

29. Loftspring MC, Johnson HL, Feng R, et al. Unconjugated bilirubin contributes to early inflammation and edema after intracerebral hemorrhage. J Cereb Blood Flow Metab 2011;31(4):1133–42.

30. Loftspring MC, Hansen C, Clark JF. A novel brain injury mechanism after intracerebral hemorrhage: the interaction between heme products and the immune system. Med Hypotheses 2010;74(1):63–6.

31. Elkins J, Veltkamp R, Montaner J, et al. Safety and efficacy of natalizumab in patients with acute ischaemic stroke (ACTION): a randomised, placebo-controlled, double-blind phase 2 trial. Lancet Neurol 2017;16(3):217–26.

32. Enlimomab Acute Stroke Trial I. Use of anti-ICAM-1 therapy in ischemic stroke: results of the Enlimomab Acute Stroke Trial. Neurology 2001;57(8):1428–34.

33. Lalancette-Hebert M, Gowing G, Simard A, et al. Selective ablation of proliferating microglial cells exacerbates ischemic injury in the brain. J Neurosci 2007;27(10):2596–605.

34. Ananda R, Roslan MHB, Wong LL, et al. Efficacy and Safety of Vagus Nerve Stimulation in Stroke Rehabilitation: A Systematic Review and Meta-Analysis. Cerebrovasc Dis 2023;52(3):239–50.

35. Engineer ND, Kimberley TJ, Prudente CN, et al. Targeted Vagus Nerve Stimulation for Rehabilitation After Stroke. Front Neurosci 2019;13:280.

36. Li L, Wang D, Pan H, et al. Non-invasive Vagus Nerve Stimulation in Cerebral Stroke: Current Status and Future Perspectives. Front Neurosci 2022;16:820665.

37. Li J, Zhang Q, Li S, et al. alpha7nAchR mediates transcutaneous auricular vagus nerve stimulation-induced neuroprotection in a rat model of ischemic stroke by enhancing axonal plasticity. Neurosci Lett 2020;730:135031.

38. Li J, Zhang K, Zhang Q, et al. PPAR-gamma Mediates Ta-VNS-Induced Angiogenesis and Subsequent Functional Recovery after Experimental Stroke in Rats. Biomed Res Int 2020;2020:8163789.

39. Haupt M, Gerner ST, Bahr M, et al. Neuroprotective Strategies for Ischemic Stroke-Future Perspectives. Int J Mol Sci 2023;24(5).

40. Cherchi L, Anni D, Buffelli M, et al. Early Application of Ipsilateral Cathodal-tDCS in a Mouse Model of Brain Ischemia Results in Functional Improvement and Perilesional Microglia Modulation. Biomolecules 2022;12(4).

41. Sheng R, Chen C, Chen H, et al. Repetitive transcranial magnetic stimulation for stroke rehabilitation: insights into the molecular and cellular mechanisms of neuroinflammation. Front Immunol 2023;14:1197422.

42. Blaschke SJ, Vlachakis S, Pallast N, et al. Transcranial Direct Current Stimulation Reverses Stroke-Induced Network Alterations in Mice. Stroke 2023. https://doi.org/10.1161/STROKEAHA.123.042808.

43. Zeiler SR, Hubbard R, Gibson EM, et al. Paradoxical Motor Recovery From a First Stroke After Induction of a Second Stroke: Reopening a Postischemic Sensitive Period. Neurorehabil Neural Repair 2016;30(8):794–800.

44. Centonze D, Rossi S, Tortiglione A, et al. Synaptic plasticity during recovery from permanent occlusion of the middle cerebral artery. Neurobiol Dis 2007; 27(1):44–53.

45. Joy MT, Carmichael ST. Encouraging an excitable brain state: mechanisms of brain repair in stroke. Nat Rev Neurosci 2021;22(1):38–53.

46. Pizzorusso T, Medini P, Berardi N, et al. Reactivation of ocular dominance plasticity in the adult visual cortex. Science 2002;298(5596):1248–51.

47. Sandvig I, Augestad IL, Haberg AK, et al. Neuroplasticity in stroke recovery. The role of microglia in engaging and modifying synapses and networks. Eur J Neurosci 2018;47(12):1414–28.

48. Clarkson AN, Huang BS, Macisaac SE, et al. Reducing excessive GABA-mediated tonic inhibition promotes functional recovery after stroke. Nature 2010;468(7321):305–9.

49. Bice AR, Xiao Q, Kong J, et al. Homotopic contralesional excitation suppresses spontaneous circuit repair and global network reconnections following ischemic stroke. Elife 2022;11.

50. Hordacre B, Austin D, Brown KE, et al. Evidence for a Window of Enhanced Plasticity in the Human Motor Cortex Following Ischemic Stroke. Neurorehabil Neural Repair 2021;35(4):307–20.

51. McDonnell MN, Stinear CM. TMS measures of motor cortex function after stroke: A meta-analysis. Brain Stimul 2017;10(4):721–34.

52. Tamakoshi K, Meguro K, Takahashi Y, et al. Comparison of motor function recovery and brain changes in intracerebral hemorrhagic and ischemic rats with similar brain damage. Neuroreport 2023;34(6):332–7.

53. Joy MT, Carmichael ST. Learning and Stroke Recovery: Parallelism of Biological Substrates. Semin Neurol 2021;41(2):147–56.

54. Masamizu Y, Tanaka YR, Tanaka YH, et al. Two distinct layer-specific dynamics of cortical ensembles during learning of a motor task. Nat Neurosci 2014;17(7): 987–94.

55. Makino H, Hwang EJ, Hedrick NG, et al. Circuit Mechanisms of Sensorimotor Learning. Neuron 2016;92(4):705–21.

56. Peters AJ, Chen SX, Komiyama T. Emergence of reproducible spatiotemporal activity during motor learning. Nature 2014;510(7504):263–7.

57. Li Q, Ko H, Qian ZM, et al. Refinement of learned skilled movement representation in motor cortex deep output layer. Nat Commun 2017;8:15834.

58. Tang E, Mattar MG, Giusti C, et al. Effective learning is accompanied by high-dimensional and efficient representations of neural activity. Nat Neurosci 2019;22(6):1000–9.

59. Biane JS, Scanziani M, Tuszynski MH, et al. Motor cortex maturation is associated with reductions in recurrent connectivity among functional subpopulations and increases in intrinsic excitability. J Neurosci 2015;35(11):4719–28.

60. Cheng MY, Wang EH, Woodson WJ, et al. Optogenetic neuronal stimulation promotes functional recovery after stroke. Proc Natl Acad Sci U S A 2014;111(35): 12913–8.

61. Wahl AS, Buchler U, Brandli A, et al. Optogenetically stimulating intact rat corticospinal tract post-stroke restores motor control through regionalized functional circuit formation. Nat Commun 2017;8(1):1187.

62. Tennant KA, Taylor SL, White ER, et al. Optogenetic rewiring of thalamocortical circuits to restore function in the stroke injured brain. Nat Commun 2017;8: 15879.

63. Mandat TS, Hurwitz T, Honey CR. Hypomania as an adverse effect of subthalamic nucleus stimulation: report of two cases. Acta Neurochir (Wien) 2006; 148(8):895–7 [discussion: 898].

64. Blomstedt P, Hariz MI. Are complications less common in deep brain stimulation than in ablative procedures for movement disorders? Stereotact Funct Neurosurg 2006;84(2–3):72–81.

65. Brown CE, Aminoltejari K, Erb H, et al. In vivo voltage-sensitive dye imaging in adult mice reveals that somatosensory maps lost to stroke are replaced over weeks by new structural and functional circuits with prolonged modes of activation within both the peri-infarct zone and distant sites. J Neurosci 2009;29(6): 1719–34.

66. Murphy TH, Corbett D. Plasticity during stroke recovery: from synapse to behaviour. Nat Rev Neurosci 2009;10(12):861–72.

67. Jones EG. Cortical and subcortical contributions to activity-dependent plasticity in primate somatosensory cortex. Annu Rev Neurosci 2000;23:1–37.

68. Raghavan P, Krakauer JW, Gordon AM. Impaired anticipatory control of fingertip forces in patients with a pure motor or sensorimotor lacunar syndrome. Brain 2006;129(Pt 6):1415–25.

69. Bolognini N, Russo C, Edwards DJ. The sensory side of post-stroke motor rehabilitation. Restor Neurol Neurosci 2016;34(4):571–86.

70. Sarlegna FR, Sainburg RL. The roles of vision and proprioception in the planning of reaching movements. Adv Exp Med Biol 2009;629:317–35.

71. Sarlegna FR, Przybyla A, Sainburg RL. The influence of target sensory modality on motor planning may reflect errors in sensori-motor transformations. Neuroscience 2009;164(2):597–610.

72. De Bruyn N, Meyer S, Kessner SS, et al. Functional network connectivity is altered in patients with upper limb somatosensory impairments in the acute phase post stroke: A cross-sectional study. PLoS One 2018;13(10):e0205693.

73. Zavaliangos-Petropulu A, Lo B, Donnelly MR, et al. Chronic Stroke Sensorimotor Impairment Is Related to Smaller Hippocampal Volumes: An ENIGMA Analysis. J Am Heart Assoc 2022;11(10):e025109.

74. Schaechter JD, Moore CI, Connell BD, et al. Structural and functional plasticity in the somatosensory cortex of chronic stroke patients. Brain 2006;129(Pt 10): 2722–33.

75. Wang L, Wang S, Zhang S, et al. Effectiveness and electrophysiological mechanisms of focal vibration on upper limb motor dysfunction in patients with subacute stroke: A randomized controlled trial. Brain Res 2023;1809:148353.

76. De Bruyn N, Saenen L, Thijs L, et al. Brain connectivity alterations after additional sensorimotor or motor therapy for the upper limb in the early-phase post stroke: a randomized controlled trial. Brain Commun 2021;3(2):fcab074.

77. Jimenez-Marin A, De Bruyn N, Gooijers J, et al. Multimodal and multidomain lesion network mapping enhances prediction of sensorimotor behavior in stroke patients. Sci Rep 2022;12(1):22400.

78. Ward NS, Brown MM, Thompson AJ, et al. Neural correlates of motor recovery after stroke: a longitudinal fMRI study. Brain 2003;126(Pt 11):2476–96.

79. Cramer SC. Repairing the human brain after stroke: I. Mechanisms of spontaneous recovery. Ann Neurol 2008;63(3):272–87.

80. Pirovano I, Mastropietro A, Antonacci Y, et al. Resting State EEG Directed Functional Connectivity Unveils Changes in Motor Network Organization in Subacute Stroke Patients After Rehabilitation. Front Physiol 2022;13:862207.

81. Lariviere S, Ward NS, Boudrias MH. Disrupted functional network integrity and flexibility after stroke: Relation to motor impairments. Neuroimage Clin 2018; 19:883–91.
82. Latifi S, Mitchell S, Habibey R, et al. Neuronal Network Topology Indicates Distinct Recovery Processes after Stroke. Cereb Cortex 2020;30(12):6363–75.
83. O'Keeffe R, Shirazi SY, Bilaloglu S, et al. Nonlinear functional muscle network based on information theory tracks sensorimotor integration post stroke. Sci Rep 2022;12(1):13029.
84. Lee J, Kim YH. Does a Cognitive Network Contribute to Motor Recovery After Ischemic Stroke? Neurorehabil Neural Repair 2023. 15459683231177604.
85. McPherson JG, Chen A, Ellis MD, et al. Progressive recruitment of contralesional cortico-reticulospinal pathways drives motor impairment post stroke. J Physiol 2018;596(7):1211–25.
86. Li S, Chen YT, Francisco GE, et al. A Unifying Pathophysiological Account for Post-stroke Spasticity and Disordered Motor Control. Front Neurol 2019;10:468.
87. Choudhury S, Shobhana A, Singh R, et al. The Relationship Between Enhanced Reticulospinal Outflow and Upper Limb Function in Chronic Stroke Patients. Neurorehabil Neural Repair 2019;33(5):375–83.
88. Paul T, Cieslak M, Hensel L, et al. The role of corticospinal and extrapyramidal pathways in motor impairment after stroke. Brain Commun 2023;5(1). fcac301.
89. Germann M, Baker SN. Evidence for Subcortical Plasticity after Paired Stimulation from a Wearable Device. J Neurosci 2021;41(7):1418–28.
90. Foysal KM, de Carvalho F, Baker SN. Spike Timing-Dependent Plasticity in the Long-Latency Stretch Reflex Following Paired Stimulation from a Wearable Electronic Device. J Neurosci 2016;36(42):10823–30.
91. Conner JM, Culberson A, Packowski C, et al. Lesions of the Basal forebrain cholinergic system impair task acquisition and abolish cortical plasticity associated with motor skill learning. Neuron 2003;38(5):819–29.
92. Conner JM, Chiba AA, Tuszynski MH. The basal forebrain cholinergic system is essential for cortical plasticity and functional recovery following brain injury. Neuron 2005;46(2):173–9.
93. Yamakawa GR, Basu P, Cortese F, et al. The cholinergic forebrain arousal system acts directly on the circadian pacemaker. Proc Natl Acad Sci U S A 2016;113(47):13498–503.
94. Berthier ML, Pujol J, Gironell A, et al. Beneficial effect of donepezil on sensorimotor function after stroke. Am J Phys Med Rehabil 2003;82(9):725–9.
95. Vitrac C, Nallet-Khosrofian L, Iijima M, et al. Endogenous dopamine transmission is crucial for motor skill recovery after stroke. IBRO Neurosci Rep 2022; 13:15–21.
96. Widmer M, Held JPO, Wittmann F, et al. Reward During Arm Training Improves Impairment and Activity After Stroke: A Randomized Controlled Trial. Neurorehabil Neural Repair 2022;36(2):140–50.
97. Li Y, Yu Z, Wu P, et al. Ability of an altered functional coupling between resting-state networks to predict behavioral outcomes in subcortical ischemic stroke: A longitudinal study. Front Aging Neurosci 2022;14:933567.
98. Raghavan P, Geller D, Guerrero N, et al. Music Upper Limb Therapy-Integrated: An Enriched Collaborative Approach for Stroke Rehabilitation. Front Hum Neurosci 2016;10:498.
99. Palumbo A, Aluru V, Battaglia J, et al. Music Upper Limb Therapy-Integrated Provides a Feasible Enriched Environment and Reduces Post-stroke

Depression: A Pilot Randomized Controlled Trial. Am J Phys Med Rehabil 2022; 101(10):937–46.

100. Jia T, Li C, Mo L, et al. Tailoring brain-machine interface rehabilitation training based on neural reorganization: towards personalized treatment for stroke patients. Cereb Cortex 2023;33(6):3043–52.

101. Liu M, Ushiba J. Brain-machine Interface (BMI)-based Neurorehabilitation for Post-stroke Upper Limb Paralysis. Keio J Med 2022;71(4):82–92.

102. Arasaki K, Igarashi O, Ichikawa Y, et al. Reduction in the motor unit number estimate (MUNE) after cerebral infarction. J Neurol Sci 2006;250(1–2):27–32.

103. Hu X, Suresh AK, Rymer WZ, et al. Assessing altered motor unit recruitment patterns in paretic muscles of stroke survivors using surface electromyography. J Neural Eng 2015;12(6):066001.

104. Mottram CJ, Heckman CJ, Powers RK, et al. Disturbances of motor unit rate modulation are prevalent in muscles of spastic-paretic stroke survivors. J Neurophysiol 2014;111(10):2017–28.

105. Yi Y, Shim JS, Oh BM, et al. Grip Strength on the Unaffected Side as an Independent Predictor of Functional Improvement After Stroke. Am J Phys Med Rehabil 2017;96(9):616–20.

106. Nowak DA, Grefkes C, Dafotakis M, et al. Dexterity is impaired at both hands following unilateral subcortical middle cerebral artery stroke. Eur J Neurosci 2007;25(10):3173–84.

107. Anker SD, Morley JE, von Haehling S. Welcome to the ICD-10 code for sarcopenia. J Cachexia Sarcopenia Muscle 2016;7(5):512–4.

108. Rosenberg IH. Sarcopenia: origins and clinical relevance. J Nutr 1997;127(5 Suppl):990S–1S.

109. Ryan AS, Dobrovolny CL, Smith GV, et al. Hemiparetic muscle atrophy and increased intramuscular fat in stroke patients. Arch Phys Med Rehabil 2002; 83(12):1703–7.

110. Scherbakov N, Sandek A, Doehner W. Stroke-related sarcopenia: specific characteristics. J Am Med Dir Assoc 2015;16(4):272–6.

111. Ryan AS, Ivey FM, Serra MC, et al. Sarcopenia and Physical Function in Middle-Aged and Older Stroke Survivors. Arch Phys Med Rehabil 2017;98(3):495–9.

112. Scherbakov N, Doehner W. Sarcopenia in stroke-facts and numbers on muscle loss accounting for disability after stroke. J Cachexia Sarcopenia Muscle 2011; 2(1):5–8.

113. Carda S, Cisari C, Invernizzi M. Sarcopenia or muscle modifications in neurologic diseases: a lexical or patophysiological difference? Eur J Phys Rehabil Med 2013;49(1):119–30.

114. De Deyne PG, Hafer-Macko CE, Ivey FM, et al. Muscle molecular phenotype after stroke is associated with gait speed. Muscle Nerve 2004;30(2):209–15.

115. Ferrandi PJ, Khan MM, Paez HG, et al. Transcriptome Analysis of Skeletal Muscle Reveals Altered Proteolytic and Neuromuscular Junction Associated Gene Expressions in a Mouse Model of Cerebral Ischemic Stroke. Genes (Basel) 2020;11(7).

116. Jagoe RT, Goldberg AL. What do we really know about the ubiquitin-proteasome pathway in muscle atrophy? Curr Opin Clin Nutr Metab Care 2001;4(3):183–90.

117. Glickman MH, Ciechanover A. The ubiquitin-proteasome proteolytic pathway: destruction for the sake of construction. Physiol Rev 2002;82(2):373–428.

118. Dent E, Morley JE, Cruz-Jentoft AJ, et al. International Clinical Practice Guidelines for Sarcopenia (ICFSR): Screening, Diagnosis and Management. J Nutr Health Aging 2018;22(10):1148–61.

119. Lauretani F, Bautmans I, De Vita F, et al. Identification and treatment of older persons with sarcopenia. Aging Male 2014;17(4):199–204.

120. Beckwee D, Delaere A, Aelbrecht S, et al. Exercise Interventions for the Prevention and Treatment of Sarcopenia. A Systematic Umbrella Review. J Nutr Health Aging 2019;23(6):494–502.

121. Theodorakopoulos C, Jones J, Bannerman E, et al. Effectiveness of nutritional and exercise interventions to improve body composition and muscle strength or function in sarcopenic obese older adults: A systematic review. Nutr Res 2017;43:3–15.

122. Yoshimura Y, Wakabayashi H, Yamada M, et al. Interventions for Treating Sarcopenia: A Systematic Review and Meta-Analysis of Randomized Controlled Studies. J Am Med Dir Assoc 2017;18(6):553 e551–e553 e516.

123. Csapo R, Alegre LM. Effects of resistance training with moderate vs heavy loads on muscle mass and strength in the elderly: A meta-analysis. Scand J Med Sci Sports 2016;26(9):995–1006.

124. Buch A, Kis O, Carmeli E, et al. Circuit resistance training is an effective means to enhance muscle strength in older and middle aged adults: A systematic review and meta-analysis. Ageing Res Rev 2017;37:16–27.

125. Emsley HC, Smith CJ, Gavin CM, et al. An early and sustained peripheral inflammatory response in acute ischaemic stroke: relationships with infection and atherosclerosis. J Neuroimmunol 2003;139(1–2):93–101.

126. Anrather J, Iadecola C. Inflammation and Stroke: An Overview. Neurotherapeutics 2016;13(4):661–70.

127. Becker KJ, Zierath D, Kunze A, et al. The contribution of antibiotics, pneumonia and the immune response to stroke outcome. J Neuroimmunol 2016;295-296: 68–74.

128. Becker KJ. Inflammation and the Silent Sequelae of Stroke. Neurotherapeutics 2016;13(4):801–10.

129. Morley W, Jackson K, Mead GE. Post-stroke fatigue: an important yet neglected symptom. Age Ageing 2005;34(3):313.

130. Beckwee D, Lefeber N, Bautmans I, et al. Muscle changes after stroke and their impact on recovery: time for a paradigm shift? Review and commentary. Top Stroke Rehabil 2021;28(2):104–11.

131. Petersen AM, Pedersen BK. The anti-inflammatory effect of exercise. J Appl Physiol (1985) 2005;98(4):1154–62.

132. Forti LN, Van Roie E, Njemini R, et al. Load-Specific Inflammation Mediating Effects of Resistance Training in Older Persons. J Am Med Dir Assoc 2016;17(6): 547–52.

133. Liberman K, Forti LN, Beyer I, et al. The effects of exercise on muscle strength, body composition, physical functioning and the inflammatory profile of older adults: a systematic review. Curr Opin Clin Nutr Metab Care 2017;20(1):30–53.

134. Forti LN, Van Roie E, Njemini R, et al. Effects of resistance training at different loads on inflammatory markers in young adults. Eur J Appl Physiol 2017; 117(3):511–9.

135. Beyer I, Njemini R, Bautmans I, et al. Inflammation-related muscle weakness and fatigue in geriatric patients. Exp Gerontol 2012;47(1):52–9.

136. Beyer I, Mets T, Bautmans I. Chronic low-grade inflammation and age-related sarcopenia. Curr Opin Clin Nutr Metab Care 2012;15(1):12–22.

137. Pedersen BK, Febbraio MA. Muscles, exercise and obesity: skeletal muscle as a secretory organ. Nat Rev Endocrinol 2012;8(8):457–65.

138. Pedersen BK. Muscular interleukin-6 and its role as an energy sensor. Med Sci Sports Exerc 2012;44(3):392–6.
139. Pedersen BK. Physical activity and muscle-brain crosstalk. Nat Rev Endocrinol 2019;15(7):383–92.
140. Norheim KL, Cullum CK, Andersen JL, et al. Inflammation Relates to Resistance Training-induced Hypertrophy in Elderly Patients. Med Sci Sports Exerc 2017; 49(6):1079–85.
141. Norheim KL, Bautmans I, Kjaer M. Handgrip strength shows no improvements in geriatric patients with persistent inflammation during hospitalization. Exp Gerontol 2017;99:115–9.
142. Bautmans I, Njemini R, Lambert M, et al. Circulating acute phase mediators and skeletal muscle performance in hospitalized geriatric patients. J Gerontol A Biol Sci Med Sci 2005;60(3):361–7.
143. Vallbo AB, Hulliger M. The dependence of discharge rate of spindle afferent units on the size of the load during isotonic position holding in man. Brain Res 1982;237(2):297–307.
144. Jalal N, Gracies JM, Zidi M. Mechanical and microstructural changes of skeletal muscle following immobilization and/or stroke. Biomech Model Mechanobiol 2020;19(1):61–80.
145. Okita M, Yoshimura T, Nakano J, et al. Effects of reduced joint mobility on sarcomere length, collagen fibril arrangement in the endomysium, and hyaluronan in rat soleus muscle. J Muscle Res Cell Motil 2004;25(2):159–66.
146. Barker D, Banks RW. The muscle spindle. In: Engel AG, Franzini-Armstrong C, editors. Myology. vol 1. 2nd edition. New York: McGraw-Hill; 1994. p. 333–60.
147. Pedrosa-Domellof F, Hellstrom S, Thornell LE. Hyaluronan in human and rat muscle spindles. Histochem Cell Biol 1998;110(2):179–82.
148. Fukami Y. Studies of capsule and capsular space of cat muscle spindles. J Physiol 1986;376:281–97.
149. Song Z, Banks RW, Bewick GS. Modelling the mechanoreceptor's dynamic behaviour. J Anat 2015;227(2):243–54.
150. Edin BB, Vallbo AB. Stretch sensitization of human muscle spindles. J Physiol 1988;400:101–11.
151. Raghavan P, Lu Y, Mirchandani M, et al. Human Recombinant Hyaluronidase Injections For Upper Limb Muscle Stiffness in Individuals With Cerebral Injury: A Case Series. EBioMedicine 2016;9:306–13.
152. Stecco A, Stecco C, Raghavan P. Peripheral mechanisms of spasticity and treatment implications. Curr Phys Med Rehabil Rep 2014;2(2):121–7.
153. Piehl-Aulin K, Laurent C, Engstrom-Laurent A, et al. Hyaluronan in human skeletal muscle of lower extremity: concentration, distribution, and effect of exercise. J Appl Physiol (1985) 1991;71(6):2493–8.
154. Brown R, Sharafi A, Slade JM, et al. Lower extremity MRI following 10-week supervised exercise intervention in patients with diabetic peripheral neuropathy. BMJ Open Diabetes Res Care 2021;9(1).
155. Menon RG, Raghavan P, Regatte RR. Quantifying muscle glycosaminoglycan levels in patients with post-stroke muscle stiffness using T1rho MRI. Sci Rep 2019;9(1):14513.
156. Padmanabhan P, Rao KS, Gulhar S, et al. Persons post-stroke improve step length symmetry by walking asymmetrically. J Neuroeng Rehabil 2020; 17(1):105.
157. Fritz S, Lusardi M. White paper: "walking speed: the sixth vital sign". J Geriatr Phys Ther 2009;32(2):46–9.

158. Studenski S, Perera S, Patel K, et al. Gait speed and survival in older adults. JAMA 2011;305(1):50–8.
159. Perera S, Patel KV, Rosano C, et al. Gait Speed Predicts Incident Disability: A Pooled Analysis. J Gerontol A Biol Sci Med Sci 2016;71(1):63–71.
160. Montero-Odasso M, Schapira M, Soriano ER, et al. Gait velocity as a single predictor of adverse events in healthy seniors aged 75 years and older. J Gerontol A Biol Sci Med Sci 2005;60(10):1304–9.
161. Lusardi MM, Fritz S, Middleton A, et al. Determining Risk of Falls in Community Dwelling Older Adults: A Systematic Review and Meta-analysis Using Posttest Probability. J Geriatr Phys Ther 2017;40(1):1–36.
162. Fini NA, Holland AE, Keating J, et al. How Physically Active Are People Following Stroke? Systematic Review and Quantitative Synthesis. Phys Ther 2017;97(7):707–17.
163. Tieges Z, Mead G, Allerhand M, et al. Sedentary behavior in the first year after stroke: a longitudinal cohort study with objective measures. Arch Phys Med Rehabil 2015;96(1):15–23.
164. Kleindorfer DO, Towfighi A, Chaturvedi S, et al. Guideline for the Prevention of Stroke in Patients With Stroke and Transient Ischemic Attack: A Guideline From the American Heart Association/American Stroke Association. Stroke 2021;52(7):e364–467.
165. Billinger SA, Arena R, Bernhardt J, et al. Physical activity and exercise recommendations for stroke survivors: a statement for healthcare professionals from the American Heart Association/American Stroke Association. Stroke 2014; 45(8):2532–53.
166. Ivey FM, Macko RF, Ryan AS, et al. Cardiovascular health and fitness after stroke. Top Stroke Rehabil 2005;12(1):1–16.
167. Tang A, Sibley KM, Thomas SG, et al. Maximal exercise test results in subacute stroke. Arch Phys Med Rehabil 2006;87(8):1100–5.
168. Mackay-Lyons MJ, Makrides L. Exercise capacity early after stroke. Arch Phys Med Rehabil 2002;83(12):1697–702.
169. Austin MW, Ploughman M, Glynn L, et al. Aerobic exercise effects on neuroprotection and brain repair following stroke: a systematic review and perspective. Neurosci Res 2014;87:8–15.
170. Ploughman M, Austin MW, Glynn L, et al. The effects of poststroke aerobic exercise on neuroplasticity: a systematic review of animal and clinical studies. Transl Stroke Res 2015;6(1):13–28.
171. Nokia MS, Lensu S, Ahtiainen JP, et al. Physical exercise increases adult hippocampal neurogenesis in male rats provided it is aerobic and sustained. J Physiol 2016;594(7):1855–73.
172. Ergul A, Valenzuela JP, Fouda AY, et al. Cellular connections, microenvironment and brain angiogenesis in diabetes: Lost communication signals in the poststroke period. Brain Res 2015;1623:81–96.
173. Moncion K, Allison EY, Al-Khazraji BK, et al. What are the effects of acute exercise and exercise training on cerebrovascular hemodynamics following stroke? A systematic review and meta-analysis. J Appl Physiol (1985) 2022;132(6): 1379–93.
174. Penna LG, Pinheiro JP, Ramalho SHR, et al. Effects of aerobic physical exercise on neuroplasticity after stroke: systematic review. Arq Neuropsiquiatr 2021; 79(9):832–43.

175. Boyne P, Billinger SA, Reisman DS, et al. Optimal Intensity and Duration of Walking Rehabilitation in Patients With Chronic Stroke: A Randomized Clinical Trial. JAMA Neurol 2023;80(4):342–51.

176. Rich B, Scadeng M, Yamaguchi M, et al. Skeletal myofiber vascular endothelial growth factor is required for the exercise training-induced increase in dentate gyrus neuronal precursor cells. J Physiol 2017;595(17):5931–43.

177. Sayyah M, Seydyousefi M, Moghanlou AE, et al. Activation of BDNF- and VEGF-mediated Neuroprotection by Treadmill Exercise Training in Experimental Stroke. Metab Brain Dis 2022;37(6):1843–53.

178. Marzolini S, Robertson AD, Oh P, et al. Aerobic Training and Mobilization Early Post-stroke: Cautions and Considerations. Front Neurol 2019;10:1187.

179. Schroder J, Truijen S, Van Criekinge T, et al. Feasibility and effectiveness of repetitive gait training early after stroke: A systematic review and meta-analysis. J Rehabil Med 2019;51(2):78–88.

180. Askim T, Dahl AE, Aamot IL, et al. High-intensity aerobic interval training for patients 3-9 months after stroke: a feasibility study. Physiother Res Int 2014;19(3):129–39.

181. Cuccurullo SJ, Fleming TK, Zinonos S, et al. Stroke Recovery Program with Modified Cardiac Rehabilitation Improves Mortality, Functional & Cardiovascular Performance. J Stroke Cerebrovasc Dis 2022;31(5):106322.

182. Cuccurullo SJ, Fleming TK, Kostis JB, et al. Impact of Modified Cardiac Rehabilitation Within a Stroke Recovery Program on All-Cause Hospital Readmissions. Am J Phys Med Rehabil 2022;101(1):40–7.

183. Cuccurullo SJ, Fleming TK, Kostis WJ, et al. Impact of a Stroke Recovery Program Integrating Modified Cardiac Rehabilitation on All-Cause Mortality, Cardiovascular Performance and Functional Performance. Am J Phys Med Rehabil 2019;98(11):953–63.

184. Dromerick AW, Geed S, Barth J, et al. Critical Period After Stroke Study (CPASS): A phase II clinical trial testing an optimal time for motor recovery after stroke in humans. Proc Natl Acad Sci U S A 2021;118(39).

185. Pruski A, Lavezza A, Ye B, et al. Feasibility of an Enhanced Therapy Model of Care for Hospitalized Stroke Patients. Am J Phys Med Rehabil 2023;102(2S Suppl 1):S19–23.

186. Langton-Frost N, Orient S, Adeyemo J, et al. Development and Implementation of a New Model of Care for Patients With Stroke, Acute Hospital Rehabilitation Intensive SErvices: Leveraging a Multidisciplinary Rehabilitation Team. Am J Phys Med Rehabil 2023;102(2S Suppl 1):S13–8.

187. Pain LAM, Baker R, Sohail QZ, et al. The three-dimensional shoulder pain alignment (3D-SPA) mobilization improves pain-free shoulder range, functional reach and sleep following stroke: a pilot randomized control trial. Disabil Rehabil 2020;42(21):3072–83.

188. Cho KH, Park SJ. Effects of joint mobilization and stretching on the range of motion for ankle joint and spatiotemporal gait variables in stroke patients. J Stroke Cerebrovasc Dis 2020;29(8):104933.

189. Lien P, Deluzio S, Adeyemo J, et al. Development and Implementation of a Standard Assessment Battery Across the Continuum of Care for Patients After Stroke. Am J Phys Med Rehabil 2023;102(2S Suppl 1):S51–5.

190. McDonald MW, Jeffers MS, Issa L, et al. An Exercise Mimetic Approach to Reduce Poststroke Deconditioning and Enhance Stroke Recovery. Neurorehabil Neural Repair 2021;35(6):471–85.

191. Raghavan P. A Unified Model for Stroke Recovery and Rehabilitation: Why Now? Am J Phys Med Rehabil 2023;102(2S Suppl 1):S3–9.
192. Jenkins L, Gonzaga S, Jedlanek E, et al. Addressing the Operational Challenges for Outpatient Stroke Rehabilitation. Am J Phys Med Rehabil 2023; 102(2S Suppl 1):S61–7.
193. Cook H, McLaughlin KH, Johnson K, et al. A Novel Way to Objectively Review Emerging Rehabilitation Technologies. Am J Phys Med Rehabil 2023;102(2S Suppl 1):S75–8.
194. Raghavan P, Gordon A, Roemmich R, et al. Treatment of Focal Muscle Stiffness with Hyaluronidase Injections. In: Raghavan P, editor. Spasticity and muscle stiffness: Restoring Form and function. 1st edition. Switzerland: Springer Nature; 2022. p. 263–86.

Biomarkers of Motor Outcomes After Stroke

Suzanne Ackerley, PhD[a,1], Marie-Claire Smith, PhD[b,1],
Harry Jordan, PhD[c], Cathy M. Stinear, PhD[c,*]

KEYWORDS

- Stroke • Motor • Prognosis • Biomarker • Transcranial magnetic stimulation
- Magnetic resonance imaging

KEY POINTS

- Neurophysiological and neuroimaging biomarkers of the motor cortex and its descending pathways are related to subsequent upper and lower limb motor outcomes after stroke.
- Prediction tools combining neurophysiological biomarkers with clinical and demographic information have been validated for upper limb motor outcomes.
- Prediction tools have been developed for lower limb and walking outcomes and combine clinical and demographic information, but do not yet incorporate biomarkers.

INTRODUCTION

Motor impairment is common after stroke, affecting around half- to three-quarters of patients.[1,2] Recovery from motor impairment mainly occurs in the first 3 months after stroke.[3–5] Further gains in activity capacity and participation can be achieved with ongoing adaptation and compensation.[6] Minimizing motor disability is essential for regaining independence in daily activities and participation in life roles.[3]

Accurate predictions of individual patients' motor outcomes can guide important decisions in the initial days after stroke, such as therapy goals and discharge destination.[7–9] Predicting motor outcomes can also help patients and their families plan and make necessary arrangements for life after stroke.

NATURE OF THE PROBLEM

Predicting motor outcomes based on clinical impression alone can be difficult. For example, 20 experienced clinicians were asked to predict upper limb functional

---

[a] School of Sport and Health Sciences, University of Central Lancashire, Preston, PR1 2HE, UK;
[b] Department of Exercise Sciences, University of Auckland, Private Bag 92019, Auckland 1023, New Zealand; [c] Department of Medicine, University of Auckland, Private Bag 92019, Auckland 1023, New Zealand
[1] Co-authors.
* Corresponding author.
E-mail address: c.stinear@auckland.ac.nz

Phys Med Rehabil Clin N Am 35 (2024) 259–276
https://doi.org/10.1016/j.pmr.2023.06.003

pmr.theclinics.com

outcome for each of their 131 patients within a week of stroke, and their overall accuracy at 6 months was only 59%.[10] Despite this, clinicians rate their clinical impression of the patient's likely functional outcome as the most important factor when deciding discharge destination from acute care.[11,12] Differences between clinicians' impressions can produce wide variations in access to rehabilitation services. For example, a 3-fold variation in the rates of discharge to inpatient rehabilitation services was found by a large study of more than 31,000 stroke patients across 918 acute hospitals in the United States.[13] This large variation persisted even when clinical characteristics and the availability of inpatient rehabilitation facilities were accounted for. These findings highlight the inaccuracy of predictions and variability in discharge decisions that arises when clinicians rely primarily on clinical impression. This variability is a potential source of inefficient allocation of rehabilitation resources, and inequitable access to rehabilitation services.[11,13] One way to reduce variability in clinical decision-making is to use decision support tools that combine clinical and demographic information with biomarkers in an evidence-based, systematic, and reproducible way.

Multivariable regression modeling has repeatedly identified several clinical and demographic variables associated with motor outcomes after stroke, including the patient's age, stroke severity evaluated with the National Institutes of Health Stroke Scale (NIHSS), and the severity of initial motor impairment. Unlike clinical variables, biomarkers provide information about underlying biological processes that are not readily discernible through clinical assessment and could be used to predict outcomes or response to treatment.[9] Biomarkers that are strongly associated with motor outcome after stroke are provided in **Box 1**. In general, patients with more normal brain structure and function experience better motor outcomes after stroke, which is not surprising. Biomarkers are particularly useful for patients with initially severe motor impairment, to identify those with latent potential for recovery. Prediction tools that systematically combine biomarker information with clinical and demographic information can improve the accuracy of clinicians' prognoses and reduce variability in their decision-making.[14,15] Desirable prediction tool characteristics are summarized in **Box 2**.

The purpose of this review is to summarize current methods for predicting motor outcomes for the upper limb, lower limb, and mobility after stroke, with a particular

---

Box 1
Biomarkers associated with motor outcomes after stroke

Neurophysiological
Motor evoked potential (MEP) status. Transcranial magnetic stimulation can be used to elicit MEPs as a biomarker of corticospinal tract function. Patients in whom MEPs can be elicited from affected muscles in the first days after stroke are considered MEP+, and generally have better UL and LL motor recovery and outcomes than patients who are MEP−.
Electroencephalography (EEG). EEG can be used to measure hemispheric symmetry of EEG power spectrum metrics in specific frequency bands, such as theta band frequency. Patients with more symmetrical EEG power spectra generally have better UL motor recovery and outcomes than those with large asymmetries.

Neuroimaging
Corticospinal tract (CST) injury. Standard care clinical MR) can be used to obtain biomarkers of stroke-related injury to the CST. Patients with more CST injury typically have poorer UL and LL motor outcomes.
Fractional anisotropy (FA). MRI can be used to obtain FA asymmetry index as a measure of microstructural integrity of the CST. When measured at the level of the posterior limb of the internal capsule, greater asymmetry between hemispheres is associated with poorer UL motor outcomes.

Box 2
Desirable characteristics of prediction tools for motor outcomes after stroke[15]

1. Designed for use within days of stroke so that predictions can inform rehabilitation and discharge planning.

2. Predict outcome at a specific later timepoint, such as 3 months post-stroke when recovery from impairment is mostly complete. This is preferable to predicting an outcome at discharge because discharge often depends on achieving a specific outcome, and the prediction can therefore become circular.

3. Predict something meaningful for the patient and their family. A binary prediction, such as a "good" or "bad" outcome, is not informative enough for patients to anticipate how stroke will affect a myriad of daily activities. At the other extreme, precisely predicting a score can lack meaning because patients find it difficult to translate an exact assessment score to real-world utility. Between these 2 extremes are categorical predictions for levels of function in daily activities, and these might be more informative for patients and families.

4. Combine a relatively small number of variables in a way that is easily remembered and used. Online apps or simple decision trees are more likely to be used by clinicians than complex regression equations.

5. Externally validated with demonstrated positive clinical impact.

---

focus on the role of biomarkers. The strengths and limitations of current methods are identified, along with recommendations for future research.

CURRENT EVIDENCE—UPPER LIMB

Upper limb (UL) impairment is a frequent consequence of stroke that affects activity capacity and performance, independence, and participation in life roles.[1,16] Early prediction of subsequent UL motor outcome can assist planning and tailoring of UL rehabilitation, and the management of patient, family, and clinician expectations. Upper limb prediction tools typically focus on UL outcome at either 3 or 6 months post-stroke, as most motor recovery occurs within this timeframe.[17] The severity of initial UL impairment along with neurophysiological and neuroimaging biomarkers have consistently been shown to predict subsequent UL motor recovery and outcomes.[18–20]

Prediction tools without biomarkers

Prediction tools have been developed that use clinical information alone to predict an individual's UL outcome after stroke. The advantage of these types of tools is that they capitalize on existing resources in terms of staff skill and time, and available equipment. **Table 1** summarizes 5 of these tools.[21–25] Some approaches use quick, simple bedside tests such as measures of upper limb strength. Other approaches incorporate selected single items from standardized assessments such as the Fugl-Meyer Upper Extremity assessment (FM-UE)[26] and the Action Research Arm Test (ARAT).[27] Many approaches use measures once, within days of stroke, whereas some use repeated measures over weeks post-stroke to make predictions iteratively.

Prediction tools without biomarkers can predict UL outcomes more accurately for patients with mild initial impairment than for patients with moderate to severe initial impairment. Patients with some finger extension or grip strength within the first few days after stroke are highly likely to recover at least some motor function by 3 to 6 months post-stroke.[21–23,28] However, prediction tools that use clinical information alone cannot accurately identify which patients with moderate to severe initial UL impairment will recover at least some UL function.[21–25,28] Repeating clinical

Table 1
Prediction tool characteristics

Tool	Reference	n	Baseline Severity	Clinical Predictors	Biomarkers	Predicted Outcome	Statistical Method	Model Type	Validation Study	Clinical Impact Study
CLINICAL Upper Limb										
EPOS-UL	Nijland et al,[21] 2010	156	NIHSS median 7, IQR 4–14 FM-UE median 21, IQR 4–56 UL MI median 39, IQR 0–76 ARAT median 1.5, IQR 0–41	FE task in FM-UE 0 or ≥ 1 within 72 h SA task in MI 0 or ≥ 9 within 72 h Both predictors also obtained on d5 and d9	None	Binarised UL dexterity at 6 m based on ARAT score < or ≥ 10	Logistic regression	Table	Yes, at 3 m[28]	No
SALGOT	Alt Murphy et al,[22] 2022	94	NIHSS median 6, IQR 3–11 FM-UE median 39, IQR 4–58	ARAT grasp 2.5 cm cube < or ≥ 2 on d3 Grip strength dynamometry 0 or > 0 kg on d3 FM-UE SA or SE within flexor synergy 0 or ≥ 1 on d3	None	One of 5 categories of UL function at 3 m based on ARAT score: full, excellent, good, limited, or poor	Logistic regression	Decision tree	No	No
Not named	Barth et al,[23] 2022	49	90% of NIHSS 0–15 59% of SAFE scores ≥ 5	SAFE score < or ≥ 5 at time of consent, mean d7, range d2 – 14 Age < or ≥ 80 y NIHSS < 9, 9, or ≥10 at 48 h	None	One of 4 categories of UL function at 3 m based on ARAT score: excellent, good, limited, and poor	Correct classification rate	Decision tree	No	No
Not named	van der Vliet et al,[24] 2020	412	NIHSS range 0–21 66% ≥ 9 on SA task in MI 45% ≥ 0 on FE task in FM-UE	FM-UE total score/s within 26 wk	None	One of 3 categories of UL impairment within 26 wk based on FM-UE score: good, moderate, or poor, with % likelihood of achieving predicted category	Longitudinal mixture (dynamic)	Web-based application	No	No

Name	Study	N	Sample characteristics	Inputs	Neurophysiology biomarker	Outcome	Model	Format	External validation	
Not named	Selles et al,[25] 2021	450	NIHSS mean 8, SD 5, FM-UE mean 25, SD 22, ARAT mean 14, SD 19, UL MI mean 38, SD 34	ARAT score/s within 26 wk, SA score/s from MI and FE score/s from FM-UE within 26 wk	None	ARAT score within 26 wk	Longitudinal mixture (dynamic)	Web-based application	No	No
CLINICAL AND NEUROPHYSIOLOGY COMBINED Upper Limb										
PREP2	Stinear et al,[39] 2017	207	95% NIHSS 0-15, 68% SAFE score ≥ 5	SAFE score < or ≥ 5 on d3, Age < or ≥ 80 y, NIHSS < or ≥ 7 on d3	FDI or ECR MEP status using TMS between d3 and 7	One of 4 categories of UL function at 3 m based on ARAT score: excellent, good, limited, or poor	CART	Decision tree	Yes	Yes[8]
Not named	Hoonhorst et al,[46] 2018	51	NIHSS not reported FM-UE median 8, IQR 3-50 UL MI arm median 18, IQR 0-70 37% had FE 53% had SA	FE task in FM-UE 0 or ≥ 1 at ≤ 48h or d11 SA task in MI 0 or ≥ 9 at ≤ 48 h or d11	ADM MEP status using TMS on ≤ 48 h or d11	Binarised UL outcome at 6m based on FM-UE score < or ≥ 22	Logistic regression ROC curve	Table	No	No
CLINICAL Lower Limb										
EPOS-LL	Veerbeek et al,[66] 2011	154	NIHSS not reported LL MI median 44.5 IQR 33-65, Berg Balance scale median 5/56 (1-23), Sitting balance yes 68%, FM-LL median 17, IQR 7-25, TCT median 62, IQR 25-87, FAC median 0, IQR 0-2, Barthel Index median 6, IQR 2-10	LL MI < or ≥ 25 TCT sitting balance < or ≥ 25 Both predictors at < 72 h, d5, and d9	None	Independent walking (FAC ≥ 4) at 6 m	Logistic regression	Table	Yes, at 3 m[65]	No

(continued on next page)

Table 1
(continued)

Tool	Reference	n	Baseline Severity	Clinical Predictors	Biomarkers	Predicted Outcome	Statistical Method	Model Type	Validation Study	Clinical Impact Study
TWIST development	Smith et al,[64] 2017	41	NIHSS median 8, range 1–11 LL MI median 48, range 0–92 FAC median 0, range 0–2	TCT < or > 40 on d7 MRC hip extension strength < or ≥ 3 on D7	None	Time taken to achieve independent walking (FAC ≥ 4) at 6 wk, 12 wk, or dependent at 12 wk	CART	Decision tree	No	No
Revised TWIST	Smith et al,[61] 2022	93	NIHSS median 8, range 1–24 LL MI median 59, range 1–100 FM-LL median 19, range 7–29	Age < or ≥ 80 y MRC knee extension strength < or ≥ 3 on d7 Berg balance test < 6, 6–15, ≥ 16 on d7	None	Time taken to achieve independent walking (FAC ≥ 4) at 4 wk, 6 wk, 9 wk, 16 wk, 26 wk, or dependent at 26 wk	Cox multivariate regression. Calibration plots and discrimination (C statistical)	Probability table Suggested interpretation	No	No

All times are relative to stroke onset.

Abbreviations: ADM, abductor digit minimi; ARAT, Action Research Arm Test; CART, classification and regression tree; e, day; ECR, extensor carpi radialis; EPOS, early prediction of functional outcome after stroke; FAC, functional ambulatory category; FDI, first dorsal interosseous; FE, finger extension; FM-LL, Fugl-Meyer Lower Limb assessment; FM-UE, Fugl-Meyer Upper Extremity assessment; IQR, interquartile range; LL, lower limb; m, months; MEP, motor-evoked potential; MI, motricity index; MRC, medical research council; NIHSS, National Institutes of Health Stroke Scale; PREP2, predict recovery potential 2; ROC, receiver operating characteristic; SA, shoulder abduction; SAFE, shoulder abduction and finger extension; SALGOT, Stroke Arm Longitudinal Study at Gothenburg University; SD, standard deviation; SE, shoulder elevation; TCT, trunk control test; TMS, transcranial magnetic stimulation; TWIST, time to walking independently after stroke; UL, upper limb.

assessments over the weeks following stroke could improve prediction accuracy for these patients.[22,24,25] But this may be too late to guide rehabilitation decision-making, and these models are currently most accurate for patients with mild initial UL impairment.[24,25] Overall, predictions based on clinical information alone are least accurate for patients with initially moderate to severe UL impairment.

From a clinical utility perspective, the Early Prediction of Functional Outcome after Stroke (EPOS)-UL model[21] is currently the only externally validated clinical prediction tool.[28] However, this model has been criticized for its binary outcome, which limits clinical meaningfulness. An extended EPOS-UL model has been explored to address this, but requires further development.[28] Three tools[22–24] offer more granular prediction categories, but are not yet validated. None of the clinical prediction tools have demonstrated positive clinical impact, and clinical implementation is not yet appropriate.

Prediction tools with biomarkers

Biomarkers of motor cortex and descending motor pathway integrity improve the accuracy of predictions for patients with moderate to severe initial UL impairment.[14,18,19,29,30]

Neurophysiological Measures

Prediction tools that include both clinical measures and neurophysiological biomarkers are summarized in **Table 1**. Electroencephalography (EEG) is a well-established tool in clinical practice, is relatively low cost, and is feasible within the acute stroke setting.[31] EEG can be used to measure cortical activity and functional connectivity after stroke.[32] Bihemispheric power spectral analysis is one of the most common and reliable analysis techniques.[33,34] Using this technique, Saes and colleagues [35] found that a measure of theta frequency symmetry obtained within 3 weeks post-stroke added prognostic value when combined with FM-UE score to predict UL impairment at 6 months post-stroke. The prognostic value of other early EEG measures, such as those derived from time-frequency analysis, evoked potentials, and EEG connectivity, is less clear.[36] A recent systematic review and meta-analysis including 12 UL-related studies concluded that EEG measures were associated with subsequent FM-UE score; however, this work is largely at the exploratory stage.[33] Currently, there are no clinical prediction tools incorporating EEG biomarkers to predict an individual's UL outcome after stroke.

Transcranial magnetic stimulation (TMS) can be used to test the functional integrity of the corticospinal tract (CST).[37] TMS is a safe, painless, noninvasive technique that can elicit a motor-evoked potential (MEP) in contralateral musculature when the CST is functionally intact. MEP status is a binary measure of MEP presence (MEP+) or absence (MEP-). MEP status can be readily obtained at a patient's bedside with no computation,[38,39] and is the simplest MEP parameter that robustly correlates with UL motor outcome.[40–42] Typically, patients in whom MEPs can be elicited from affected UL muscles in the first days after stroke (MEP+) have better UL functional outcomes than MEP– patients.[39–42] Importantly, patients with initially severe UL impairment who are MEP + are likely to have a good motor outcome, and this potential may go unrecognized without the UL MEP status biomarker.[14,39] MEP absence in affected UL muscles in the first week after stroke indicates a patient is unlikely to regain fine motor control of the hand, which relies on a functional CST.[29] MEP– patients may regain gross movements of the UL, and even hand opening and closing, but not dexterous hand movement.[43] Several studies have found that combining UL MEP status with clinical assessments typically produces more accurate predictions than using either type of predictor alone.[19,39]

To date, 2 UL prediction tools have combined TMS biomarkers with clinical assessments for predicting an individual's likely UL outcome. In 2017, Stinear and colleagues [39] developed the PREP2 prediction tool, which predicts an individual's UL outcome at 3 months in 1 of 4 categories: excellent, good, limited, or poor. The tool begins with the SAFE score, which is the combined Medical Research Council (MRC) strength grades for shoulder abduction and finger extension. If the SAFE score is greater than or equal to 5 by day 3 post-stroke it is combined with the patient's age to predict an excellent or good UL outcome. If the SAFE score is less than 5, then TMS is needed to determine UL MEP status within 7 days of stroke. Patients who are MEP+ are predicted to have a good UL outcome. For MEP– patients, a binarized NIHSS score (<7, ≥ 7) obtained on day 3 post-stroke predicts either a limited or poor UL outcome.

Overall, PREP2 was accurate for 75% of patients, and most accurate for limited and poor predictions (85% and 90%, respectively).[39] Misclassification was most common between good and excellent categories, with predictions generally too optimistic. All MEP– patients had a limited or poor outcome, confirming the importance of CST functional integrity for achieving good functional outcomes.[39] Importantly, PREP2 predictions remained accurate for 80% of patients at 2 years post-stroke.[44]

A criticism of PREP2 is that the timeframes for obtaining clinical and biomarker measures may not be feasible in all health care settings. If PREP2 is used outside the recommended timeframe at 2 weeks post-stroke then prediction accuracy falls from 75% to 60%, highlighting that the prediction tool needs to be used at the appropriate time to retain accuracy.[45] A strength of PREP2 is that it has been validated, and has demonstrated positive effects on clinical care such as increasing therapist confidence, enabling tailoring of therapy content, and shortening the length of inpatient stay.[8]

Hoonhorst and colleagues[46] predicted the likelihood of achieving some return of dexterity (FM-UE ≥ 22) at 6 months post-stroke. The model included binarized finger extension strength based on the relevant FM-UE item (0, ≥ 1), and binarized shoulder abduction strength using the relevant Motricity Index item (0, ≥ 9). These clinical measures were combined with abductor digiti minimi (ADM) MEP status obtained within 2 days and again at 11 days post-stroke. The models combining the clinical measures with ADM MEP status at these 2 timepoints had good overall accuracy, with areas under the curve of 0.83 and 0.91, respectively. The combined model was more accurate than ADM MEP status alone, but only at 11 days post-stroke, and it was no more accurate than a model using clinical measures alone. The authors concluded ADM MEP status is not required due to a negligible improvement in prediction accuracy. However, this could reflect the wide range of participants' initial UL impairment (FM-UE scores 3–50). Upper limb MEP status is of most value for patients with moderate to severe initial UL impairment. The inclusion of patients with mild impairment may have diluted the predictive value of UL MEP status in the regression model. This highlights one of the potential limitations of regression models, where all variables are required to predict outcomes for all patients. However, some predictors, such as UL MEP status, are only relevant for a subset of patients. The models produced by Hoonhorst and colleagues are displayed as tables with probabilities of achieving favorable UL outcomes for all combinations of finger extension and shoulder abduction scores along with UL MEP status, but the predicted outcome is binary and its clinical meaningfulness is therefore questionable.

In summary, the most promising neurophysiological biomarker is UL MEP status obtained with TMS. Upper limb MEP status alone though appears to be an insufficient predictor of UL motor outcome. Combining UL MEP status with clinical measures improves prediction accuracy, particularly in tools where UL MEP status is only required for patients with moderate to severe initial UL impairment. To date, PREP2 is the only UL prediction tool to be validated and implemented within clinical practice, with evidence of positive clinical impact. However, TMS is not currently part of standard clinical care for stroke.

Neuroimaging Measures

Several biomarkers obtained from structural and functional neuroimaging are associated with UL motor outcome after stroke. In general, greater disruption to typical brain structure or patterns of activation is associated with worse UL outcomes.[14]

Standard care clinical MRI can provide biomarkers of the structural integrity of the cortex and white matter pathways, and multivariable regression modeling has consistently identified associations between these biomarkers and motor outcomes. Lesion volume is broadly associated with motor outcomes, whereas lesion location and injury to the CST are biomarkers with more specific relevance to UL motor outcome.[18,36,47] Typically, greater CST injury measured with neuroimaging in the first few days after stroke is associated with worse UL motor recovery and outcome at 3 months post-stroke.[47–49] In patients with severe initial UL impairment, Feng and colleagues[47] found FM-UE score at 3 months post-stroke was more strongly associated with initial weighted lesion load than initial FM-UE score. In contrast, in patients with moderate to severe initial UL impairment, Lim and colleagues[50] found FM-UE score at greater than or equal to 2 months post-stroke was more strongly associated with initial FM-UE than initial CST injury. Differences in methodology, the cut-off for classifying severe stroke (FM-UE $\leq$ 10 vs < 35, respectively), and the different outcome timeframes may account for discrepancies. CST injury, when combined with initial FM-UE score, only accounted for about 10% of the variance in UL impairment outcome in patients with moderate to severe initial UL impairment.[50]

MRI can also be used to obtain biomarkers of white matter microstructure characteristics of the CST. Diffusion tensor imaging (DTI) can derive metrics such as fractional anisotropy (FA), mean diffusivity, radial diffusivity and axial diffusivity, which have moderate to strong relationships with UL recovery and outcome.[18,19] DTI measures of structures such as the posterior limb of the internal capsule (PLIC) at both the acute stage[51,52] and 2 weeks post-stroke[53] are significant predictors of UL motor outcome at 3 months post-stroke. Typically, greater PLIC FA asymmetry is associated with less favorable UL motor recovery and outcomes.[29,53] CST axial diffusivity measured within 24 hours after stroke may prove to be an alternative biomarker to FA for predicting UL motor outcome in the hyperacute phase.[54] The relevance of injury to nonprimary motor cortex CST projections is less well-studied. However, relationships have been identified between UL motor outcome and measures of sensorimotor tract lesion load,[39] fibers originating from the premotor cortex,[55,56] and cerebellar and corpus callosum tracts.[57] There is also some evidence that structural MRI biomarkers may outperform clinical assessment in prediction accuracy,[19,53] but this may depend on how soon after stroke the images are acquired.[51] Further research into structural biomarkers is warranted; however, implementation in clinical care may be difficult if nonstandard imaging techniques are used that currently require specialized skills to extract biomarker values.

Functional MRI (fMRI) provides another source of biomarkers, relating cortical activity and connectivity to motor outcomes after stroke. For instance, greater activation in the ipsilesional primary motor cortex, ipsilesional premotor cortex, and contralesional cerebellum activation while performing paretic UL motor tasks within the first week post-stroke are related to better UL outcome.[36,58] The predictive value of resting state fMRI remains unclear.[19,59]

In general, associations between neuroimaging biomarkers and UL motor outcome are observed at a group level using regression modeling. However, the ability to use these biomarkers to make accurate predictions for individual patients is limited by high variability and no clear cut-off values. Neuroimaging biomarkers may hold more value when combined with clinical and/or demographic information, or other biomarkers, compared to when used alone.[18,19]

The optimal imaging biomarker may vary depending on UL MEP status.[57] The original PREP prediction tool in 2012 was the first approach to include a neuroimaging biomarker, PLIC FA asymmetry index, in a sequential manner following SAFE score and UL MEP status to predict an individual's UL motor outcome.[53] The PLIC FA asymmetry index was used to predict either a limited or poor outcome for MEP− patients. Overall accuracy was moderate at 64%, and PREP has been superseded by PREP2[39] and therefore is not included in **Table 1**. The subsequent development of PREP2 found that sensorimotor tract lesion load was a more accurate predictor than CST lesion load and PLIC FA asymmetry index.[39] Further, PREP2 replaced sensorimotor tract lesion load with day 3 NIHSS score, as the latter had equivalent prediction accuracy and is easier to obtain.

In summary, neuroimaging biomarkers of CST injury and white matter integrity are related to subsequent UL motor outcomes. To date, there has been little integration of neuroimaging biomarkers within clinical prediction tools for UL motor outcome, and there are currently no validated tools incorporating neuroimaging biomarkers. Further prospective studies combining promising neuroimaging biomarkers with clinical and demographic information or other biomarkers are recommended.

CURRENT EVIDENCE—LOWER LIMB

The likelihood of recovering independent walking has significant implications for discharge planning and long-term support needs after stroke. Thus, most lower limb (LL) prediction studies focus on the binary outcome of independent walking or not rather than walking pattern, speed, or endurance. The Functional Ambulation Categories (FAC) is the most commonly used outcome assessment with a category of greater than or equal to 4/5 indicating independent walking. Age,[60-63] initial stroke severity,[60,62] LL strength,[61,63-66] and trunk control or balance[61,63-66] are consistently identified as variables associated with subsequent independent walking after stroke. These variables have typically been identified through large-scale regression models, providing a basis from which to develop prediction tools.

Prediction tools for independent walking after stroke fall into 2 categories: predicting achievement of independent walking by a specific timepoint post-stroke such as 3 or 6 months[65]; or predicting time taken to achieve independent walking in weeks or months.[61] Tools that predict independent walking at discharge from rehabilitation are not considered in this review, as discharge criteria often relate to mobility, creating a circular argument (see **Box 1**).[15]

Prediction Tools Without Biomarkers

Two prediction tools using only clinical and/or demographic variables to predict independent walking are outlined in **Table 1**. The EPOS-LL model predicts the probability of independent walking by 3 months post-stroke using the sitting component of the Trunk Control Test (TCT) and the lower limb Motricity Index (LL-MI).[65] EPOS-LL is currently the only externally validated prediction tool for the lower limb.[65] The ability to sit for 30 seconds unsupported (TCT) and an LL-MI score $\geq 25/100$ predicts independent walking by 3 months post-stroke with up to 86% accuracy.[65] EPOS-LL used multiple assessments over time from 1 to 9 days post-stroke and predictions improved with time post-stroke. Model accuracy at day 1 post-stroke was 64% but increased to 83% at day 3 post-stroke and 86% by day 9. Although EPOS-LL performs well overall, its specificity ranges from 55% to 73%, which indicates the tool is less able to identify those patients who will not achieve independent walking than those who will. The EPOS-LL study did not include age as a potential variable despite older age being identified as a factor in remaining nonambulant or taking longer to achieve independent walking after stroke.[65] It is also unclear whether patients were allowed to use walking aids for the FAC assessment at 3 months post-stroke.

The EPOS-LL development and validation studies had different outcome timepoints of 6 months (development)[66] and 3 months (validation)[65] post-stroke with very similar findings This supports previous work identifying that most patients who achieve independent walking do so within the first 3 months post-stroke,[60–63] with a much smaller number achieving independent walking between 3 and 6 months.[61]

The TWIST (Time to Walking Independently after Stroke) studies also identified trunk control and lower limb strength as important clinical predictors for independent walking.[61,64] The TWIST prediction tool uses clinical and demographic variables at 1 week post-stroke to predict time taken to achieve independent walking after stroke.[61,64] TWIST combines age (<80 years), knee extension strength greater than or equal to 3 out of 5 (MRC strength grades) and a Berg Balance Test score of less than 6, 6 to 15, or greater than or equal to 15 out of 56 to predict the likelihood of independent walking at 4, 6, 9, 16, and 26 weeks post-stroke.[61] TWIST performs well overall with accuracy ranging from 83% to 86%. However, specificity and negative predictive value at 6 months post-stroke were poor due to a very small number of participants achieving independent walking between 16 and 26 weeks post-stroke.[61] The TWIST prediction tool has been internally validated with bootstrapping and goodness of fit calculations.

The TWIST and EPOS-LL studies had relatively large sample sizes (93 and 124, respectively) and viewed together, these studies indicate that similar variables predict both independent walking at 3 months post-stroke and time taken to achieve independent walking. Age and standing balance (Berg Balance Test) are predictors in TWIST but not EPOS-LL, indicating these may be important factors for achieving independent walking in the first weeks post-stroke but may have less influence on achievement of walking at 3 or 6 months.

Neurophysiological Measures

Similar to the UL, the relationships between EEG and walking outcomes are at an early stage of exploration. A recent meta-analysis and systematic review identified only 2 studies investigating EEG as a predictor for walking outcomes with contradictory results.[33] There are currently no prediction tools for walking outcomes incorporating EEG biomarkers.

TMS can be used to assess the functional integrity of the CST to the LL. Lower limb MEPs are usually recorded from the paretic tibialis anterior muscle. The predictive value of LL MEPs is not clear due to small sample sizes[64,67,68] and few studies obtaining MEP status within 10 days of stroke.[64,69] In general, patients with LL MEPs experience better walking outcomes than those without MEPs.[67,68,70,71] There are no prediction tools developed for the LL that include MEP status.

Only one study has combined LL MEP status or MRI measures with clinical variables in the process of developing a prediction tool.[64] The TWIST development study combined LL MEP status, CST lesion load, and a range of demographic and clinical variables in a single analysis. Sitting balance and hip extensor strength were stronger predictors of time taken to achieve independent walking than either LL MEP status or CST lesion load. Caution should be used in interpreting these results as the sample size was very small (TMS n = 25; MRI n = 30). There are also some possible technical and neuroanatomical explanations for this finding that CST biomarkers do not add value over clinical predictors for walking after stroke.

There are unique challenges with LL TMS. The LL motor cortex is situated within the medial longitudinal fissure and is therefore more difficult to effectively stimulate. From a neuroanatomical perspective, motor control of the lower limb is less reliant on CST function than the UL, and LL MEP status may therefore be less relevant. The most important clinical predictors for independent walking after stroke are trunk control (sitting balance) and proximal leg strength. Axial and proximal lower limb muscles are controlled by bilateral descending pathways, which support recovery of independent walking despite disruption to the CST.[72–74] Further work combining TMS with clinical and demographic variables should be conducted with larger sample sizes.

Neuroimaging Measures

Very few studies have used MRI measures early after stroke to predict walking outcomes. Sample sizes are small and study design is highly variable, making it difficult to draw conclusions. Overall, participants with less structural CST damage measured with DTI achieve better walking outcomes at 6 months post-stroke.[75–78] One of these studies also identified a relationship between the ratio of ipsilesional-to-contralesional CST FA at the level of the pons and walking performance (FAC) at 6 months.[77] An intact CST predicts independent walking; however, walking outcomes for patients with damage to the CST can be highly variable. There are currently no prediction tools for walking recovery after stroke that combine MRI and clinical measures.

As control of walking is not solely reliant on CST integrity, imaging studies have begun to explore non-CST neural pathways as potential biomarkers for walking recovery.[78] Independent walking is associated with FA measures of ipsilesional CST, ipsilesional corticoreticulospinal tract, and contralesional cerebellar peduncles.[78] These findings indicate that subcortical motor networks contribute to walking recovery after stroke. The contributions of cortical and subcortical networks beyond the CST warrant further investigation.

DISCUSSION

Accurate predictions for motor outcomes after stroke can improve rehabilitation planning by clinical teams and help patients and their families adjust to life after stroke. This review has found that predictions can be made for patients with initially mild upper limb impairment using clinical and demographic information. However, CST biomarkers are needed to make accurate predictions for patients with initially moderate to severe upper limb impairment, and these biomarkers can be combined with clinical and demographic information in prediction tools. Upper limb MEP status is a simple and robust CST biomarker that has been incorporated in the PREP2 prediction tool. PREP2 has been validated and implemented, with demonstrable clinical impact. The role of CST biomarkers is less clear for predicting independent walking after stroke, as clinical and demographic information can be combined in prediction tools to accurately predict both whether and when a patient will safely walk independently again. However, there is relatively less literature on biomarkers for walking recovery, sample sizes are small, and study design is variable. Future research could usefully explore neuroimaging biomarkers of non-M1 CST white matter projections, particularly for walking outcomes after stroke. Measures of non-motor functions such as vision, sensation, attention, and cognition could also be further investigated to see whether they improve the accuracy of prediction tools for motor outcomes.[79,80]

The implementation of prediction tools needs to be considered during their development and validation.[81,82] Implementation is likely to be easier when prediction tools have the characteristics summarized in **Box 2**. Prediction tools also need to be applicable to a wide range of patients, with evidence of accuracy and relative advantage over clinical judgment. Further considerations are clinicians' appetite for change, and the resources and training needed to support accurate and sustainable use of prediction tools in clinical practice. Although therapists typically agree that having prediction information is valuable,[82,83] there are barriers to implementing the biomarkers identified in this review. TMS is not widely available, and MRI measures require sophisticated analyses. Therapists identify the need for specific equipment and training, along with a lack of time, as barriers to implementation,[82,84] and addressing these barriers early in tool development can facilitate subsequent use in routine clinical care. Identifying adaptable components of prediction tools, such as the time windows for obtaining predictor information, may also facilitate implementation. Finally, implementation goes beyond the use of a tool to generate a prediction; it requires the thoughtful communication and effective use of prediction information to guide clinical care. There is some evidence that therapists have concerns about providing prediction information to patients,[84] and these concerns need to be addressed through training and support to enable effective implementation.

SUMMARY

CST biomarkers obtained within days of stroke are strongly related to subsequent motor outcomes. MEP status is particularly important for patients with initially moderate to severe UL impairment, and can be efficiently obtained and interpreted using the PREP2 prediction tool. In contrast, CST biomarkers have not yet been incorporated in prediction tools for independent walking outcomes, as these can be predicted using clinical and demographic variables.

CLINICS CARE POINTS

- Predicting motor outcomes using clinical information alone is often inaccurate for patients with initially moderate-severe motor impairment, and contributes to potentially inefficient and inequitable use of rehabilitation resources.

- The UL MEP status biomarker obtained within 1 week of stroke can accurately identify whether a patient with initially moderate-severe UL motor impairment will recover individuated finger movement by 3 months post-stroke.

- Prediction tools for UL motor outcome are more accurate when they combine clinical and demographic variables with the MEP status biomarker, particularly for patients with moderate to severe initial UL impairment.

- At present, CST biomarkers do not add value to clinical prediction tools for recovery of independent walking.

DISCLOSURE

The authors have no disclosures.

REFERENCES

1. Langhorne P, Coupar F, Pollock A. Motor recovery after stroke: a systematic review. Lancet Neurol 2009;8(8):741–54.
2. Simpson LA, Hayward KS, McPeake M, et al. Challenges of Estimating Accurate Prevalence of Arm Weakness Early After Stroke. Neurorehabil Neural Repair 2021;35(10):871–9.
3. Langhorne P, Bernhardt J, Kwakkel G. Stroke rehabilitation. Lancet 2011; 377(9778):1693–702.
4. Duncan PW, Lai SM, Keighley J. Defining post-stroke recovery: implications for design and interpretation of drug trials. Neuropharmacology 2000;39(5):835–41.
5. Duncan PW, Goldstein LB, Matchar D, et al. Measurement of motor recovery after stroke. Outcome assessment and sample size requirements. Stroke 1992;23(8): 1084–9.
6. Levin MF, Kleim JA, Wolf SL. What do motor "recovery" and "compensation" mean in patients following stroke? Neurorehabilitation Neural Repair 2009;23(4):313–9.
7. Stinear CM. Prediction of recovery of motor function after stroke. Lancet Neurol 2010;9(12):1228–32.
8. Stinear CM, Byblow WD, Ackerley SJ, et al. Predicting Recovery Potential for Individual Stroke Patients Increases Rehabilitation Efficiency. Stroke 2017;48(4): 1011–9.
9. Boyd LA, Hayward KS, Ward NS, et al. Biomarkers of stroke recovery: Consensus-based core recommendations from the Stroke Recovery and Rehabilitation Roundtable. Int J Stroke 2017;12(5):480–93.
10. Nijland RH, van Wegen EE, Harmeling-van der Wel BC, et al. Accuracy of Physical Therapists' Early Predictions of Upper-Limb Function in Hospital Stroke Units: The EPOS Study. Phys Ther 2013;93(4):460–9.
11. Cormier DJ, Frantz MA, Rand E, et al. Physiatrist referral preferences for postacute stroke rehabilitation. Medicine 2016;95(33):e4356.
12. Kennedy GM, Brock KA, Lunt AW, et al. Factors influencing selection for rehabilitation after stroke: a questionnaire using case scenarios to investigate physician perspectives and level of agreement. Arch Phys Med Rehabil 2012;93(8):1457–9.
13. Xian Y, Thomas L, Liang L, et al. Unexplained Variation for Hospitals' Use of Inpatient Rehabilitation and Skilled Nursing Facilities After an Acute Ischemic Stroke. Stroke 2017;48(10):2836–42.
14. Stinear CM. Prediction of motor recovery after stroke: advances in biomarkers. Lancet Neurol 2017;16(10):826–36.
15. Stinear CM, Smith MC, Byblow WD. Prediction Tools for Stroke Rehabilitation. Stroke 2019;50(11):3314–22.
16. Veerbeek JM, Kwakkel G, van Wegen EE, et al. Early prediction of outcome of activities of daily living after stroke: a systematic review. Stroke 2011;42(5):1482–8.
17. Stinear CM, Byblow WD. Predicting and accelerating motor recovery after stroke. Curr Opin Neurol 2014;27(6):624–30.
18. Boyd LA, Hayward KS, Ward NS, et al. Biomarkers of Stroke Recovery: Consensus-Based Core Recommendations from the Stroke Recovery and Rehabilitation Roundtable. Neurorehabilitation Neural Repair 2017;31(10–11):864–76.
19. Kim B, Winstein C. Can Neurological Biomarkers of Brain Impairment Be Used to Predict Poststroke Motor Recovery? A Systematic Review. Neurorehabilitation Neural Repair 2017;31(1):3–24.
20. Coupar F, Pollock A, Rowe P, et al. Predictors of upper limb recovery after stroke: a systematic review and meta-analysis. Clin Rehabil 2012;26(4):291–313.

21. Nijland RH, van Wegen EE, Harmeling-van der Wel BC, et al. Presence of finger extension and shoulder abduction within 72 hours after stroke predicts functional recovery: early prediction of functional outcome after stroke: the EPOS cohort study. Stroke 2010;41(4):745–50.
22. Alt Murphy M, Al-Shallawi A, Sunnerhagen KS, et al. Early prediction of upper limb functioning after stroke using clinical bedside assessments: a prospective longitudinal study. Sci Rep 2022;12(1):22053.
23. Barth J, Waddell KJ, Bland MD, et al. Accuracy of an Algorithm in Predicting Upper Limb Functional Capacity in a United States Population. Arch Phys Med Rehabil 2022;103(1):44–51.
24. van der Vliet R, Selles RW, Andrinopoulou ER, et al. Predicting Upper Limb Motor Impairment Recovery after Stroke: A Mixture Model. Ann Neurol 2020;87(3): 383–93.
25. Selles RW, Andrinopoulou ER, Nijland RH, et al. Computerised patient-specific prediction of the recovery profile of upper limb capacity within stroke services: the next step. J Neurol Neurosurg Psychiatry 2021;92(6):574–81.
26. Fugl-Meyer AR, Jaasko L, Leyman I, et al. The post-stroke hemiplegic patient. 1. a method for evaluation of physical performance. Scand J Rehabil Med 1975; 7(1):13–31.
27. Van der Lee JH, De Groot V, Beckerman H, et al. The intra- and interrater reliability of the action research arm test: a practical test of upper extremity function in patients with stroke. Arch Phys Med Rehabil 2001;82(1):14–9.
28. Veerbeek JM, Pohl J, Luft AR, et al. External validation and extension of the Early Prediction of Functional Outcome after Stroke (EPOS) prediction model for upper limb outcome 3 months after stroke. PLoS One 2022;17(8):e0272777.
29. Byblow WD, Stinear CM, Barber PA, et al. Proportional recovery after stroke depends on corticomotor integrity. Ann Neurol 2015;78(6):848–59.
30. Hayward KS, Schmidt J, Lohse KR, et al. Are we armed with the right data? Pooled individual data review of biomarkers in people with severe upper limb impairment after stroke. Neuroimage Clin 2017;13:310–9.
31. Wu J, Srinivasan R, Burke Quinlan E, et al. Utility of EEG measures of brain function in patients with acute stroke. Journal of neurophysiology 2016;115(5): 2399–405.
32. van Putten MJ, Hofmeijer J. EEG Monitoring in Cerebral Ischemia: Basic Concepts and Clinical Applications. J Clin Neurophysiol 2016;33(3):203–10.
33. Vatinno AA, Simpson A, Ramakrishnan V, et al. The Prognostic Utility of Electroencephalography in Stroke Recovery: A Systematic Review and Meta-Analysis. Neurorehabilitation Neural Repair 2022;36(4–5):255–68.
34. Keser Z, Buchl SC, Seven NA, et al. Electroencephalogram (EEG) With or Without Transcranial Magnetic Stimulation (TMS) as Biomarkers for Post-stroke Recovery: A Narrative Review. Front Neurol 2022;13:827866.
35. Saes M, Meskers CGM, Daffertshofer A, et al. Are early measured resting-state EEG parameters predictive for upper limb motor impairment six months poststroke? Clin Neurophysiol 2021;132(1):56–62.
36. Zhang JJ, Sanchez Vidana DI, Chan JN, et al. Biomarkers for prognostic functional recovery poststroke: A narrative review. Front Cell Dev Biol 2022;10: 1062807.
37. Hallett M. Transcranial magnetic stimulation: a primer. Neuron 2007;55(2):187–99.
38. Kuo YL, Lin DJ, Vora I, et al. Transcranial magnetic stimulation to assess motor neurophysiology after acute stroke in the United States: Feasibility, lessons learned, and values for future research. Brain Stimul 2022;15(1):179–81.

39. Stinear CM, Byblow WD, Ackerley SJ, et al. PREP2: A biomarker-based algorithm for predicting upper limb function after stroke. Ann Clin Transl Neurol 2017;4(11): 811–20.

40. Escudero JV, Sancho J, Bautista D, et al. Prognostic value of motor evoked potential obtained by transcranial magnetic brain stimulation in motor function recovery in patients with acute ischemic stroke. Stroke 1998;29(9):1854–9.

41. Karatzetzou S, Tsiptsios D, Terzoudi A, et al. Transcranial magnetic stimulation implementation on stroke prognosis. Neurol Sci 2022;43(2):873–88.

42. Bembenek JP, Kurczych K, Karli Nski M, et al. The prognostic value of motor-evoked potentials in motor recovery and functional outcome after stroke - a systematic review of the literature. Funct Neurol 2012;27(2):79–84.

43. Schambra HM, Xu J, Branscheidt M, et al. Differential Poststroke Motor Recovery in an Arm Versus Hand Muscle in the Absence of Motor Evoked Potentials. Neurorehabilitation Neural Repair 2019;33(7):568–80.

44. Smith MC, Ackerley SJ, Barber PA, et al. PREP2 Algorithm Predictions Are Correct at 2 Years Poststroke for Most Patients. Neurorehabilitation Neural Repair 2019;33(8):635–42.

45. Lundquist CB, Nielsen JF, Arguissain FG, et al. Accuracy of the Upper Limb Prediction Algorithm PREP2 Applied 2 Weeks Poststroke: A Prospective Longitudinal Study. Neurorehabilitation Neural Repair 2021;35(1):68–78.

46. Hoonhorst MHJ, Nijland RHM, van den Berg PJS, et al. Does Transcranial Magnetic Stimulation Have an Added Value to Clinical Assessment in Predicting Upper-Limb Function Very Early After Severe Stroke? Neurorehabilitation Neural Repair 2018;32(8):682–90.

47. Feng W, Wang J, Chhatbar PY, et al. Corticospinal tract lesion load: An imaging biomarker for stroke motor outcomes. Ann Neurol 2015;78(6):860–70.

48. Lin DJ, Cloutier AM, Erler KS, et al. Corticospinal Tract Injury Estimated From Acute Stroke Imaging Predicts Upper Extremity Motor Recovery After Stroke. Stroke 2019;50(12):3569–77.

49. Doughty C, Wang J, Feng W, et al. Detection and Predictive Value of Fractional Anisotropy Changes of the Corticospinal Tract in the Acute Phase of a Stroke. Stroke 2016;47(6):1520–6.

50. Lim JY, Oh MK, Park J, et al. Does Measurement of Corticospinal Tract Involvement Add Value to Clinical Behavioral Biomarkers in Predicting Motor Recovery after Stroke? Neural Plast 2020;2020:8883839.

51. Puig J, Pedraza S, Blasco G, et al. Acute damage to the posterior limb of the internal capsule on diffusion tensor tractography as an early imaging predictor of motor outcome after stroke. AJNR Am J Neuroradiol 2011;32(5):857–63.

52. Puig J, Blasco G, Terceno M, et al. Predicting Motor Outcome in Acute Intracerebral Hemorrhage. AJNR Am J Neuroradiol 2019;40(5):769–75.

53. Stinear CM, Barber PA, Petoe M, et al. The PREP algorithm predicts potential for upper limb recovery after stroke. Brain 2012;135(Pt 8):2527–35.

54. Moulton E, Magno S, Valabregue R, et al. Acute Diffusivity Biomarkers for Prediction of Motor and Language Outcome in Mild-to-Severe Stroke Patients. Stroke 2019;50(8):2050–6.

55. Boccuni L, Meyer S, D'Cruz N, et al. Premotor dorsal white matter integrity for the prediction of upper limb motor impairment after stroke. Sci Rep 2019;9(1):19712.

56. Saltao da Silva MA, Baune NA, Belagaje S, et al. Clinical Imaging-Derived Metrics of Corticospinal Tract Structural Integrity Are Associated With Post-stroke Motor Outcomes: A Retrospective Study. Front Neurol 2022;13:804133.

57. Lee J, Kim H, Kim J, et al. Multimodal Imaging Biomarker-Based Model Using Stratification Strategies for Predicting Upper Extremity Motor Recovery in Severe Stroke Patients. Neurorehabil Neural Repair. Mar 2022;36(3):217–26.
58. Rehme AK, Volz LJ, Feis DL, et al. Individual prediction of chronic motor outcome in the acute post-stroke stage: Behavioral parameters versus functional imaging. Hum Brain Mapp. Nov 2015;36(11):4553–65.
59. Rosso C, Lamy JC. Prediction of motor recovery after stroke: being pragmatic or innovative? Curr Opin Neurol 2020;33(4):482–7.
60. Kennedy C, Bernhardt J, Churilov L, et al. Factors associated with time to independent walking recovery post-stroke. J Neurol Neurosurg Psychiatry 2021; 92(7):702–8.
61. Smith MC, Barber AP, Scrivener BJ, et al. The TWIST Tool Predicts When Patients Will Recover Independent Walking After Stroke: An Observational Study. Neurorehabilitation Neural Repair 2022;36(7):461–71.
62. Kwah LK, Harvey LA, Diong J, et al. Models containing age and NIHSS predict recovery of ambulation and upper limb function six months after stroke: an observational study. J Physiother 2013;59(3):189–97.
63. Preston E, Ada L, Stanton R, et al. Prediction of Independent Walking in People Who Are Nonambulatory Early After Stroke: A Systematic Review. Stroke 2021; 52(10):3217–24.
64. Smith MC, Barber PA, Stinear CM. The TWIST Algorithm Predicts Time to Walking Independently After Stroke. Neurorehabilitation Neural Repair 2017;31(10–11): 955–64.
65. Veerbeek JM, Pohl J, Held JPO, et al. External Validation of the Early Prediction of Functional Outcome After Stroke Prediction Model for Independent Gait at 3 Months After Stroke. Front Neurol 2022;13:797791.
66. Veerbeek JM, Van Wegen EE, Harmeling-Van der Wel BC, et al. Is accurate prediction of gait in nonambulatory stroke patients possible within 72 hours poststroke? The EPOS study. Neurorehabilitation Neural Repair 2011;25(3):268–74.
67. Piron L, Piccione F, Tonin P, et al. Clinical correlation between motor evoked potentials and gait recovery in poststroke patients. Arch Phys Med Rehabil 2005; 86(9):1874–8.
68. Chang MC, Do KH, Chun MH. Prediction of lower limb motor outcomes based on transcranial magnetic stimulation findings in patients with an infarct of the anterior cerebral artery. Somatosens Mot Res 2015;1–5.
69. Hendricks HT, Pasman JW, van Limbeek J, et al. Motor evoked potentials of the lower extremity in predicting motor recovery and ambulation after stroke: a cohort study. Arch Phys Med Rehabil 2003;84(9):1373–9.
70. Kim BR, Moon WJ, Kim H, et al. Transcranial Magnetic Stimulation and Diffusion Tensor Tractography for Evaluating Ambulation after Stroke. Journal of stroke 2016;18(2):220–6.
71. Hwang P, Sohn MK, Jee S, et al. Transcranial Motor Evoked Potentials of Lower Limbs Can Prognosticate Ambulation in Hemiplegic Stroke Patients. Ann Rehabil Med 2016;40(3):383–91.
72. Cho HM, Choi BY, Chang CH, et al. The clinical characteristics of motor function in chronic hemiparetic stroke patients with complete corticospinal tract injury. NeuroRehabilitation 2012;31(2):207–13.
73. Jang SH, Chang CH, Lee J, et al. Functional role of the corticoreticular pathway in chronic stroke patients. Stroke; a journal of cerebral circulation 2013;44(4): 1099–104.

74. Dawes H, Enzinger C, Johansen-Berg H, et al. Walking performance and its recovery in chronic stroke in relation to extent of lesion overlap with the descending motor tract. Exp Brain Res 2008;186(2):325–33.
75. Cho SH, Kim DG, Kim DS, et al. Motor outcome according to the integrity of the corticospinal tract determined by diffusion tensor tractography in the early stage of corona radiata infarct. Neurosci Lett 2007;426(2):123–7.
76. Jang SH, Bai D, Son SM, et al. Motor outcome prediction using diffusion tensor tractography in pontine infarct. Ann Neurol 2008;64(4):460–5.
77. Kim EH, Lee J, Jang SH. Motor outcome prediction using diffusion tensor tractography of the corticospinal tract in large middle cerebral artery territory infarct. NeuroRehabilitation 2013;32(3):583–90.
78. Soulard J, Huber C, Baillieul S, et al. Motor tract integrity predicts walking recovery: A diffusion MRI study in subacute stroke. Neurology 2020;94(6):e583–93.
79. Lundquist CB, Nielsen JF, Brunner IC. Prediction of Upper Limb use Three Months after Stroke: A Prospective Longitudinal Study. J Stroke Cerebrovasc Dis 2021;30(11):106025.
80. Barth J, Lohse KR, Bland MD, et al. Predicting later categories of upper limb activity from earlier clinical assessments following stroke: an exploratory analysis. J NeuroEng Rehabil 2023;20(1):24.
81. Connell LA, Smith MC, Byblow WD, et al. Implementing biomarkers to predict motor recovery after stroke. NeuroRehabilitation 2018;43(1):41–50.
82. Connell LA, Chesworth B, Ackerley S, et al. Implementing the PREP2 Algorithm to Predict Upper Limb Recovery Potential After Stroke in Clinical Practice: A Qualitative Study. Phys Ther 2021;(5):101.
83. Kiaer C, Lundquist CB, Brunner I. Knowledge and application of upper limb prediction models and attitude toward prognosis among physiotherapists and occupational therapists in the clinical stroke setting. Top Stroke Rehabil 2021;28(2):135–41.
84. Lundquist CB, Pallesen H, Tjornhoj-Thomsen T, et al. Exploring physiotherapists' and occupational therapists' perceptions of the upper limb prediction algorithm PREP2 after stroke in a rehabilitation setting: a qualitative study. BMJ Open 2021;11(4):e038880.

Motor Learning Following Stroke

Mechanisms of Learning and Techniques to Augment Neuroplasticity

Lauren Winterbottom, MS, MM, OTR/l [a,b,*],
Dawn M. Nilsen, EdD, OTR/L, FAOTA [b,c]

KEYWORDS

• Motor learning • Neuroplasticity • Training • Stroke rehabilitation

KEY POINTS

• Sensorimotor impairments after stroke, such as weakness, spasticity, and decreased interjoint coordination, often cause limited use of the more affected side in daily activities.
• Motor learning (ML), or improvement in the ability to perform a skill, results in experience-dependent neuroplasticity, which is critical for those with motor deficits after stroke.
• Theories of motor control and ML inform stroke rehabilitation interventions by providing insight into the development of coordination and the effects of multiple factors on skill acquisition.
• Instructional language, augmented feedback, and practice conditions impact ML and should be carefully considered in interventions focused on skill reacquisition after stroke.
• Adjunctive strategies such as mental practice and neurostimulation techniques have been shown to improve ML for stroke survivors when combined with motor training.

INTRODUCTION

Sensorimotor deficits following stroke often result in loss of independence and are a leading cause of long-term disability.[1,2] These impairments can include weakness, spasticity, and reduced interjoint coordination. Loss of normal muscle tone and function can result in reduced functional range of motion, leading to soft tissue abnormalities such as tendon shortening and contracture.[3] Limb movements are characterized

[a] Department of Rehabilitation & Regenerative Medicine, Columbia University, 180 Fort Washington Avenue, HP1, Suite 199, New York, NY 10032, USA; [b] Department of Biobehavioral Sciences, Teachers College, Columbia University, New York, NY, USA; [c] Department of Rehabilitation & Regenerative Medicine, Columbia University, 617 West 168th Street, 3rd Floor, Room 305, New York, NY 10032, USA
* Corresponding author.
E-mail address: lbw2136@cumc.columbia.edu

Phys Med Rehabil Clin N Am 35 (2024) 277–291
https://doi.org/10.1016/j.pmr.2023.06.004
1047-9651/24/© 2023 Elsevier Inc. All rights reserved.

by abnormal velocity profiles with reduced movement speed and smoothness and are often limited by co-contraction and difficulty decoupling movements between joints.[4] Abnormal flexor synergy patterns limit functional reaching space, leading to compensation with the trunk to access objects in the environment.[3] Impaired proximal control of the arm leads to an overhand grasping strategy, and dexterity is often limited by flexor coupling between the fingers and thumb.[3] Sensory impairments, such as loss of touch and proprioception, can also limit function and lead to increased difficulty engaging in daily activities.[3,5]

Motor recovery, which is often a goal in stroke rehabilitation, refers to the return of normal movement patterns that were present before the stroke.[6] This can be differentiated from compensation, which involves the development of new movement patterns that typically have lower efficiency and quality of movement.[7,8] The amount of motor recovery that occurs varies between individuals and is associated with clinical factors such as stroke severity, time poststroke, corticospinal tract integrity, poststroke depression, comorbidities, genetics, and quality of rehabilitation.[9] As an individual attempts to regain independence after stroke, there is potential for both motor recovery and the development of compensatory movements. As functional skills are relearned, new neural connections are created through synaptogenesis based on experience.[6] Movement compensations are commonly used to overcome daily obstacles. This can lead to learned nonuse, in which the more affected limb is not engaged functionally, or learned "bad-use," in which maladaptive movement patterns are developed and become habitual.[10,11] Further disability can then occur in the more affected side due to lack of use and preference for the more functional limb. These changes in behavior drive neuroplasticity mechanisms to further limit use of the more affected side, as new movement patterns become neurologically ingrained.[6] Although skills can be relearned after stroke, increased numbers of repetitions are often needed for skill improvement compared with healthy individuals.[12] Additionally, spasticity may obstruct skill reacquisition.[13] To address these issues, motor learning (ML) principles have been used to guide stroke rehabilitation interventions to further enhance neural reorganization and support recovery.[4,6,14,15]

DEFINITIONS OF MOTOR LEARNING AND SKILL ACQUISITION

ML can be defined as a change in one's ability to perform a skill that results from practice or experience and can be demonstrated by improvements in speed and accuracy.[16] As performance becomes more stable in response to internal and external stressors, it can be generalized to different environments and situations, becoming less cognitively demanding with improved automaticity.[16] Although learning cannot be directly measured, ML is often inferred through retention and transfer tests. Motor skill retention is tested after a period of no practice to determine the persistence of the skill. Transfer tests determine the adaptability of the skill to new conditions by testing a variation of the skill or by testing it in a new context.[16,17] According to Krakauer and colleagues, different types of ML include sequence learning, novel skill acquisition, motor adaptation, and improvements in motor acuity.[18] Much of adult ML involves assembling new sequences of movements from coordination patterns that have already stabilized.[19] Daily activities are composed of sequences of motor skills that are linked together in order to achieve a task goal.[18,20,21] Coordination patterns for these underlying motor skills (grasp, reach, and transport) are acquired during childhood and then are incorporated sequentially to complete complex daily activities.[19,21] Cognitive processes are also required to efficiently organize performance and ensure that task goals are effectively met.[18,20] ML can also involve the acquisition of novel movements in which coordinative structures have not yet been developed.[16,18,19] This requires the learner to navigate numerous movement options to determine an efficient and effective method of executing the task.[22] In contrast, motor adaptation refers to involuntary adjustments that are implicitly made to maintain motor performance in response to perturbations from the environment.[18] Finally, ML can reflect improvements in motor acuity, or movement quality, such as accuracy and precision.[18] Kinematic measures can be used to quantify movement quality and compare normal patterns of movement with those that are impaired.[8]

CONSIDERING THEORIES OF MOTOR CONTROL AND MOTOR LEARNING IN STROKE REHABILITATION

Many stroke rehabilitation interventions are informed by theories of motor control and ML, which aim to explain the production of coordinated movement and the process of skill acquisition within the context of various types of motor skills in diverse environments.[15,16,23] Here, we provide an overview of selected theories; for a full account of motor control and ML theories, please refer to Magill and Anderson[16] or Schmidt and colleagues.[24] Dynamical systems theory is a relevant theory of motor control for stroke rehabilitation. This theory states that coordinated movement patterns emerge through self-organization in response to interactions among multiple systems. Stable, energy-efficient coordination patterns are developed, which the individual will return to, following perturbation from the environment.[16,25] Skilled movement occurs through the development of functional motor synergies, where stable patterns of behavior emerge and are adapted based on the task goal.[26] Newell's complementary theory proposed that optimal coordination patterns result from the constraints of the individual, the task, and the environment; although some of these movement patterns are developed at an early age, others can be learned through intensive practice.[16,19,27] Similarly, in Gibson's theory of affordances, the individual's perception of the environment guides the development of coordinated movement patterns, based on the fit between the environmental characteristics and the individual performing the task.[16,28] This is relevant for stroke rehabilitation as lack of fit between the natural environment and the motor capacity of the individual may lead to limited arm use during daily task performance, resulting in further reductions in arm function.[29]

Theories of ML have also focused on the process of skill acquisition, which is crucial for individuals after stroke who must relearn to perform daily activities. Different models have been proposed to describe the stages of learning a new motor skill. Fitts and Posner developed a classic 3-stage model that includes cognitive, associative, and autonomous stages, whereas Gentile describes 2 stages of learning (**Fig. 1**).[30,31] In both models, early stages are characterized by greater cognitive demand as the performer must learn the basic movements required for the task while determining relevant environmental characteristics. Explicit learning processes (ie, verbalizable knowledge) are involved in understanding the goal of the task while implicit processes guide production of appropriate forces to complete smooth, efficient movements.[32] Importantly, for individuals with stroke, explicit instructions may interfere with implicit learning and have a negative impact on skill acquisition, so instructions and cues should be carefully considered.[33] In later stages of learning, movements have increased consistency and automaticity; reduced cognitive demand and improved efficiency allow for generalization to different conditions and situations.[16,30,31] Although the early stages of ML are more commonly studied after stroke,[17] it is important that the later stages of learning be attained; increased use of the more affected side during daily performance is unlikely

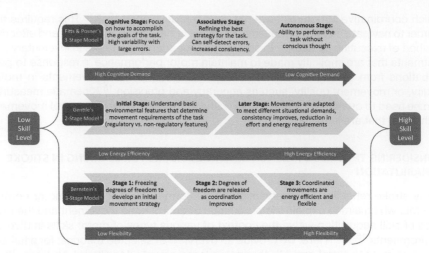

Fig. 1. Stages of ML.[a]Fitts and Posner.[30] [b]Gentile.[31] [c]Bernstein.[22]

unless skills can be completed with a satisfactory level of effectiveness and efficiency.[29,34,35]

Bernstein focused on the development of coordination during skill acquisition, noting that when learning a novel skill, learners reduce (or "freeze") degrees of freedom to limit the number of potential movements, resulting in movements with less efficiency and flexibility (see **Fig. 1**).[22] As coordination develops, functional motor synergies enable adaptation to different environments and contexts.[26] Based on these ideas, Newell suggested that ML is hierarchical, and skill optimization is preceded by the development of coordination and control.[19] Although healthy adults have already developed functional synergy patterns needed to carry out common tasks, new coordinative structures must be developed when learning novel skills, such as those in sports. Recently, Otte and colleagues proposed a new framework for skill development in sports that integrates Newell's stages of ML with the concept of periodization, in which training variables are systematically organized to optimize performance according to skill level, cognitive effort, and environmental demands.[36] This framework incorporates ML principles into a longitudinal training paradigm that addresses coordination, skill adaptability, and performance.[36] Although there are clear differences between sports training and motor recovery after stroke, both involve the development of functional synergy patterns that enable effective and efficient performance of a variety of skills in complex real-world situations. Specifically, for upper limb use after stroke, functional movement primitives must be performed with adequate coordination to be able to complete the wide variety of skills that comprise complex daily tasks (**Fig. 2**).[21]

Additionally, the importance of intrinsic motivation in ML has recently been emphasized in the OPTIMAL theory of ML, in which ML is enhanced by supporting autonomy, expectations for success, and focus on the task goal.[37] As individuals with stroke have reported decreased motivation to use their more affected arm in daily life,[34] incorporation of factors that support intrinsic motivation may be beneficial in stroke rehabilitation.[23,38]

NEUROPLASTICITY AND MOTOR LEARNING

Regardless of the stage of learning, the process of learning involves changes in neural connections in the brain. Thus, what we do in stroke rehabilitation needs to be

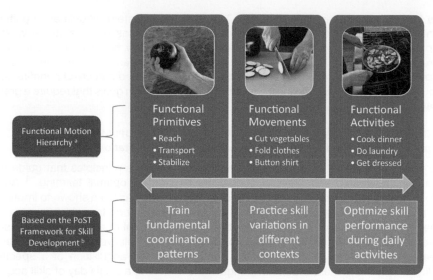

Fig. 2. General structure of a practice method for upper limb rehabilitation after stroke. [a]Schambra and colleagues.[21] [b]Otte and colleagues.[36]

carefully considered in light of neuroplasticity. Neuroplasticity refers to the ability of the nervous system to reorganize based on both internal and external experiences.[39] During the critical period after stroke, there is heightened potential for neuroplasticity, and motor recovery can occur both spontaneously and through functional use of the limb.[7] Neural plasticity mechanisms can also induce the development of maladaptive synergies if compensatory movement patterns are learned.[3] To counteract learned nonuse and encourage neuroplasticity that supports motor recovery, ML principles, such as specificity, intensity, frequency, salience, optimal level of difficulty, and feedback, have commonly been applied to stroke rehabilitation interventions.[6,15] Animal studies have suggested that repetitive training of a novel motor skill stimulates neural growth and reorganization of the primary motor cortex, whereas repetition of habitual movement patterns does not.[40,41] Task-specific training in animal studies leads to synaptogenesis, dendritic branching and spine formation, elimination and selective stabilization, and new long-range neural connections.[42,43] Similarly, longitudinal studies of skill acquisition in humans have found that ML results in increased gray matter density in the brain.[42] These findings have informed interventions such as constraint-induced movement therapy (CIMT), which focus on forced use of the more affected limb through task-specific, intensive practice to guide neuroplasticity toward the recovery of motor function.[11] CIMT has been shown to increase gray matter volume in bilateral sensory and motor areas of the brain, along with the hippocampus, which was correlated with increased functional use of the upper limb.[44] More recently, transcranial direct current stimulation (tDCS) combined with motor training resulted in improved ML and increased cortical gray matter volume.[42,45]

Dopamine also plays an important role in neuroplasticity related to motor control, memory, and learning. Dopaminergic neurons from the ventral tegmental area (VTA) that project to limbic and cortical regions via mesocorticolimbic pathways are associated with reward.[46] Animal studies have suggested that stimulation of the dopamine system may improve ML after stroke via dopaminergic projections from the VTA to the primary motor cortex.[47,48] Hypoactivation of the dopamine system after stroke has been linked with impaired ML.[48,49] The dopamine system modulates cognitive control, or the ability to pursue long-term goals. In diseases such as stroke where dopamine transmission is reduced, perceived efforts may be judged to outweigh perceived rewards, reducing motivation for continued engagement.[50] Thus, increasing dopamine transmission may improve motivation by increased perceived benefits and reducing perceived cost, making it easier to pursue long-term goals that require a great deal of effort.[50,51]

TECHNIQUES TO AUGMENT MOTOR LEARNING AND NEUROPLASTICITY
Application of Motor Learning Principles in Stroke Rehabilitation

ML research with healthy adults has determined numerous principles that guide instruction, feedback, and practice conditions to support optimal learning.[16] After stroke, task-specific practice using the more affected arm has been shown to improve ML and increase activation of the contralateral primary motor cortex, which is not seen when general arm use is increased.[52] Although a great deal of research has investigated the efficacy of stroke rehabilitation interventions, relatively few studies have measured the effects of individual ML principles on the acquisition of a specific skill.[15,17,53] Most of these studies investigate the effects of a single day of skill acquisition on next-day retention for individuals with chronic stroke, often excluding those with cognitive deficits or severe motor impairments.[17] More commonly, ML principles that are advantageous for healthy individuals have been applied in complex interventions aimed at improving general measures of function and capacity.[54] However, as research has also demonstrated differences in skill acquisition between healthy individuals and individuals with stroke,[12,33,55] the benefits of using several ML principles with individuals after stroke are unclear. **Table 1** includes examples of ML principles that have been investigated with individuals after stroke. See Gregor and colleagues for a more detailed analysis.[17]

Dosage, Intensity, and Repetition

In stroke rehabilitation, dosage can refer to the number of hours of practice, the number of repetitions completed, or frequency and duration of practice sessions.[15] Intensity can be defined as the number of repetitions completed within a given unit of time, including the length and number of sessions and their distribution over time.[4] According to Bernstein, repetition is essential because it allows the learner to discover new ways of solving the motor problem; each repetition should be performed with focus on updating and improving the skilled movement.[56] Compared with healthy individuals, individuals with motor impairments after stroke require many more repetitions to acquire new movement patterns.[12] In animal studies of ML, hundreds of repetitions are achieved by depriving the animals of food and then offering a food reward for successful task completion in a setting that prevents compensation, leading to skill acquisition and cortical reorganization.[40,41] Research with human subjects post-stroke has found that repetitive practice of one task can transfer to improvements in other tasks.[57] However, there is not clear evidence that increasing the number of repetitions during task-specific training improves motor function, especially in chronic stroke.[53,54] Thus, precise dosage recommendations for ML after stroke have yet to be determined.[4]

Strategies to Augment Motor Learning (Mental Practice/Motor Imagery, Action Observation, Mirror Therapy, Aerobic Exercise, Sleep)

Specific strategies can be combined with task practiced to enhance ML. Mental practice, or the use of motor imagery to cognitively practice a skill without performing

Table 1
Motor learning principles investigated in individuals after stroke

ML Principle	Definition	Application with Stroke
Verbal cues	**Short phrases that direct attention to relevant aspects of the task or key movement patterns[16]**	
Explicit instructions	Instructions that increase verbalizable knowledge of the task, such as verbal and written information and rules[16,33]	Explicit information has a negative effect on ML after stroke[17,33]
Implicit instructions	Instructions that do not increase conscious awareness of the task being learned, such as movement analogies[16]	
External focus of attention	Instructions that direct attention to the goal of the task[37]	No significant differences were found between instructions with external or internal attentional focus after stroke[55]
Internal focus of attention	Instructions that direct attention to body movements[37]	
Augmented feedback	**Information about skill performance that is provided from an external source that adds to the natural sensory feedback available to the performer[16]**	
Knowledge of results (KR)	Information about the outcome of the task performance[16]	Both KR and KP may improve ML after stroke[15,17]
Knowledge of performance (KP)	Information about movement characteristics related to task performance[16]	
Biofeedback	Information about physiologic processes such as muscle activity[16]	Biofeedback may enhance gait retraining after stroke[79]
Feedback frequency	Schedule with which feedback is given; lower frequency of feedback improves ML in healthy adults[80]	No significant difference was found between 100% and 67% feedback schedules[17,80]
Practice conditions	**Variables that influence the way a task is practiced[16]**	
Specificity	ML is influenced by the characteristics of the task, including available sensory feedback, the environment, and cognitive requirements[16]	Practicing a single motor task can transfer to improvements in untrained tasks[57]
Variability	Changes in the context and movement requirements of the skill that is practiced[16]	The benefits of variable practice compared with constant practice are unclear after stroke[15,17]
Constant practice	Only one variation of the skill is practiced[16]	
Variable practice	Multiple skill variations are practiced[16]	

(continued on next page)

Table 1
(continued)

ML Principle	Definition	Application with Stroke
Practice distribution	The spacing of the practice schedule such the amount of time between sessions or trials and the number and length of sessions[16]	The benefits of massed practice compared with distributed practice are unclear after stroke[15]
Massed practice	Practice schedule with a short amount of rest between practice trials where each session involves more trials/longer duration[16]	
Distributed practice	Practice schedule with more time between sessions or trials; sessions are shorted and spaced over a longer period of time[16]	
Difficulty	Task difficulty and complexity is progressively increased to provide an optimal level of challenge[15]	Progressively increasing task difficulty may promote ML after stroke[15,17]
Problem-solving	Use of problem-solving strategies and guided discovery for skill acquisition[68]	Combining problem-solving with task-specific training may improve transfer to untrained tasks[68]
Manipulating degrees of freedom	Limiting the number of joints that can simultaneously move to simplify movement options[16]	Use of a trunk restraint improves reaching performance after stroke[53]
Manipulating error	Error can be increased (error augmentation) or minimized (error minimization) during training to elicit adaptation[81]	Error augmentation during split-belt treadmill training may improve step length symmetry[81]

physical movements, can augment ML and recovery when combined with physical practice for individuals with stroke.[15,17,58] Similarly, action observation involves watching a video demonstrating skilled task performance before practicing the task and has also been shown to promote ML and motor recovery.[15,17,59] Mirror therapy, which involves placing the more affected limb in a mirror box while the mirror reflection of the less affected arm is observed, has also been shown to improve upper limb recovery.[60] Aerobic exercise, such as high-intensity interval training, and sleep following motor practice can also lead to improvements in ML.[17]

Modalities to Augment Motor Learning (Transcranial Direct Current Stimulation, Repetitive Transcranial Magnetic Stimulation, Intermittent Theta Burst Stimulation, Vagus Nerve Stimulation)

Noninvasive brain stimulation techniques such as tDCS and repetitive transcranial magnetic stimulation (rTMS) modulate cortical excitability and can enhance ML when combined with rehabilitation.[17,61,62] Intermittent theta burst stimulation (iTBS) is a newer type of rTMS that may also improve ML and upper limb function after stroke.[17,63] Vagus nerve stimulation (VNS), involving a surgically implanted device, is another emerging treatment that may improve upper limb function when combined with rehabilitation and has been shown to induce plasticity in the motor cortex of rodents.[64,65]

Psychosocial Factors

Stroke rehabilitation interventions often require high levels of motivation and engagement, which may be difficult for individuals with stroke to maintain.[34] Studies that have used extrinsic rewards such as money have demonstrated improved outcomes in motor adaptation, retention, and sensorimotor capacity.[66,67] Participation in intrinsically motivating activities, such as those that facilitate autonomy and problem-solving, may also support engagement in self-directed practice and high-intensity interventions.[23,38] Interventions that encourage problem-solving and decision-making during skill acquisition can transfer to improvements in untrained tasks and improve self-efficacy.[68] Additionally, structuring interventions so that they provide frequent experiences of success during practice may improve motivation and support recovery.[69] Social engagement and confidence in upper limb use have also recently been linked with the amount the more affected arm is used in daily activities, highlighting the importance social context and self-efficacy.[15,70]

DISCUSSION

Theories of motor control and ML inform many stroke rehabilitation interventions in order to drive neuroplasticity and support skill acquisition.[15] More information is needed on how people with poststroke sensorimotor impairments respond to specific ML principles.[17] Continued exploration of the most effective practice conditions for skill reacquisition following stroke can guide the development of complex interventions and ensure that the correct mechanisms of action are emphasized. Ideally, interventions would both improve underlying motor deficits and increase the skilled use of the more affected side during the performance of daily activities. However, interventions that focus on improving motor impairment often do not improve functional performance, whereas interventions that are focused on the performance of functional activities may have less impact on motor impairment.[14] Task-specific training in natural environments may promote compensatory strategies that lead to the development of maladaptive movement patterns.[15] Repetition of these movement patterns can cause them to become further ingrained and habitual.[4,38] These motor habits may develop within weeks after stroke and can limit future use of the arm even as motor function continues to improve.[71]

In order for skill development to progress once habits have formed, habits must be continually broken and replaced with improved iterations of the skill, which is known as deliberate practice.[72] Deliberate practice is associated with the development of expertise and requires professional instruction to guide optimal skill development.[18,72] Frameworks for skill acquisition in sports organize multiple levels of training within long-term programming, which may support continued skill development by focusing on both fundamental skills and application of those skills during performance.[36] In contrast, stroke rehabilitation interventions often attempt to solve a complex problem by addressing a single mechanism of action.[38] It is possible that multifaceted frameworks for stroke rehabilitation could help guide long-term skill development and support both motor recovery and functional limb use. Longitudinal studies on complex skill development after stroke are needed to assess both movement quality as well as effectiveness and efficiency of real-world skill performance.[8]

In practice, therapy doses after stroke are quite low,[73] and individuals with stroke may think that their services do not provide adequate support for recovery. For instance, they may be told to "just use" their more affected arm without being given any type of program for home practice or adequate feedback.[74] Systematic methods of practice could potentially improve efficiency during therapy time by setting up programming to support long-term self-directed practice. New technologies, such as tele-health, have the potential to support daily practice routines by monitoring activity, providing feedback, and creating environmental adaptations that offer increased opportunities for successful practice.[75] Integrating strategies that enhance ML after stroke, such as mental practice and action observation, into practice routines may also support skill acquisition and recovery.[58,59] Additionally, expanding access to neurostimulation techniques (tDCS, rTMS, VNS) and systematically integrating them into clinical practice may help improve effectiveness of current ML interventions, particularly for individuals with chronic stroke.[61,62,65]

Psychosocial factors such as motivation and self-efficacy may also help drive ML and neuroplasticity. Although motivation is frequently identified as an important factor,[6,15,38] less is known about the effects of motivation on rehabilitation outcomes. For example, although virtual reality and active video gaming interventions are designed to be motivating, constructs related to motivation are infrequently measured, and motivational outcomes are rarely compared among groups.[76] Intrinsic motivation, in which activities are performed for the sake of enjoyment and interest, may also be important for ML after stroke because it encourages curious exploration of the environment and is associated with the dopaminergic rewards system.[37,51] A study of healthy older adults found that giving participants control over the amount they practiced a novel motor task led to improvements on retention and transfer tests.[77] Similarly, when learning a novel surgical skill, medical students who were focused on skill proficiency outperformed those who were prescribed amounts of practice, even though the skill was practiced for similar amounts of time and repetitions.[78] Giving participants control over practice conditions may help elicit intrinsic motivation and stimulate dopaminergic pathways.[37,51] However, although this concept has been applied in complex stroke interventions,[23] the specific effects of self-controlled practice on poststroke ML are largely unknown.

SUMMARY

Sensorimotor impairments after stroke pose a significant barrier to functional independence. Motor control and ML theories, and the training principles derived from them (ie, verbal cues, augmented feedback, and practice conditions), inform many stroke rehabilitation interventions promoting neuroplasticity and skill acquisition. Evidence suggests that task-specific practice improves ML after stroke and that it may be possible to augment ML by engaging stroke survivors in specific strategies (eg, mental practice, action observation) or through the application of noninvasive brain stimulation. Psychosocial factors such as motivation and self-efficacy may affect ML after stroke, although further research in this area is warranted.

CLINICS CARE POINTS

- Task-specific training improves ML after stroke, although specific dosage recommendations are currently unknown.
- It is important to address movement quality during motor training to prevent compensatory movements from becoming habitual.
- Although more research is needed to determine effects of different practice variables on ML for stroke survivors, clinicians should be aware that explicit instructions may reduce ML, while augmented feedback may enhance it.
- Strategies such as mental practice and action observation can be combined with physical practice to enhance ML.
- Neurostimulation techniques augment ML when combined with motor training.

DISCLOSURE

The authors report there are no competing interests to declare.

REFERENCES

1. Guidetti S, Ytterberg C, Ekstam L, et al. Changes in the impact of stroke between 3 and 12 months post-stroke, assessed with the Stroke Impact Scale. J Rehabil Med 2014;46(10):963–8.
2. Virani SS, Alonso A, Aparicio HJ, et al. Heart Disease and Stroke Statistics— 2021 Update. Circulation 2021;143(8):e254–743.
3. Roby-Brami A, Jarrassé N, Parry R. Impairment and Compensation in Dexterous Upper-Limb Function After Stroke. From the Direct Consequences of Pyramidal Tract Lesions to Behavioral Involvement of Both Upper-Limbs in Daily Activities. Front Hum Neurosci 2021;15. https://doi.org/10.3389/fnhum.2021.662006.
4. Levin MF, Demers M. Motor learning in neurological rehabilitation. Disabil Rehabil 2021;43(24):3445–53.
5. Ingemanson ML, Rowe JR, Chan V, et al. Somatosensory system integrity explains differences in treatment response after stroke. Neurology 2019;92(10):e1098–108.
6. Kleim JA, Jones TA. Principles of experience-dependent neural plasticity: implications for rehabilitation after brain damage. J Speech Lang Hear Res 2008;51(1): S225–39.
7. Joy MT, Carmichael ST. Encouraging an excitable brain state: mechanisms of brain repair in stroke. Nat Rev Neurosci 2021;22(1):38–53.
8. Saes M, Mohamed Refai MI, van Beijnum BJF, et al. Quantifying Quality of Reaching Movements Longitudinally Post-Stroke: A Systematic Review. Neurorehabilitation Neural Repair 2022;36(3):183–207.

9. Alawieh A, Zhao J, Feng W. Factors affecting post-stroke motor recovery: Implications on neurotherapy after brain injury. Behav Brain Res 2018;340:94–101.

10. Raghavan P. Upper Limb Motor Impairment After Stroke. Phys Med Rehabil Clin N Am 2015;26(4):599–610.

11. Taub E, Wolf SL. Constraint Induced Movement Techniques To Facilitate Upper Extremity Use in Stroke Patients. Top Stroke Rehabil 1997;3(4):38–61.

12. Cirstea MC, Ptito A, Levin MF. Arm reaching improvements with short-term practice depend on the severity of the motor deficit in stroke. Exp Brain Res 2003; 152(4):476–88.

13. Subramanian SK, Feldman AG, Levin MF. Spasticity may obscure motor learning ability after stroke. J Neurophysiol 2018;119(1):5–20.

14. Kitago T, Krakauer JW. Motor learning principles for neurorehabilitation. Handb Clin Neurol 2013;110:93–103.

15. Maier M, Ballester BR, Verschure PFMJ. Principles of Neurorehabilitation After Stroke Based on Motor Learning and Brain Plasticity Mechanisms. Front Syst Neurosci 2019;13;74.

16. Magill RA, Anderson DI. Motor learning and control: concepts and applications. 12th edition. New York, NY: McGraw-Hill; 2021.

17. Gregor S, Saumur TM, Crosby LD, et al. Study Paradigms and Principles Investigated in Motor Learning Research After Stroke: A Scoping Review. Arch Rehabil Res Clin Transl 2021;3(2):100111.

18. Krakauer JW, Hadjiosif AM, Xu J, et al. Motor Learning. Compr Physiol 2019;9(2): 613–63.

19. Newell KM. Coordination, control and skill. In: Goodman D, Wilberg RB, Franks IM, editors. Differing perspectives in motor learning, memory, and control. Amsterdam: Elsevier Science; 1985. p. 295–317.

20. Bernspång B, Fisher AG. Differences between persons with right or left cerebral vascular accident on the Assessment of Motor and Process Skills. Arch Phys Med Rehabil 1995;76(12):1144–51.

21. Schambra HM, Parnandi A, Pandit NG, et al. A Taxonomy of Functional Upper Extremity Motion. Front Neurol 2019;10. https://doi.org/10.3389/fneur.2019.00857.

22. Bernstein NA. The co-ordination and regulation of movements. Oxford: Pergamon Press; 1967.

23. Lewthwaite R, Winstein CJ, Lane CJ, et al. Accelerating Stroke Recovery: Body Structures and Functions, Activities, Participation, and Quality of Life Outcomes From a Large Rehabilitation Trial. Neurorehabilitation Neural Repair 2018;32(2): 150–65.

24. Schmidt RA, Lee TD, Winstein CJ, et al. Motor control and learning: a behavioral emphasis. 6th edition. Champaign, IL: Human Kinetics; 2019.

25. Kelso JAS. Relative timing in brain and behavior: Some observations about the generalized motor program and self-organized coordination dynamics. Hum Mov Sci 1997;16(4):453–60.

26. Latash ML. One more time about motor (and non-motor) synergies. Exp Brain Res 2021;239(10):2951–67.

27. Newell KM. Constraints on the development of coordination. In: Wade MG, Whiting HTA, editors. Motor development in children: aspects of coordination and control. The Hague, The Netherlands: Nijhoff; 1986. p. 341–60.

28. Gibson JJ. The ecological approach to visual perception. Boston, MA: Houghton Mifflin; 1979.

29. Ballester BR, Winstein C, Schweighofer N. Virtuous and Vicious Cycles of Arm Use and Function Post-stroke. Front Neurol 2022;13. https://doi.org/10.3389/fneur.2022.804211.

30. Fitts PM, Posner MI. Human performance. Belmont, CA: Brooks/Cole; 1967.

31. Gentile AM. A Working Model of Skill Acquisition with Application to Teaching. Quest 1972;17(1):3–23.

32. Gentile AM. Movement Science: Implicit and Explicit Processes during Acquisition of Functional Skills. Scand J Occup Ther 1998;5(1):7–16.

33. Boyd LA, Winstein CJ. Explicit Information Interferes with Implicit Motor Learning of Both Continuous and Discrete Movement Tasks After Stroke. J Neurol Phys Ther 2006;30(2):46–57.

34. Meadmore KL, Hallewell E, Freeman C, et al. Factors affecting rehabilitation and use of upper limb after stroke: views from healthcare professionals and stroke survivors. Top Stroke Rehabil 2019;26(2):94–100.

35. Grajo L, Boisselle A, DaLomba E. Occupational Adaptation as a Construct: A Scoping Review of Literature. Open J Occup Ther 2018;6(1). https://doi.org/10.15453/2168-6408.1400.

36. Otte FW, Millar SK, Klatt S. Skill Training Periodization in "Specialist" Sports Coaching—An Introduction of the "PoST" Framework for Skill Development. Front Sports Act Living 2019;1. https://doi.org/10.3389/fspor.2019.00061.

37. Wulf G, Lewthwaite R. Optimizing performance through intrinsic motivation and attention for learning: The OPTIMAL theory of motor learning. Psychon Bull Rev 2016;23(5):1382–414.

38. Sánchez N, Winstein CJ. Lost in Translation: Simple Steps in Experimental Design of Neurorehabilitation-Based Research Interventions to Promote Motor Recovery Post-Stroke. Front Hum Neurosci 2021;15:644335.

39. Cramer SC, Sur M, Dobkin BH, et al. Harnessing neuroplasticity for clinical applications. Brain 2011;134(Pt 6):1591–609.

40. Plautz EJ, Milliken GW, Nudo RJ. Effects of repetitive motor training on movement representations in adult squirrel monkeys: role of use versus learning. Neurobiol Learn Mem 2000;74(1):27–55.

41. Kleim JA, Barbay S, Nudo RJ. Functional Reorganization of the Rat Motor Cortex Following Motor Skill Learning. J Neurophysiol 1998;80(6):3321–5.

42. Sampaio-Baptista C, Sanders ZB, Johansen-Berg H. Structural Plasticity in Adulthood with Motor Learning and Stroke Rehabilitation. Annu Rev Neurosci 2018; 41(1):25–40.

43. Xu T, Yu X, Perlik AJ, et al. Rapid formation and selective stabilization of synapses for enduring motor memories. Nature 2009;462(7275):915–9.

44. Gauthier LV, Taub E, Perkins C, et al. Remodeling the brain: plastic structural brain changes produced by different motor therapies after stroke. Stroke 2008; 39(5):1520–5.

45. Allman C, Amadi U, Winkler AM, et al. Ipsilesional anodal tDCS enhances the functional benefits of rehabilitation in patients after stroke. Sci Transl Med 2016; 8(330):330re1.

46. Speranza L, di Porzio U, Viggiano D, et al. Dopamine: The Neuromodulator of Long-Term Synaptic Plasticity, Reward and Movement Control. Cells 2021; 10(4). https://doi.org/10.3390/cells10040735.

47. Gower A, Tiberi M. The Intersection of Central Dopamine System and Stroke: Potential Avenues Aiming at Enhancement of Motor Recovery. Front Synaptic Neurosci 2018;10. https://doi.org/10.3389/fnsyn.2018.00018.

48. Bradley CL, Damiano DL. Effects of Dopamine on Motor Recovery and Training in Adults and Children With Nonprogressive Neurological Injuries: A Systematic Review. Neurorehabilitation Neural Repair 2019;33(5):331–44.
49. Widmer M, Lutz K, Luft AR. Reduced striatal activation in response to rewarding motor performance feedback after stroke. Neuroimage Clin 2019;24:102036.
50. Cools R, Fröböse M, Aarts E, et al. Dopamine and the motivation of cognitive control. Handb Clin Neurol 2019;163:123–43.
51. Di Domenico SI, Ryan RM. The Emerging Neuroscience of Intrinsic Motivation: A New Frontier in Self-Determination Research. Front Hum Neurosci 2017;11:1–14.
52. Boyd LA, Vidoni ED, Wessel BD. Motor learning after stroke: is skill acquisition a prerequisite for contralesional neuroplastic change? Neurosci Lett 2010;482(1):21–5.
53. Hayward KS, Barker RN, Carson RG, et al. The effect of altering a single component of a rehabilitation programme on the functional recovery of stroke patients: a systematic review and meta-analysis. Clin Rehabil 2014;28(2):107–17.
54. Lang CE, Strube MJ, Bland MD, et al. Dose response of task-specific upper limb training in people at least 6 months poststroke: A phase II, single-blind, randomized, controlled trial. Ann Neurol 2016;80(3):342–54.
55. Kal E, Houdijk H, van der Kamp J, et al. Are the effects of internal focus instructions different from external focus instructions given during balance training in stroke patients? A double-blind randomized controlled trial. Clin Rehabil 2019; 33(2):207–21.
56. Bernstein NA. On dexterity and its development. In: Latash ML, Turvey MT, editors. Dexterity and its development. Mahwah, NJ: Erlbaum; 1996. p. 3–244.
57. Schaefer SY, Patterson CB, Lang CE. Transfer of Training Between Distinct Motor Tasks After Stroke. Neurorehabilitation Neural Repair 2013;27(7):602–12.
58. Nilsen DM, Gillen G, Gordon AM. Use of mental practice to improve upper-limb recovery after stroke: a systematic review. Am J Occup Ther 2010;64(5):695–708.
59. Borges LR, Fernandes AB, Oliveira Dos Passos J, et al. Action observation for upper limb rehabilitation after stroke. Cochrane Database Syst Rev 2022;8(8): CD011887.
60. Thieme H, Morkisch N, Mehrholz J, et al. Mirror therapy for improving motor function after stroke. Cochrane Database Syst Rev 2018;7(7):CD008449.
61. Van Hoornweder S, Vanderzande L, Bloemers E, et al. The effects of transcranial direct current stimulation on upper-limb function post-stroke: A meta-analysis of multiple-session studies. Clin Neurophysiol 2021;132(8):1897–918.
62. Starosta M, Cichoń N, Saluk-Bijak J, et al. Benefits from Repetitive Transcranial Magnetic Stimulation in Post-Stroke Rehabilitation. J Clin Med 2022;11(8):2149.
63. Huang W, Chen J, Zheng Y, et al. The Effectiveness of Intermittent Theta Burst Stimulation for Stroke Patients With Upper Limb Impairments: A Systematic Review and Meta-Analysis. Front Neurol 2022;13.
64. Morrison RA, Hulsey DR, Adcock KS, et al. Vagus nerve stimulation intensity influences motor cortex plasticity. Brain Stimul 2019;12(2):256–62.
65. Dawson J, Liu CY, Francisco GE, et al. Vagus nerve stimulation paired with rehabilitation for upper limb motor function after ischaemic stroke (VNS-REHAB): a randomised, blinded, pivotal, device trial. Lancet 2021;397(10284):1545–53.
66. Quattrocchi G, Greenwood R, Rothwell JC, et al. Reward and punishment enhance motor adaptation in stroke. J Neurol Neurosurg Psychiatry 2017;88(9): 730–6.
67. Widmer M, Held JPO, Wittmann F, et al. Reward During Arm Training Improves Impairment and Activity After Stroke: A Randomized Controlled Trial. Neurorehabilitation Neural Repair 2022;36(2):140–50.

68. McEwen S, Polatajko H, Baum C, et al. Combined Cognitive-Strategy and Task-Specific Training Improve Transfer to Untrained Activities in Subacute Stroke: An Exploratory Randomized Controlled Trial. Neurorehabilitation Neural Repair 2015;29(6):526–36.

69. Rowe JB, Chan V, Ingemanson ML, et al. Robotic Assistance for Training Finger Movement Using a Hebbian Model: A Randomized Controlled Trial. Neurorehabilitation Neural Repair 2017;31(8):769–80.

70. Chen YA, Lewthwaite R, Schweighofer N, et al. Essential Role of Social Context and Self-Efficacy in Daily Paretic Arm/Hand Use After Stroke: An Ecological Momentary Assessment Study With Accelerometry. Arch Phys Med Rehabil 2023;104(3):390–402.

71. Lang CE, Waddell KJ, Barth J, et al. Upper Limb Performance in Daily Life Approaches Plateau Around Three to Six Weeks Post-stroke. Neurorehabilitation Neural Repair 2021;35(10):903–14.

72. Du Y, Krakauer JW, Haith AM. The relationship between habits and motor skills in humans. Trends Cogn Sci 2022;26(5):371–87.

73. Young BM, Holman EA, Cramer SC. STRONG Study Investigators. Rehabilitation Therapy Doses Are Low After Stroke and Predicted by Clinical Factors. Stroke 2023;54(3):831–9.

74. Purton J, Sim J, Hunter SM. Stroke survivors' views on their priorities for upper-limb recovery and the availability of therapy services after stroke: a longitudinal, phenomenological study. Disabil Rehabil 2022;1–11.

75. Dobkin BH. A Rehabilitation-Internet-of-Things in the Home to Augment Motor Skills and Exercise Training. Neurorehabilitation Neural Repair 2017;31(3):217–27.

76. Rohrbach N, Chicklis E, Levac DE. What is the impact of user affect on motor learning in virtual environments after stroke? A scoping review. J NeuroEng Rehabil 2019;16(1):79.

77. Lessa HT, Chiviacowsky S. Self-controlled practice benefits motor learning in older adults. Hum Mov Sci 2015;40:372–80.

78. Willis RE, Richa J, Oppeltz R, et al. Comparing three pedagogical approaches to psychomotor skills acquisition. Am J Surg 2012;203(1):8–13.

79. Spencer J, Wolf SL, Kesar TM. Biofeedback for Post-stroke Gait Retraining: A Review of Current Evidence and Future Research Directions in the Context of Emerging Technologies. Front Neurol 2021;12. https://doi.org/10.3389/fneur.2021.637199.

80. Winstein CJ, Merians AS, Sullivan KJ. Motor learning after unilateral brain damage. Neuropsychologia 1999;37(8):975–87.

81. Dzewaltowski AC, Hedrick EA, Leutzinger TJ, et al. The Effect of Split-Belt Treadmill Interventions on Step Length Asymmetry in Individuals Poststroke: A Systematic Review With Meta-Analysis. Neurorehabilitation Neural Repair 2021;35(7):563–75.

Health Care Disparities in Stroke Rehabilitation

Audrie A. Chavez, MD, MPH[a], Kent P. Simmonds, DO, PhD, MPH[b],
Aardhra M. Venkatachalam, MPH, CCRC (MS2)[c],
Nneka L. Ifejika, MD, MPH[b,d,]*

KEYWORDS

- Stroke • Disparities • Rehabilitation • Functional outcomes

KEY POINTS

- To date, no rehabilitative-focused interventions to address disparities in stroke outcomes have been identified.
- There is a gap in literature for disseminated rehabilitative stroke interventions.
- There has been a significant increase in rehabilitation representation in stroke disparity literature between 2008 and 2022.

INTRODUCTION

Despite significant strides in clinical practice, stroke remains the fifth leading cause of death and a leading case of disability within the United States.[1] Stroke outcomes are influenced by a variety of factors related to lifestyle, education, access to care, and resources available to patients that facilitate functional recovery. The United States is composed of a highly heterogeneous population with known inequities between multiple types of groups. To date, the majority of work has focused on investigating disparities primarily by differences in race/ethnicity, age, and sex.[2] Other less explored facets of disparities include income, geography (rural vs urban), disability, sexual orientation, immigrant status, religion, mental health status, English as a second language, technology access, and insurance type.[2]

[a] Brain Injury Medicine Fellow, Spaulding Rehabilitation, Harvard University, Cambridge, MA, USA; [b] Department of Physical Medicine and Rehabilitation, UT Southwestern Medical Center, Dallas, TX, USA; [c] Ross University School of Medicine, Miramar, FL; [d] Department of Neurology, UT Southwestern Medical Center, 5323 Harry Hines Boulevard, Stop 9055, Dallas, TX 75390-9055, USA
* Corresponding author.
E-mail address: Nneka.Ifejika@utsouthwestern.edu
Twitter: @stilettoscience (N.L.I.)

Phys Med Rehabil Clin N Am 35 (2024) 293–303
https://doi.org/10.1016/j.pmr.2023.06.030
1047-9651/24/© 2023 Elsevier Inc. All rights reserved.

REVIEW OF STROKE DISPARITIES LITERATURE

A literature review was conducted to assess the body of stroke disparity literature published between 2008 and 2022. The search was conducted, and articles were cross-referenced across PubMed, OVID, ResearchGate, and Google Scholar, which resulted in an initial n = 527 articles. This number included original research, editorials, and conference proceedings. The authors narrowed down the search for a final count of 345 original research articles to calculate percentages of articles published on stroke type and disparity category. Although analyses for original research generally included disparity demographics such as age, sex, and race/ethnicity as covariables, only articles that included disparity variables for the main/secondary hypotheses were included in the final count, to emphasize the focus of the reported investigation on stroke disparities.

Disparity categories that had 5% or greater representation in the literature have been listed in **Fig. 1**. Of the articles that investigated disparity by stroke type, 43% of articles looked at multiple stroke types, 23% acute ischemic stroke only, 14% intra-cerebral hemorrhage only, 10% subarachnoid hemorrhage (SAH) only, and 5% other strokes (lacunar, transient ischemic attack [TIA], etc.). Thirty-seven percent of articles focused on race/ethnicity, 17% on age, 15% on sex, 12% on socioeconomic status (SES), and 9% by insurance status. Other disparity categories that had less than 5% representation in the literature (ie, geography, sexual orientation, language barriers, medical communication, stroke literacy, immigrant status, mental health) were grouped together and represented as "other" (~10%).

Between the years 2008 and 2022, an average of 23 articles were published on stroke disparity annually; articles which represented rehabilitation data made up 10% of stroke disparity literature in 2008 (2 out of 20 papers), but has risen up to as much as 44% of total published stroke disparity literature by year since 2016 (12 out of 27 papers). These articles largely focused on identification of disparities in reha-bilitation disposition and functional outcomes. At the time of this literature search, no articles focusing on rehabilitation-based health disparity interventions were identified, although there has been a significant increase in interventional studies targeting pre-venting stroke incidence in high-risk groups by focusing on stroke-related risk factors.

Of note, the conducted review was not able to account for any programs or inter-ventions that may have been conducted but were not disseminated in an academic

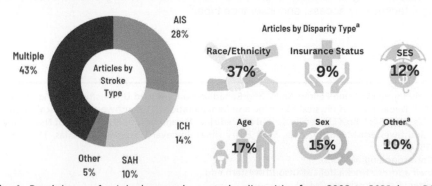

Fig. 1. Breakdown of original research on stroke disparities from 2008 to 2022 (n = 345). AIS, acute ischemic stroke; ICH, intracerebral hemorrhage; SAH, subarachnoid hemorrhage; SES, socioeconomic status. [a]Other = Language barriers, medical communication, stroke lit-eracy, immigrant status.

medium (conference, journal, American Heart Association [AHA] guidelines, etc.). If present, this could lead to a gap in representation of efforts made to overcome stroke disparity in the body of academic literature.

DISPARITIES IN STROKE-RELATED RISK FACTORS

Racial and ethnic minorities are projected to make up nearly 40% of the US population by 2030, heightening the importance of addressing health-related disparities affecting stroke survivors.[3] A large body of literature has focused on identifying disparities in risk factors associated with stroke incidence, often focusing on differences in hypertension, type 2 diabetes mellitus (DM), low-density lipoprotein (LDL) cholesterol, and tobacco use. Regarding race/ethnicity, the black population has the largest incidence of hypertension in the United States; elevated blood pressure accounts for 50% of the excess stroke risk among the black population compared with non-Hispanic whites (NHWs).[4] DM rates are highest in the Hispanic population followed closely by the black population when compared with NHWs.[4] Although a large study using data from the National Health and Nutrition Examination Survey (NHANES) study showed the highest mean LDL cholesterol values in the NHW population, Mexicans had the lowest rate of cholesterol screening at 59.3% compared to a rate of 71.8% in NHWs.[4] Beyond racial/ethnic differences in the prevalence of risk factors, there are also differences in the medical management in many of these medical conditions considered as primary risk factors. Data from the Reasons for Geographic and Racial Differences in Stroke (REGARDS) study showed that even after controlling for access to medical care, disparities exist in individuals with DM who are prescribed a statin with women and black patients having a lower prescription frequency compared with NHWs.[4] Tobacco use is also more prevalent among certain groups including native American/Alaskan natives, lesbian, gay, bisexual, and transgender populations, and individuals with low SES–often linked to underrepresented ethnic minorities.[4] Beyond race/ethnicity, there are marked sex differences as women with DM have a 27% higher relative risk of stroke compared with males with DM even after controlling for baseline differences in other major cardiovascular risk factors.[5]

The combination of higher stroke incidence and poor management of conditions considered primary risk factors contributes to minority populations having more severe strokes and higher levels of subsequent disability compared with NHWs.[6–14] Age-adjusted incidence rates for first time stroke have been shown to be higher in black and Hispanic individuals compared with NHWs, particularly in younger age groups.[4,15,16] Existing disparities in stroke-related risk factors compounded with a higher stroke incidence and disease burden affect the potential for recovery in the continuum of post-stroke rehabilitative care. These variables will be further explored in the following sections.

DISPARITIES IN THE ACUTE STROKE SETTING: STROKE TYPE, TREATMENT, AND FUNCTIONAL STATUS

Within the United States, the overall prevalence of stroke subtypes is as follows: 87% ischemic, 10% hemorrhagic, and 3% SAH.[4] However, the prevalence of these subtypes is not uniform across various racial/ethnic groups. Prior data have shown that Native Americans[17] and African Americans[18] have similar subtype rates to the overall population, but Hispanics may have higher rates of hemorrhagic stroke (as high as 48% in the Barrow Stroke Database) and SAH.[19,20]

Ischemic stroke patients with a large vessel occlusion (LVO) lose 2.5 million neurons every minute ensuring that timely arrival to a stroke center for treatment is a mainstay of mitigating post-stroke disability.[21] A Get With the Guidelines-Stroke study including over 1000 hospitals published in 2012 (n = 413,147 with symptom onset time and hospital presentation time) showed that a predictor for early arrival to the hospital for acute stroke treatment was race–NHW patients were more likely to have earlier arrival times, whereas black and Hispanic patients had later arrival times. Differences in arrival times may be due to lower levels of health literacy, less awareness of stroke symptoms, and lack of education on the importance of the need for rapid presentation to emergency departments.[22] However, another study that included 14 hospitals, both university and community affiliated (n = 1159), did not find a significant relationship between ethnicity and time to presentation after acute stroke.[23] A lack of significant differences in the second study may be due to geographic differences in the 2 study populations.

In addition to later arrival times, black patients also have lower intravenous thrombolysis treatment rates with tissue plasminogen activator (t-PA) when compared with NHW patients.[24–26] This difference persists even after controlling for confounding factors (age, gender, type of insurance, and stroke severity) and restricting analysis to those without contraindications to t-PA.[24–26] Although there has been some improvement in this discrepancy over time from 2008 to 2017,[25] a 2011 study by Ifejika-Jones and colleagues[27] demonstrated ischemic stroke patients who receive intravenous t-PA were more likely to go home immediately following the acute hospitalization, despite having higher stroke severity on arrival. There have been mixed results in the literature comparing t-PA rates in Asian and Hispanic patients compared with NHWs.[24–26] Part of the challenge is that there are often only a small number of ethnic minorities included in the analysis.[24–26] Beyond racial/ethnic differences in t-PA treatment rates, a study of 54,334 ischemic stroke patients found disparities in the rate of hemorrhagic complications, with increased prevalence among black and Asian patients compared with NHWs.[28]

In patients with LVO undergoing revascularization via mechanical thrombectomy (MT), treatment disparities persisted. Black patients were less likely to receive this evidence-based, Food and Drug Administration (FDA) approved treatment option for anterior circulation acute ischemic stroke.[25,29] Similarly to t-PA, there have been mixed results in the literature with some demonstrating no significant difference and some showing lower rates of MT when comparing Hispanic to NHW patients.[25,26,29] Stroke survivors with Medicaid health insurance or no health insurance were also less likely to receive MT.[26] Some study variability can be attributed to low sample sizes of racial/ethnic minorities as well as regional differences and access to academic/teaching hospitals.

Sex disparities in access to acute stroke treatment have also been studied. A review by Reeves and colleagues[30] found mixed results in time to presentation when comparing men to women; 5 studies showed delayed presentation to the acute hospital for women, one showed earlier presentation. They also found that women were more likely to have delays in emergency department evaluation compared with men. This review also found that women were less likely to receive diagnostic studies such as echocardiography and carotid imaging during their hospital stay.[30]

A recent study by Jones and colleagues[31] reviewed prospective data in young patients (ages 18–50 years) who suffered an acute ischemic stroke and found that black and Hispanic patients were significantly less likely to have good functional outcome (modified Rankin score of 0–1) at discharge from acute care after adjusting for age, history of prior ischemic stroke, congestive heart failure, hypertension, diabetes, end-stage renal disease, smoking, National Institutes of Health Stroke Scale on arrival, t-PA given, and endovascular treatment with MT.

DISPARITIES IN REHABILITATIVE STROKE CARE: ACUTE/SUBACUTE REHABILITATION, COMMUNITY-BASED REHABILITATIVE CARE, AND FUNCTIONAL OUTCOMES

Acute stroke patients benefit from rehabilitation therapeutics across the continuum of care–ranging from the intensive care unit to outpatient follow-up visits in the community. Although recovery trajectories for stroke patients often plateau around 1 year, many patients will require chronic management of numerous medical complications as well as high levels of functional debility.[32] Rehabilitation care focuses on maximizing recovery and minimizing complications; however, a substantial body of evidence continues to identify disparities in the type, timing, and duration of rehabilitation care that stroke patients receive. Most disparities studies have focused on race/ethnicity, sex, and geographic differences in rehabilitation care. For example, a large study of 11,862 stroke patients used data from the Behavior Risk Factor Surveillance System (BRFSS) to identify that women and NHW (vs black) patients were less likely to report receiving *any* type of stroke rehabilitation care.[33]

Following acute hospitalization, most stroke patients are discharged to a form of post-acute care (PAC) for further medical management and/or rehabilitation therapies for residual debility. PAC takes place at a variety of settings with large differences in the extent of medical management, amount of nursing care, and time intensity of rehabilitation therapies provided in each of these settings. Patients may receive inpatient PAC at Inpatient Rehabilitation Facilities (IRFs) or Skilled Nursing Facilities (SNFs) or from home in the form of outpatient visits and/or home health. Regarding receipt of PAC, a large study of 849,780 stroke survivors used data from Get With The Guidelines-Stroke to find that patients who were black or female were more likely to receive *some type* of PAC. For the comparison of discharge to a facility versus home, several large studies found that patients who are black (vs white), female, or live in urban settings are more likely to be discharged to a rehabilitation facility.[34,35] Hispanics and those who were uninsured were more likely to be discharged home even after controlling for illness severity.[35]

Among patients discharged to facility-based PAC, several large studies have shown that patients who are female, older, rural (vs urban), and have lower SES were less likely to be discharged to IRFs (vs SNFs); these differences persisted even after adjustment of multiple potential confounding variables.[35–37] A large Medicare-based study with data from 1999 found that proximity to rehabilitation facilities was a stronger driver than other clinical characteristics demonstrating that the further one lived from an IRF and the closer one lived to a SNF, the less likely they were to end up at an IRF.[38] Results for race/ethnicity have been mixed, particularly for the comparison of black (vs NHW). Fewer studies have investigated differences among Hispanic patients, but one study focused on comparing Mexican American (MA) to NHW patients found that NHWs were more likely to get inpatient rehabilitation (73%) compared with males (30%).[39]

When comparing level of intensity (SNF vs IRF), black patients, women, and individuals of lower SES were more likely to receive less intensive facility based treatment (ie, SNF care).[35] However, a Northeast regional study did not find significant racial differences in those referred to an institutional rehabilitation facility.[37]

Access to IRF versus SNF care does not necessarily mitigate disparities. A study of 1066 stroke patients who received rehabilitation at 11 inpatient rehabilitation facilities across the United States found that among all stroke patients, significant racial/ethnic differences first emerged at 3 months when the majority of patients would be discharged back the community.[40] Mechanistic differences in the pathophysiology of stroke etiology may affect some of these differences, as black (vs white) patients had lower functional scores on admission to IRFs with the differences possibly due to black (vs white) patients having more severe hemorrhagic strokes.[40] Hispanics have also been shown to have lower Functional Independence Measure scores on IRF admission, with one study demonstrating lower admission scores when compared with white and black patients.[41]

Importantly, there is fluidity in PAC transitions; heterogeneous recovery trajectories may facilitate the need for patients to receive different intensities of rehabilitation across different PAC settings. A large study by Skolarus and colleagues[42] used Medicare data to track transitions across post-acute care settings among 186,168 patients. Stroke patients received rehabilitation in an average of 2 settings (interquartile range [IQR]: 1–5). This same study also estimated the total number of minutes of physical, occupational, and speech therapies that patients received in the first year after their stroke, finding black (vs white) patients received a higher number of total therapy minutes (897.8 vs 743.4; $P < 0.01$). However, after adjustments for demographics, comorbidities, intravenous thrombolysis, and markers of stroke severity, there was no racial difference in therapy utilization in this patient population. Similar findings were seen in an academic-based rehabilitation setting in Texas using Get with the Guidelines-Stroke data which did not demonstrate a difference in rehabilitation duration (total therapy minutes) during the acute stroke hospitalization after controlling for confounding factors such as stroke severity, age, and comorbidities.[43]

LANGUAGE BARRIERS

Since 2014, the American Heart Association has identified health equity in stroke care as a priority area in systems of care for secondary ischemic stroke prevention and addressing language differences is an important aspect.[44] Language barriers can lead to mistrust of health care providers as well as limitations in access to quality rehabilitation care. In a 2021 study by Nguyen and colleagues,[45] as a large safety net hospital, the use of translation services was associated with a significant decrease in rehabilitation duration among adults over age 65 years, including stroke patients.

Clark and colleagues[46] conducted systematic reviews showing the association between English proficiency and improved outcomes in preventive aspects of stroke care. In 20 selected articles (n = 891 unique articles in original search), patients with Limited English Proficiency (LEP) also experienced a lower quality of life post-stroke; language barriers negatively affect access to care in rehabilitation and clinicians' ability to provide quality care. LEP and English groups show similar mortality despite greater length of stay and greater proportions of stroke rehab units dedicated for LEP patients. Equitable stroke rehabilitation care was equated to a high degree of interpreter availability. Patients can benefit from tailored education regarding stroke symptom recognition, secondary stroke prevention management, and from access to translated written educational material for their care across the rehabilitation continuum to address inequities that can lead to impacts on care and functional outcomes.[46]

DISPARITIES IN FUNCTIONAL OUTCOMES FOR SURVIVORS OF STROKE

There is limited data on racial/ethnic disparities in long-term functional outcomes after stroke, as most research is focused on the first 90 days. A study published by the Brain Attack Surveillance in Corpus Christi (BASIC) group in 2015 found after multivariable adjustment, post-stroke quality of life (QOL) at 90 days was lower for Mexican-Americans than NHWs overall and in the physical domain, with no ethnic differences found in the psychosocial domain. Age modified the associations between ethnicity and post-stroke QOL–differences were present in older (age 69+ in overall post-stroke QOL and physical QOL scores) but not in younger ages.[47] However, another study found that Hispanics were less likely to report physical difficulties with ambulation, whereas black patients reported more difficulties than NHWs.[48]

A large multicenter study of stroke patients at IRFs found compared with older patients (age > 65 years), younger patients were more likely to be independent at discharge, be discharged to their prior residence, and return to work. Notably, younger patients also had longer lengths of IRF stay and were more likely to receive community rehabilitation, potentially indicating higher goals of rehabilitation care were required to return patients to their prior level of function.[49]

Reeves and colleagues[30] reported although men have greater age-specific stroke incidence and mortality, women had worse functional outcomes and reduced QOL post-stroke with 34% of women disabled at 6 months (Barthel index <60) compared with only 16% of men. However, a large IRF based study found no sex differences in the length of stay or functional discharge scores among 20,143 stroke patients, indicating that the gender outcome differences may be accounted for in patients discharged to other rehabilitation levels or home.[50]

INTERVENTIONS FOCUSED ON REHABILITATIVE STROKE DISPARITIES

Identifying the role and importance of disparities across the continuum of stroke-related care drives research in the field to address these inequities. The majority of this research has remained focused on stroke prevention, including modifiable risk factors (which disproportionately affect ethnic/racial minorities),[51] stroke education, and symptom identification. Examples of these include a Corpus Christi (large Hispanic population) based education program to teach middle school children how to recognize symptoms of stroke and call 911[52] and Swipe out Stroke (SOS) which involves the use of a smartphone-based mobile application to reduce obesity in high-risk minority stroke patients.[51]

Although disparities extend into the rehabilitation spectrum, which was the area of focus for this article, there were no identified interventional research articles to address these inequities at this stage.

SUMMARY

Stroke-related disparities are present along the continuum of care starting with non-modifiable health determinants, modifiable risk factors, acute stroke treatment, access to rehabilitation services, and functional outcomes. This has appropriately resulted in increased research to identify disparities along the continuum of care that can be addressed with targeted interventions. We identified no rehabilitative focused interventions to address disparities; therefore, this is a field with critical needs. Rehabilitation providers provide care to stroke survivors across the continuum, positioning them to address this call to research and continue to improve stroke-related outcomes through purposeful care equity. Rehabilitation providers also care for these patients chronically and at times for the duration of the remainder of these patients lives providing a unique opportunity to contribute to important data in long-term functional outcomes and disparities that exist across different time points. Negative repercussions of stroke disparities go beyond the individual patient and can be self-perpetuating. For example, a stroke patient who does not have insurance coverage may not be able to use rehabilitation services, and may not be able to return to work, which further contributes to their poor SES. This cycle not only affects current patients, but also future generations. Additional calls to research include diversifying the workforce, including unconscious bias training for health care workers (recognizing and mitigating), and quality improvement projects that include aspects of culture and community for the targeted populations.[53]

CLINICS CARE POINTS

- Health care disparities in stroke rehabilitation decrease the probability of optimal functional recovery.
- Clinicians should be prepared to identify and address these disparities and to acknowledge the importance of providing equitable access to rehabilitation therapeutics.
- Providing patients and families the opportunity to address their concerns regarding disparities, including bridging potential language barriers, is a key compoent of improving satisfaction with the transition to post-stroke rehabilitation.

SOURCES OF FUNDING

Dr N.L. Ifejika's current work: UT Southwestern/Texas Health Resources Clinical Scholar Award (#4). Dr N.L. Ifejika previous work: Center for Clinical and Translational Sciences at the McGovern Medical School at UTHealth, funded by NIH/NCATS Clinical and Translational Award UL1 TR000371 and KL2 TR000370. The content is solely the responsibility of the authors and does not necessarily represent the official views of the National Center for Research Resources or the NIH. Dr N.L. Ifejika's preliminary work: NIH/NINDS Diversity Supplement to P50 NS 044227, the University of Texas Specialized Program of Translational Research in Acute Stroke (SPOTRIAS).

DISCLOSURE

All authors have no commercial or financial conflicts of interest. N.L. Ifejika's funding sources have been listed above. All other authors have no funding sources to disclose.

REFERENCES

1. Tsao CW, Aday AW, Almarzooq ZI, et al. Heart disease and stroke statistics—2023 update: a report from the American Heart Association. Circulation 2023; 147(8):e93–621.
2. Hubbard K, Huang DT. National Center for Health Statistics. Healthy People 2020 Final Review. 2021. Available at: https://stacks.cdc.gov/view/cdc/111173.
3. Cruz-Flores S, Rabinstein A, Biller J, et al. Racial-ethnic disparities in stroke care: the american experience. Stroke 2011;42(7):2091–116.
4. Benjamin EJ, Muntner P, Alonso A, et al. Heart disease and stroke statistics—2019 update: a report from the american heart association. Circulation 2019; 139(10):e56–66.
5. Peters SAEP, Huxley RRP, Woodward MP. Diabetes as a risk factor for stroke in women compared with men: a systematic review and meta-analysis of 64 cohorts, including 775 385 individuals and 12 539 strokes. The Lancet (British edition) 2014;383(9933):1973–80.
6. Xie J, Wu EQ, Zheng ZJ, et al. Impact of stroke on health-related quality of life in the noninstitutionalized population in the United States. Stroke 2006;37(10): 2567–72.

7. Ottenbacher KJ, Campbell J, Kuo YF, et al. Racial and ethnic differences in post-acute rehabilitation outcomes after stroke in the United States. Stroke 2008;39(5): 1514–9.

8. Ellis C, Boan AD, Turan TN, et al. Racial differences in poststroke rehabilitation utilization and functional outcomes. Arch Phys Med Rehabil 2015;96(1):84–90.

9. Lisabeth LD, Sánchez BN, Baek J, et al. Neurological, functional, and cognitive stroke outcomes in mexican Americans. Stroke 2014;45(4):1096–101.

10. Kuhlemeier KV, Stiens SA. Racial disparities in severity of cerebrovascular events. Stroke 1994;25(11):2126–31.

11. Bhandari VK, Kushel M, Price L, et al. Racial disparities in outcomes of inpatient stroke rehabilitation. Arch Phys Med Rehabil 2005;86(11):2081–6.

12. Burke JF, Feng C, Skolarus LE. Divergent poststroke outcomes for black patients: Lower mortality, but greater disability. Neurology 2019;93(18):e1664–74.

13. Garcia JJ, Warren KL. Race/ethnicity matters: differences in poststroke inpatient rehabilitation outcomes. Ethn Dis 2019;29(4):599–608.

14. Skolarus LE, Feng C, Burke JF. Exploring factors contributing to race differences in poststroke disability. Stroke 2020;51(6):1813–9.

15. Morgenstern LB, Smith MA, Lisabeth LD, et al. Excess stroke in Mexican Americans compared with non-hispanic whites - the brain attack surveillance in corpus christi project. Am J Epidemiol 2004;160(4):376–83.

16. White H, Boden-Albala B, Wang C, et al. Ischemic stroke subtype incidence among whites, blacks, and hispanics. Circulation 2005;111(10):1327–31.

17. Zhang Y, Galloway JM, Welty TK, et al. Incidence and risk factors for stroke in American Indians - The strong heart study. Circulation 2008;118(15):1577–84.

18. Owolabi M, Sarfo F, Howard VJ, et al. Stroke in indigenous Africans, African Americans, and European Americans. Stroke 2017;48(5):1169–75.

19. Frey JL, Jahnke HK, Bulfinch EW. Differences in Stroke between white, hispanic, and native American patients. Stroke 1998;29(1):29–33.

20. Sacco RL, Hauser WA, Mohr JP. Hospitalized stroke in blacks and hispanics in northern manhattan. Stroke 1991;22(12):1491–6.

21. Saver JL. Time is brain–quantified. Stroke 2006;37(1):263–6.

22. Tong D, Reeves MJ, Hernandez AF, et al. Times from symptom onset to hospital arrival in the get with the guidelines–stroke program 2002 to 2009. Stroke 2012; 43(7):1912–7.

23. Barsan WG, Brott TG, Broderick JP, et al. Time of hospital presentation in patients with acute stroke. Arch Intern Med 1993;153(22):2558–61.

24. Johnston SC, Fung LH, Gillum LA, et al. Utilization of intravenous tissue-type plasminogen activator for ischemic stroke at academic medical centers. Stroke 2001; 32(5):1061–8.

25. Otite FO, Saini V, Sur NB, et al. Ten-year trend in age, sex, and racial disparity in tPA (Alteplase) and thrombectomy use following stroke in the United States. Stroke 2021;52(8):2562–70.

26. Rinaldo L, Rabinstein AA, Cloft H, et al. Racial and ethnic disparities in the utilization of thrombectomy for acute stroke. Stroke 2019;50(9):2428–32.

27. Ifejika-Jones NL, Harun N, Mohammed-Rajput NA, et al. Thrombolysis with intravenous tissue plasminogen activator predicts a favorable discharge disposition in patients with acute ischemic stroke. Stroke 2011;42(3):700–4.

28. Mehta RH, Cox M, Smith EE, et al. Race/ethnic differences in the risk of hemorrhagic complications among patients with ischemic stroke receiving thrombolytic therapy. Stroke 2014;45(8):2263–9.

29. Esenwa C, Lekoubou A, Bishu KG, et al. Racial differences in mechanical thrombectomy utilization for ischemic stroke in the United States. Ethn Dis 2020; 30(1):91–6.
30. Reeves MJ, Bushnell CD, Howard G, et al. Sex differences in stroke: epidemiology, clinical presentation, medical care, and outcomes. Lancet Neurol 2008; 7(10):915–26.
31. Jones EM, Okpala M, Zhang X, et al. Racial disparities in post-stroke functional outcomes in young patients with ischemic stroke. J Stroke Cerebrovasc Dis 2020;29(8):104987.
32. Winstein CJ, Stein J, Arena R, et al. Guidelines for adult stroke rehabilitation and recovery: a guideline for healthcare professionals from the American heart association/American stroke association. Stroke 2016;47(6):e98–169.
33. Ross JS, Halm EA, Bravata DM. Use of stroke secondary prevention services: are there disparities in care? Stroke 2009;40(5):1811–9.
34. Prvu Bettger J, McCoy L, Smith EE, et al. Contemporary trends and predictors of postacute service use and routine discharge home after stroke. J Am Heart Assoc 2015;4(2):e001038.
35. Freburger JK, Holmes GM, Ku L-JE, et al. Disparities in postacute rehabilitation care for stroke: an analysis of the state inpatient databases. Arch Phys Med Rehabil 2011;92(8):1220–9.
36. Xian Y, Thomas L, Liang L, et al. Unexplained variation for hospitals' use of inpatient rehabilitation and skilled nursing facilities after an acute ischemic stroke. Stroke 2017;48(10):2836–42.
37. Stein J, Bettger JP, Sicklick A, et al. Use of a standardized assessment to predict rehabilitation care after acute stroke. Arch Phys Med Rehabil 2015;96(2):210–7.
38. Buntin MB, Garten AD, Paddock S, et al. How much is postacute care use affected by its availability? Health Serv Res 2005;40(2):413–34.
39. Morgenstern LB, Sais E, Fuentes M, et al. Mexican Americans receive less intensive stroke rehabilitation than non-hispanic whites. Stroke 2017;48(6):1685–7.
40. Simmonds KP, Luo Z, Reeves M. Race/ethnic and stroke subtype differences in poststroke functional recovery after acute rehabilitation. Arch Phys Med Rehabil 2021;102(8):1473–81.
41. Chiou-Tan FY, Keng MJ Jr, Graves DE, et al. Racial/ethnic differences in FIM™ scores and length of stay for underinsured patients undergoing stroke inpatient rehabilitation. Am J Phys Med Rehabil 2006;85(5):415–23.
42. Skolarus LE, Feng C, Burke JF. No racial difference in rehabilitation therapy across all post-acute care settings in the year following a stroke. Stroke 2017; 48(12):3329–35.
43. Chavez AA, Abraham AM, Venkatachalam AM, et al. Differences in postacute rehabilitation recommendations by ethnicity at an urban comprehensive stroke center. Am J Phys Med Rehabil 2022;101(12):1104–10.
44. Kleindorfer DO, Towfighi A, Chaturvedi S, et al. 2021 Guideline for the prevention of stroke in patients with stroke and transient ischemic attack: a guideline from the American Heart Association/American Stroke association. Stroke 2021; 52(7):e364–467.
45. Nguyen DQ, Ifejika NL, Reistetter TA, et al. Factors associated with duration of rehabilitation among older adults with prolonged hospitalization. J Am Geriatr Soc 2021;69(4):1035–44.
46. Clark JR, Shlobin NA, Batra A, et al. The relationship between limited English proficiency and outcomes in stroke prevention, management, and rehabilitation: a systematic review. Front Neurol 2022;13:77.

47. Reeves SL, Brown DL, Baek J, et al. Ethnic differences in poststroke quality of life in the Brain Attack Surveillance in Corpus Christi (BASIC) project. Stroke 2015; 46(10):2896–901.
48. Tshiswaka DI, Seals S, Raghavan P. Correlates of physical function among stroke survivors: an examination of the 2015 BRFSS. Public Health 2018;155: 17–22.
49. Purvis T, Hubbard IJ, Cadilhac DA, et al. Age-related disparities in the quality of stroke care and outcomes in rehabilitation hospitals: the Australian national audit. J Stroke Cerebrovasc Dis 2021;30(5):105707.
50. MacDonald SL, Hall RE, Bell CM, et al. Sex differences in the outcomes of adults admitted to inpatient rehabilitation after stroke. PM&R 2022;14(7):779–85.
51. Ifejika NL, Bhadane M, Cai CC, et al. Use of a smartphone-based mobile app for weight management in obese minority stroke survivors: pilot randomized controlled trial with open blinded end point. JMIR Mhealth Uhealth 2020;8(4): e17816.
52. Morgenstern LB, Gonzales NR, Maddox KE, et al. A randomized, controlled trial to teach middle school children to recognize stroke and call 911: the kids identifying and defeating stroke project. Stroke 2007;38(11):2972–8.
53. Sacco RL. Stroke disparities: from observations to actions. Stroke 2020;51(11): 3392–405.

Telerehabilitation Following Stroke

Steven C. Cramer, MD[a,b,*], Brittany M. Young, MD, PhD[a,b],
Anne Schwarz, PT, PhD[a,b], Tracy Y. Chang, MD[a,b],
Michael Su, MD[a,b]

KEYWORDS

- Stroke • Motor • Telehealth • Rehabilitation • Therapy

KEY POINTS

- Stroke remains a major cause of disability.
- Intensive rehabilitation therapy can improve outcomes.
- Most patients receive low doses of rehabilitation therapy.
- Telehealth methods can overcome obstacles to delivering intensive therapy after stroke.
- Telerehabilitation enables a holistic approach that includes assessment, education, prevention, and activity-based therapy.

STROKE REMAINS A MAJOR CAUSE OF HUMAN DISABILITY

Stroke is a major cause of human disability. In middle- and high-income countries, stroke is the leading neurologic cause of lost disability-adjusted life years.[1] The mean survival after stroke is 7 years, with ~85% of patients living more than 1 year after stroke onset.[2] Most patients thus survive their stroke and live with enduring disability for many years.

The number of stroke survivors has increased over time, in part due to declining stroke mortality rates, which has further increased the global stroke-related disability burden. As the population ages, these issues are projected to further increase in magnitude.

Some patients with ischemic stroke are helped by acute reperfusion therapies; however, these are not indicated for most such patients. For example, among 318,127 acute stroke admissions in the United States from October, 2014 to March, 2018, only 15.7% received intravenous (IV) recombinant tissue plasminogen activator, and 5.4% underwent mechanical thrombectomy.[3] Furthermore, approximately half of

[a] Department of Neurology, UCLA, Los Angeles, CA, USA; [b] California Rehabilitation Institute, 2070 Century Park East, Los Angeles, CA 90067-1907, USA
* Corresponding author. Dept. Neurology, UCLA, 710 Westwood Plaza, Reed C239, Los Angeles, CA 90095-1769.
E-mail address: sccramer@mednet.ucla.edu

Phys Med Rehabil Clin N Am 35 (2024) 305–318
https://doi.org/10.1016/j.pmr.2023.06.005
1047-9651/24/© 2023 Elsevier Inc. All rights reserved.

the patients receiving either of these acute reperfusion therapies show significant long-term disability.[4,5] Moreover, patients with hemorrhagic stroke are not eligible for reperfusion. Additional approaches to treating stroke, which can be accessed by a majority of patients, are needed.

What can be done to help patients with persisting deficits after the acute reperfusion time window is closed? Animal studies provide strong evidence that many classes of restorative therapy can improve outcomes after stroke, and some of these therapies seem promising in human trials to date.[6-8] These restorative therapies do not aim to reduce acute injury but instead focus on promoting clinically useful plasticity within brain areas that survive the acute insult. Although there are many forms of restorative therapy under review, this review focuses on telerehabilitation (TR).

HIGH DOSES OF REHABILITATION THERAPY IMPROVE OUTCOMES AFTER STROKE

Interdisciplinary rehabilitation therapy is the standard of care in the weeks following a stroke and often includes physical therapy (PT), occupational therapy (OT), and speech–language therapy (ST). Strong evidence suggests that rehabilitation interventions that use movement- and activity-based treatments are associated with reduced mortality and increased functional independence.[9] Level 1 A evidence indicates that greater intensity of OT and PT improves functional outcomes after stroke.[10]

Increasing evidence suggests that higher dose and intensity of movement therapy after stroke lead to better outcomes[11-14]; the same may be true for ST.[15] Some specific programs have demonstrated remarkable results, for example, with provision of constraint-induced movement therapy,[16] an intense clinic-based outpatient program,[17] and a massive doses of arm motor therapy[18]—each associated with substantial benefit. Two recent trials did find no outcome differences when additional rehabilitation therapy was introduced in the chronic phase[19,20]; however, some argue that the doses evaluated in these trials were too low. The quality of rehabilitation therapy is also important, with effects increased when therapy is challenging, motivating, and engaging.[21-23]

Advantages of activity-based therapies include that (1) they can be provided in a variety of settings (eg, clinic or home[24]); (2) adverse events are generally uncommon and mild; (3) regulatory concerns are smaller than with many drugs or devices; and (4) significant benefits are seen whether provided early or late poststroke.

MOST PATIENTS DO NOT RECEIVE HIGH DOSES OF REHABILITATION THERAPY AFTER STROKE

Currently, rehabilitation services are the primary mechanism by which functional recovery is promoted after acute stroke. Another major focus is prevention plus medical management of comorbidities and poststroke complications. The quality and quantity of such services vary across treatment settings (inpatient rehabilitation facility [IRF], skilled nursing home, or home health).

Although high doses of rehabilitation therapy can improve outcomes after stroke, few patients receive this in clinical practice.[25,26] Reasons include limited health insurance coverage, shortage of regional rehabilitation care, problems traveling to a provider, and poor compliance with assignments.

The amount of rehabilitation therapy received with usual care in the United States is generally small and inconsistent. During the acute stroke admission, the dose of OT and PT provided to a patient varies widely across hospitals.[27] After discharge, there is also substantial variation in the type, dose, and setting of rehabilitation therapy,[28,29] despite the fact that it can improve functional status and quality of life and help with psychological outcomes.[9,29]

In the United States, Medicare pays for few outpatient OT and PT sessions,[30] and outpatient stroke rehabilitation is overall sparse. Among 23,413 US patients less than 30 days poststroke in acute care and community settings, Medicare claims disclosed that 59% did not see an OT or PT at all.[31] Among 6743 US stroke survivors, telephone survey disclosed that 67% did not receive any outpatient rehabilitation therapy following their stroke.[29] Young and colleagues[32] found that among 510 US patients, therapy counts were overall low in the 3-month following acute stroke admission, with mean number of sessions being 12.1 for PT, 9.7 for OT, and 6.0 for ST.[32] Importantly, 35.0% of patients received no PT; 48.8% no OT, and 61.7% no ST.

Furthermore, even when patients do access standard of care stroke rehabilitation, the amount of therapy provided is limited,[25,26] averaging just 32 arm movements/session,[25] vastly lower than the 600 to 924 movements/session needed to promote plasticity and recovery in animal studies.[33–35]

TELEHEALTH CAN OVERCOME BARRIERS TO PROVIDING HIGH REHABILITATION DOSES

Stroke leads to disability, and intensive rehabilitation therapy can help, but most patients do not receive this—what can be done? A telehealth approach may offer solutions that offset limitations to accessing high-dose therapy.

TR has been defined as the "delivery of rehabilitation services via information and communication technologies (that) encompasses a range of rehabilitation and habilitation services that include assessment, monitoring, prevention, intervention, supervision, education, consultation, and counseling."[36]

TR can address the unmet need resulting from rehabilitation therapy doses.[37] It can be delivered both synchronously (live therapist–patient interactions) and asynchronously (patient works alone; therapist later reviews patient data) and follows the same basic principles of traditional person-to-person rehabilitation. Such telehealth therapy increases access to rehabilitation therapy[29] and so provides a powerful alternative to the brick-and-mortar approach of delivering rehabilitation services.

TR can overcome several specific barriers that currently limit the dose of rehabilitation therapy after stroke by (1) increasing access to care, important in regions with providers shortages, while reducing the need for impaired patients to travel; (2) boosting motivation, which overcomes low compliance common with stroke rehabilitation[38–40] by using functional games, which promote patient participation in health care[41–44]; (3) reducing costs[45]; and (4) promoting performance of high rehabilitation doses. Patients can repeat TR assignments hundreds of times. A TR approach also supports accountability, as the actual amount of home activity can be reviewed by a therapist and discussed with the patient—a powerful tool to enhance patient compliance.

Overall, studies support the feasibility and potential utility of this approach. One meta-analysis reported that all 18 studies of poststroke motor TR improved motor disabilities.[46] Other reviews report that greater TR usage results in greater benefit,[47] although to date many studies have been small and uncontrolled[46–49] and there is high variability in the approach to TR-based therapy.

Laver and colleagues[50] reviewed 22 randomized controlled stroke trials of 1937 patients receiving TR. Concerns included that many studies had inadequate reporting quality, selective outcome reporting, and incomplete outcome data. Therapy targets varied across studies and included depression, upper extremity (UE) training, mobility retraining, communication therapy, and a discharge support program. The technology used also varied and included telephone, videoconferencing, desktop videophones, video recordings, email, an online chat program, an online resource room, an in-home messaging device, and a dedicated TR device. Overall, this meta-analysis reported that there is only low- or moderate-level evidence testing whether TR is a more effective or similarly effective way to provide rehabilitation.

However, asking "Does TR work?" may be an oversimplification—combining too many things under a single label—and is like asking "Do pills work?" Combining widely different TR approaches that use fundamentally different forms of technology across studies with very different treatment targets and therapeutic regimens may not be the best way to evaluate progress in this nascent field. Details are provided below for one specific approach to TR that is focused on UE motor deficits after stroke.

A TELEREHABILITATION APPROACH TO TREATING UPPER EXTREMITY MOTOR DEFICITS AFTER STROKE

We have developed a TR system and method, the details of which are useful to illustrate general points about using telehealth to improve outcomes in the setting of neurologic disease. Our system targets UE motor deficits, a frequent contributor to poststroke disability; few patients fully recover from arm weakness after a stroke, with the remainder demonstrating persistent impairments directly linked to larger activity limitations, greater participation restrictions, lower quality of life, and decreased well-being.[9,51,52] TR efforts targeting other diseases or other deficits (eg, language, hemineglect, or cognition) have also been studied but are not further considered here.

Hardware: For our TR system, hardware consists of an Internet-enabled computer, table, and chair, plus 11 gaming input devices (eg, buttons, grip, pinch, joystick, accelerometer), ensuring TR usability across a range of UE impairments (**Fig. 1**). There is no keyboard, as no computer operations are required by subjects. Therapists can incorporate additional standard exercise equipment.

Software

Therapist-facing software in our TR system, accessed through a Web portal, is used by a licensed OT or PT to generate and supervise treatment. A graphical interface is

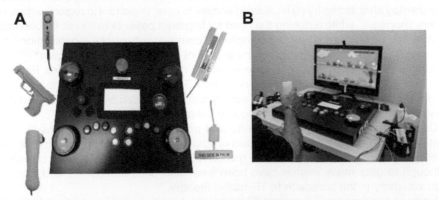

Fig. 1. The telerehabilitation system hardware includes (*A*) a table with large buttons, small buttons, joystick, trackball, trackpad, and dial, to which five gameplay devices are connected (wand, gaming pistol, pinch gauge, squeeze gauge, and accelerometer) and (*B*) an Internet-connected computer with camera/speakers, 3 foot × 3 foot table, and chair (not shown).

used to drag therapy elements (eg, functional games and exercises) to populate each session, adjusting the challenge level and duration for each. This portal allows therapists to review patient performance and usage data, at any time, and from any secure location. TR does not compete with a therapist but instead extends what they can do.

Patient-facing software is used to drive treatment sessions. Our current approach provides 36 TR sessions, 6/wk for 6 weeks, half supervised by an OT or PT who joins by videoconference and half unsupervised and so completed autonomously. Each session is 70-minute long and includes 65 min/d of functional games and exercises plus 5 min/d of stroke education—all of which require UE movements. Each TR session has five elements:

1. *Daily testing* (**Fig. 2**): Sessions start with daily assessments, which generate a digital record of progress and help therapists monitor patients on unsupervised days. Our current daily testing protocol has four components: proximal UE motor, distal UE motor, shoulder pain, and fatigue.
2. *UE exercises*: A total of 114 UE exercises are available, each 1 to 5 minute long and consisting of a video showing repetitions of the assigned movement.

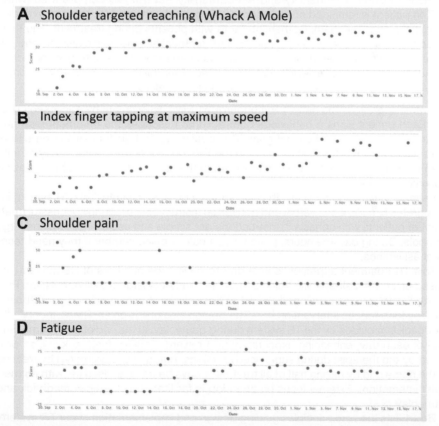

Fig. 2. Daily testing occurs for each patient at the start of each TR session. These data are from a patient with baseline UE motor Fugl–Meyer score of 31/66 who began TR 19 days after stroke onset: (*A*) proximal UE movement (# targets), (*B*) distal UE movement (in Hz), (*C*) shoulder pain, and (*D*) fatigue. (With permission from Edwards et al,[56] https://pubmed.ncbi.nlm.nih.gov/36876946/.)

3. *Functional training through games*: There are 35 functional games, each of which can be 1 to 5 minute long. These stress motor control features by varying demands on movement speed, range of motion, squeeze strength, pinch strength, visuomotor tracking, unilateral versus bilateral movement, memory, cognitive function, and so forth. The details of game play are adjusted by the therapist, for example, during the *Whack-A-Mole game*, higher difficulty level means a larger area where targets can appear and less time to hit the target. Therapists also select from 11 input devices used for game play, for example, the patient can control the vertical position of the flying bird in the *Flappy-Bird game* using the grip force cylinder, pinch force cube, or trackpad.

4. *Stroke education*: Stroke patients often have limited knowledge about their disease and its prevention. This education module targets risk factors, prevention, stroke effects, diet, and exercise. Each day, patients use their paretic UE to answer multiple-choice questions delivered via a Jeopardy game format, an approach known to foster learning,[53] and receive feedback on their answers. This education significantly increases patients' knowledge on stroke-related topics.[54,55]

5. *Videoconferences*: During supervised sessions, the therapist joins the patient using Health Insurance Portability and Accountability Act (HIPAA)-compliant software. The patient is reminded of an upcoming videoconference via 30 minutes of audiovisual alerts. The therapist then interacts with patients during treatment. The therapist can score specific assessments. Our protocol has therapists discuss how UE movements practiced during TR can be extended to functional activity in the home. Adverse events are reviewed and addressed. Therapists write an electronic progress note in the TR Web portal after each videoconference.

Overall approach: The patient first undergoes a live assessment by a licensed OT or PT. Each patient signs a behavioral contract that describes the treatment plan and states a personalized functional goal. The patient has a training session on use of the system, which is then set up either in the IRF room or home. Therapy may be initiated in an IRF[56] before the system is set up in the home for subsequent use, easing transition of care.

Patients initiate and progress through successive assignments. This TR system incorporates simultaneous verbal and nonverbal instructions, enabling successful treatment of patients with aphasia.[54] Instructions are simple and use a large font and large symbols. During daytime hours, patients can call a hotline number if they need technical assistance.

This TR treatment approach is intended to drive large numbers of UE movements based on an UE task-specific training manual[57] and Accelerated Skill Acquisition Program,[19] using games developed as part of prior stroke studies that used game-based therapy for a robotic intervention.[58,59] The design also builds on OPTIMAL theory[60,61]: feedback is provided by the TR system during gameplay, at the end of each game, and end of each day, enhancing expectancy and reward. Positive feedback is also provided by the therapist during supervised sessions. Autonomy is promoted by treating in the home and by having half of all treatment days be unsupervised (ie, with no therapist interaction). External focus on attention is facilitated by therapist feedback and gameplay.

Box 1 lists the core principles guiding design and implementation of our TR system. Physical and technological barriers to system use are minimized, with no need for computer literacy.[55] This approach drives high-intensity practice, exceeding[54,55] the number of UE movements necessary for motor cortex plasticity found in animal studies,[33–35] a value greater than 20× higher than what is provided during standard

---

Box 1
Our core principles for effective telerehabilitation

1. Easy to access and easy to use

2. Promotes high-intensity movement practice

3. Engages numerous brain circuits

4. Gamification

5. OT and PT have a central role, for socialization and for supervision

---

of care OT and PT.[25] The biological model underlying this TR program is that the performance of UE movement during TR activates numerous motor-related networks, including attention, somatosensory, visuomotor, reward, and cognitive circuits, each of which drives motor cortex activity, which converges on signaling in ipsilesional motor cortices and their efferent corticospinal tracts, especially that from primary motor cortex. For example, in the *Clay Shooting game*, the patient uses the UE to track an on-screen flying clay pigeon, activating dorsal and lateral reaching systems.[62] In the *Target game*, squeezing a force transducer keeps an on-screen cursor within increasingly narrow brackets, activating sensorimotor and reward circuits.[63] In the *Slot Machine game*, the patient times button pushes to line up the same image on three successive reels, activating error-detection networks.[64] The use of games motivates patients to engage in enjoyable play behavior that involves therapeutically relevant movements, overcoming the low compliance common with stroke rehabilitation.[38–40] Activities that are challenging, motivating, and engaging[21,22] promote neural plasticity. Finally, a licensed OT or PT plays a central role in administering TR, providing supervision, socialization, and guidance to integrate TR-related gains into activities of daily life.

Pilot study: Our first study evaluated a home-based TR system in patients with hemiparetic stroke occurring an average of 6 months prior.[55] Enrollees received 28 days of TR, 60 minute/d each day. Patients performed therapy on 97.9% of assigned days and rated the system favorably. Arm movements during TR averaged 879/d. Arm motor status significantly improved, with UE Fugl–Meyer (UE-FM) increasing an average of 4.8 points and half of the patients showing clinically important gains. In parallel, other findings included that TR-based stroke education significantly increased patients' knowledge about stroke. Telehealth scoring of depression score was validated. Blood pressure and pulse were recorded by patients using the home TR system and validated against live in-clinic measures. This TR approach did not require computer skills, which were measured using a validated scale and which were found to be unrelated to motor gains or system use. These and other key findings from our TR program are listed in **Box 2**.

Multisite national non-inferiority trial: Subsequently, a randomized, assessor-blinded, non-inferiority 11-site phase II trial[54] was performed, testing the hypothesis that therapy targeting arm movement delivered via home-based TR would produce substantial benefits that are comparable to dose-matched therapy delivered live in-clinic. Patients (*n* = 124) with stroke a mean of 4 months prior and arm motor deficits (mean UE-FM = 43/66) were randomized to receive intensive arm motor therapy, 36 sessions each 70 minutes long: (1) in-home via TR versus (2) in-clinic.

Compliance was 98.3% in the TR group. Change in UE-FM score from baseline to 1-month post-therapy was 8.4 ± 7.0 points in the in-clinic group versus 7.9 ± 6.7 points in the TR group; the covariate-adjusted UE-FM score change was higher in the TR

> **Box 2**
> **Clinical care points: 25 key findings from our telerehabilitation research program**
>
> 1. Engaging in 70-min/d of intensive activity targeting the UE via TR produces greater than 1000 arm movements/d.[54]
>
> 2. The 70-minute TR sessions produce more UE movements (1031)[54] than do 60-minute TR sessions (879).[55]
>
> 3. Treatment-related gains from TR are larger with 6 weeks of therapy[54] compared with 4 week.[55]
>
> 4. Intensive daily therapy for 6 weeks is safe, reduces UE impairment, and improves UE function.[54,66]
>
> 5. Benefits generalize outside the TR system, often improving global function.[66]
>
> 6. Benefits from in-home TR are comparable to dose-matched therapy provided in the clinic.[54]
>
> 7. Treatment gains are related to social network integrity.[69]
>
> 8. Concomitant daily stroke education increases knowledge about stroke.[54,55]
>
> 9. Concomitant stroke prevention is feasible,[55] for example, TR can remotely monitor daily blood pressure.
>
> 10. Can treat UE and LE deficits in parallel.[67]
>
> 11. Screening for depression after stroke via TR is valid.[55,67]
>
> 12. Ability to use this TR system does not depend on computer skills.[55]
>
> 13. Patients on one side of the United States can be treated by a therapist on the other side.[56]
>
> 14. Very high compliance across 6 weeks of daily TR.[54–56]
>
> 15. A TR system module can be used to drive daily ingestion of a pill.[67]
>
> 16. Delivers actionable reports.[67]
>
> 17. The TR system guides patients to independently score patient-reported outcomes.[67]
>
> 18. Treatment-related benefits may be limited by factors such as spasticity and visual field deficits.[68]
>
> 19. Can be initiated during the early weeks poststroke.[56]
>
> 20. More than doubled the rehabilitation therapy dose received as usual care early after stroke.[56]
>
> 21. Eases transitions of care: treatment may start in the hospital and finish at home.[56]
>
> 22. Treatment in the home may continue uninterrupted despite a new COVID-19 infection.[56]
>
> 23. Patients and caregivers report gains in UE function, cognitive abilities, and emotional well-being.[70]
>
> 24. Promotes both external and internal motivation.[70]
>
> 25. Videoconferences were regarded highly, enabling direct feedback and reducing isolation.[70]

group (0.06 points; 95% CI 2.14, 2.26); the non-inferiority margin fell outside this 95% CI, indicating that TR is not inferior to in-clinic therapy. Motor gains remained significant when analyzing only patients recruited less than 90 days poststroke or greater than 90 days. Gains were also significant on the Box and Blocks Test, a functional measure. Shoulder pain was reported in 9.7% of patients, and none had to pause therapy. Stroke knowledge scores increased significantly. Patients' averaged 1031 UE movements/d during TR which is 33-times higher than standard of care.[25]

These TR benefits extended to gains in global function. Among patients starting TR greater than 90 days poststroke, when scores on the modified Rankin Scale (mRS), a measure of global function, are at a plateau,[65] and 39.5% showed mRS improvement by at least 1 level.[66]

Study of expanded TR: Next, a pilot study examined expanded TR in patients and average of 4 months poststroke.[67] Patients received 1 hour of therapy/d, 6 d/wk, for 12 weeks; also, some games/exercises targeted the lower extremity (LE). FM motor scores increased by an average of six points in the UE and one point in the LE. Real household objects, instrumented with a wireless sensor, could be used to drive TR game play, an approach that can increase object affordance and task ecology.

In addition, this study examined the feasibility of having patients take a daily experimental pill; the ability of a TR system to incorporate such a module could enable future pharmacologic trials by ensuring a study medication is ingested in a manner that is linked to training, enabling experience-dependent plasticity. This module performed well in this pilot study, as a placebo pill was taken by patients on 91% of assigned days.

This study generated several other findings regarding expansion of TR. Automatic actionable reports were generated, reliably notifying study personnel when critical values were reached. Telehealth scoring of aphasia assessment was validated in relation to live testing. A key question was whether patients would continue to do TR each day when the TR regimen was extended to 12 weeks; noncompliance doubled during weeks 7 to 12, possibly related to the protocol-directed reduction in therapist interactions during this period. We confirmed that some scales can be scored by patients on unsupervised days without therapist assistance, for example, the Generalized Anxiety Disorder-7 scale. A game using augmented reality was successfully implemented in the home through this system.

Predictors of benefit from this telerehabilitation program: Although the average patient response to TR in the national trial was substantial, significant intersubject variability nonetheless occurred, prompting examination of predictors of response to TR.[68] Female sex, less spasticity, and less visual field defects predicted greater motor gains.

Initiation of telerehabilitation early poststroke, in an inpatient rehabilitation facility: We next sought to assess whether this TR dose could be initiated early after stroke, during IRF admission. A single-arm, two-site pilot study[56] enrolled 19 patients with hemiparetic stroke to receive the same TR dose (36 70-minutes sessions over 6 weeks), started during IRF admission and continued at home. Therapy was not completed in 3/19 due to sepsis, no space in the home for the TR system, and injury outside of study procedures. The 16 patients who completed therapy had average age 61.3 years and mean baseline UE-FM score = 35.9/66. TR was started an average of 28.3 days poststroke. Median compliance was 100%; patient satisfaction was 93%. Patients on one side of the United States were treated by a therapist on the other side. Two patients developed COVID-19 during study participation and nonetheless continued TR. There were no study-related adverse events. Post-intervention UE-FM improvement averaged 18.1 points; Box & Blocks Test (BBT) was 22.4 blocks. The dose of rehabilitation therapy received as usual care during this 6-week interval was 33.9 ± 20.3 hours; adding TR more than doubled this to 73.6 ± 21.8 hours. This study demonstrates (1) safety and feasibility of recruiting patients with hemiparetic stroke from an IRF, (2) ability to provide intensive TR early after stroke, and (3) seamless continuity of TR from IRF to home.

Benefits from TR are related to social factors: As above, the mechanism of the TR involves strengthening activity in, and output of, motor-related neural circuits. These circuits are modulated by psychosocial factors. Patients often experience a contraction of social networks following stroke, which can worsen disability: social isolation is associated with poorer physical outcomes and more depression following stroke, and high social support levels are associated with better functional recovery.

In collaboration with Dr Amar Dhand, we quantified social networks for patients receiving TR to evaluate social factors related to treatment gains.[69] Social network structural metrics were associated with treatment-related gains in motor status and mood: patients with larger and more closely-knit social networks showed greater functional gains and greater decline in depressive symptoms, underscoring the potential importance of social factors for achieving benefit from TR.

A qualitative study: perspectives of patients and their caregivers: We interviewed 13 patients with subacute stroke who completed TR in the national trial,[54] along with their caregivers.[70] Patients mostly reported positive experiences, describing gains in UE function, cognitive abilities, and emotional well-being. One caregiver noted: "It was a great help mentally." They also perceived the system easy to learn and easy to use, with all patients commenting that being able to conduct rehabilitation at home made rehabilitation more accessible. One patient noted: "it was very convenient. You could go over there in your robe or pajamas…"

Functional games were enjoyable and challenging. The importance of technical support was noted. Family members' support helped patients engaged in their TR assignments. Patients emphasized the importance of personalizing the challenge level and visualizing progress.

Benefits generalized outside the TR system, for example, one patient noted that "my arm started getting a little stronger…I could reach more…and I started reaching for the refrigerator with my right hand and door knobs." This might explain the gains in global function (mRS score) seen in nearly half of enrollees receiving 6 weeks of TR, as above.[66]

Among the system components, all patients rated the videoconferences highly, as this enabled direct feedback and encouragement from therapists. Patients felt less isolated and established a personal connection with their therapist.

The TR experience provided both external and internal motivation. Externally, communicating with therapists three times/wk held patients accountable for their assigned exercises and functional games. Internally, witnessing their progress over time helped patients maintain continued use of TR. They specifically noticed progress when (1) playing games faster, easier, and with higher scores; (2) receiving feedback from therapists; and (3) observing improvement in activities of daily living.

THE FUTURE OF TELEREHABILITATION

The current review describes the vast unmet need for intensive rehabilitation therapy and outlines the potential for a TR approach to meet this need and thereby improve functional outcomes. Further studies are needed to understand how benefits from home-based TR generalize. Algorithms can be developed to modify challenge level of TR activities in response to changes in patient performance over time. Our approach focuses on UE motor deficits after stroke, but ultimately a multidisciplinary TR approach is needed, across neurologic conditions. Reimbursement for TR also requires attention, for a wide range of TR services, for all health care providers who treat stroke survivors.

DISCLOSURE

Dr S.C. Cramer serves as a consultant for Abbvie, Constant Therapeutics, BrainQ, Myomo, MicroTransponder, Neurolutions, Panaxium, NeuExcell, Elevian, Helius, Omniscient, Brainsgate, Nervgen, Battelle, and TRCare.

FUNDING

Dr Cramer is supported by grants from NIH (UH3-NS121565, U01-NS120910, R01-HD095457, 2U01-NS086872, R01-HD062744, R01-NS115845), the Department of Veterans Affairs (1 I01 RX003662), and the Patient-Centered Outcomes Research Institute.

REFERENCES

1. Johnston SC, Hauser SL. Neurological disease on the global agenda. Ann Neurol 2008;64(1):A11–2.
2. Lloyd-Jones D, Adams RJ, Brown TM, et al. Heart disease and stroke statistics–2010 update: a report from the American Heart Association. Circulation 2010; 121(7):e46–215.
3. Rinaldo L, Cloft HJ, Rangel Castilla L, et al. Utilization rates of tissue plasminogen activator and mechanical thrombectomy in patients with acute stroke and underlying malignancy. J Neurointerv Surg 2019;11(8):768–71.
4. Hacke W, Donnan G, Fieschi C, et al. Association of outcome with early stroke treatment: pooled analysis of ATLANTIS, ECASS, and NINDS rt-PA stroke trials. Lancet 2004;363(9411):768–74.
5. Goyal M, Menon BK, van Zwam WH, et al. Endovascular thrombectomy after large-vessel ischaemic stroke: a meta-analysis of individual patient data from five randomised trials. Lancet 2016;387(10029):1723–31.
6. Cramer SC. Treatments to Promote Neural Repair after Stroke. J Stroke 2018; 20(1):57–70.
7. Cramer SC. Recovery After Stroke. Continuum 2020;26(2):415–34.
8. Lin DJ, Finklestein SP, Cramer SC. New Directions in Treatments Targeting Stroke Recovery. Stroke 2018;49(12):3107–14.
9. Winstein CJ, Stein J, Arena R, et al. Guidelines for Adult Stroke Rehabilitation and Recovery: A Guideline for Healthcare Professionals From the American Heart Association/American Stroke Association. Stroke 2016;47(6):e98–169.
10. Teasell R, Hussein N. Background concepts in stroke rehabilitation. The Evidence-based review of stroke rehabilitation. Available at: www.ebrsr.com. Accessed May 8, 2023.
11. Kwakkel G, van Peppen R, Wagenaar RC, et al. Effects of augmented exercise therapy time after stroke: a meta-analysis. Stroke 2004;35(11):2529–39.
12. Lohse KR, Lang CE, Boyd LA. Is more better? Using metadata to explore dose-response relationships in stroke rehabilitation. Stroke 2014;45(7):2053–8.
13. Schneider EJ, Lannin NA, Ada L, et al. Increasing the amount of usual rehabilitation improves activity after stroke: a systematic review. J Physiother 2016;62(4): 182–7.
14. Winstein C, Kim B, Kim S, et al. Dosage Matters. Stroke 2019;50(7):1831–7.
15. Brady MC, Kelly H, Godwin J, et al. Speech and language therapy for aphasia following stroke. Cochrane Database Syst Rev 2016;(6):CD000425.

16. Wolf SL, Winstein CJ, Miller JP, et al. Effect of constraint-induced movement therapy on upper extremity function 3 to 9 months after stroke: the EXCITE randomized clinical trial. JAMA 2006;296(17):2095–104.

17. Ward NS, Brander F, Kelly K. Intensive upper limb neurorehabilitation in chronic stroke: outcomes from the Queen Square programme. J Neurol Neurosurg Psychiatry 2019;90(5):498–506.

18. McCabe J, Monkiewicz M, Holcomb J, et al. Comparison of robotics, functional electrical stimulation, and motor learning methods for treatment of persistent upper extremity dysfunction after stroke: a randomized controlled trial. Randomized Controlled Trial. Arch Phys Med Rehabil 2015;96(6):981–90.

19. Winstein CJ, Wolf SL, Dromerick AW, et al. Effect of a Task-Oriented Rehabilitation Program on Upper Extremity Recovery Following Motor Stroke: The ICARE Randomized Clinical Trial. JAMA 2016;315(6):571–81.

20. Lang CE, Strube MJ, Bland MD, et al. Dose response of task-specific upper limb training in people at least 6 months poststroke: A phase II, single-blind, randomized, controlled trial. Ann Neurol 2016;80(3):342–54.

21. Woldag H, Hummelsheim H. Evidence-based physiotherapeutic concepts for improving arm and hand function in stroke patients: a review. J Neurol 2002; 249(5):518–28.

22. Kleim JA, Jones TA. Principles of experience-dependent neural plasticity: implications for rehabilitation after brain damage. J Speech Lang Hear Res 2008; 51(1):S225–39.

23. Cramer SC, Riley JD. Neuroplasticity and brain repair after stroke. Curr Opin Neurol 2008;21(1):76–82.

24. Chen Y, Abel KT, Janecek JT, et al. Home-based technologies for stroke rehabilitation: A systematic review. Int J Med Inform 2019;123:11–22.

25. Lang CE, Macdonald JR, Reisman DS, et al. Observation of amounts of movement practice provided during stroke rehabilitation. Arch Phys Med Rehabil 2009;90(10):1692–8.

26. Bernhardt J, Chan J, Nicola I, et al. Little therapy, little physical activity: rehabilitation within the first 14 days of organized stroke unit care. J Rehabil Med 2007;39(1):43–8.

27. Kumar A, Adhikari D, Karmarkar A, et al. Variation in Hospital-Based Rehabilitation Services Among Patients With Ischemic Stroke in the United States. Phys Ther 2019;99(5):494–506.

28. Newhouse JP, Garber AM. Geographic variation in Medicare services. N Engl J Med 2013;368(16):1465–8.

29. Ayala C, Fang J, Luncheon C, et al. Use of Outpatient Rehabilitation Among Adult Stroke Survivors — 20 States and the District of Columbia, 2013, and Four States, 2015. Morb Mortal Wkly Rep 2018;67:575–8.

30. Pergolotti M, Lavery J, Reeve BB, et al. Therapy Caps and Variation in Cost of Outpatient Occupational Therapy by Provider, Insurance Status, and Geographic Region. Am J Occup Ther 2018;72(2). 7202205050p1-7202205050p9.

31. Freburger JK, Li D, Fraher EP. Community Use of Physical and Occupational Therapy After Stroke and Risk of Hospital Readmission. Arch Phys Med Rehabil 2018;99(1):26–34.

32. Young BM, Holman EA, Cramer SC, et al. Rehabilitation Therapy Doses Are Low After Stroke and Predicted by Clinical Factors. Stroke 2023;54(3):831–9.

33. Jeffers MS, Karthikeyan S, Gomez-Smith M, et al. Does Stroke Rehabilitation Really Matter? Part B: An Algorithm for Prescribing an Effective Intensity of Rehabilitation. Neurorehab Neural Repair 2018;32(1):73–83.

34. Nudo R, Wise B, SiFuentes F, et al. Neural substrates for the effects of rehabilitative training on motor recovery after ischemic infarct. Science 1996;272:1791–4.
35. Plautz E, Milliken G, Nudo R. Effects of repetitive motor training on movement representations in adult squirrel monkeys: role of use versus learning. Neurobiol Learn Mem 2000;74(1):27–55.
36. Brennan D, Tindall L, Theodoros D, et al. A blueprint for telerehabilitation guidelines. Int J Telerehabil 2010;2(2):31–4.
37. Richmond T, Peterson C, Cason J, et al. American Telemedicine Association's Principles for Delivering Telerehabilitation Services. Int J Telerehabil 2017; 9(2):63–8.
38. Duncan PW, Horner RD, Reker DM, et al. Adherence to postacute rehabilitation guidelines is associated with functional recovery in stroke. Stroke 2002;33(1): 167–77.
39. Jurkiewicz MT, Marzolini S, Oh P. Adherence to a home-based exercise program for individuals after stroke. Top Stroke Rehabil 2011;18(3):277–84.
40. Touillet A, Guesdon H, Bosser G, et al. Assessment of compliance with prescribed activity by hemiplegic stroke patients after an exercise programme and physical activity education. Comparative Study. Annals of physical and rehabilitation medicine 2010;53(4):250–7, 257-257.
41. Baranowski T, Buday R, Thompson DI, et al. Playing for real: video games and stories for health-related behavior change. Am J Prev Med 2008;34(1):74–82.
42. Brox E, Fernandez-Luque L, Tøllefsen T. Healthy Gaming – Video Game Design to promote Health. Appl Clin Inf 2011;2:128–42.
43. Hansen MM. Versatile, immersive, creative and dynamic virtual 3-D healthcare learning environments: a review of the literature. Review. J Med Internet Res 2008;10(3):e26.
44. Thompson D, Baranowski T, Buday R, et al. Serious Video Games for Health How Behavioral Science Guided the Development of a Serious Video Game. Simulat Gaming 2010;41(4):587–606.
45. Llorens R, Noe E, Colomer C, et al. Effectiveness, usability, and cost-benefit of a virtual reality-based telerehabilitation program for balance recovery after stroke: a randomized controlled trial. Arch Phys Med Rehabil 2015;96(3):418–425 e2.
46. Sarfo FS, Ulasavets U, Opare-Sem OK, et al. Tele-Rehabilitation after Stroke: An Updated Systematic Review of the Literature. J Stroke Cerebrovasc Dis 2018. https://doi.org/10.1016/j.jstrokecerebrovasdis.2018.05.013.
47. Jansen-Kosterink S, In 't Veld RH, Hermens H, et al. A Telemedicine Service as Partial Replacement of Face-to-Face Physical Rehabilitation: The Relevance of Use. Telemed J e Health 2015;21(10):808–13.
48. Agostini M, Moja L, Banzi R, et al. Telerehabilitation and recovery of motor function: a systematic review and meta-analysis. J Telemed Telecare 2015;21(4): 202–13.
49. Chen J, Jin W, Zhang X, et al. Telerehabilitation approaches for stroke patients: systematic review and meta-analysis of randomized controlled trials. J Stroke Cerebrovasc Dis 2015;24:2660–8.
50. Laver KE, Adey-Wakeling Z, Crotty M, et al. Telerehabilitation services for stroke. Cochrane Database Syst Rev 2020;1:CD010255.
51. Stewart JC, Cramer SC. Patient-reported measures provide unique insights into motor function after stroke. Stroke 2013;44(4):1111–6.
52. Wyller TB, Sveen U, Sodring KM, et al. Subjective well-being one year after stroke. Clin Rehabil 1997;11(2):139–45.

53. Wirth LA, Breiner J. Jeopardy: using a familiar game to teach health. J Sch Health 1997;67(2):71–4.
54. Cramer SC, Dodakian L, Le V, et al. Efficacy of Home-Based Telerehabilitation vs In-Clinic Therapy for Adults After Stroke: A Randomized Clinical Trial. JAMA Neurol 2019;76:1079–87.
55. Dodakian L, McKenzie AL, Le V, et al. A Home-Based Telerehabilitation Program for Patients With Stroke. Neurorehabil Neural Repair 2017;31(10–11):923–33.
56. Edwards D, Kumar S, Brinkman L, et al. Telerehabilitation Initiated Early in Post-Stroke Recovery: A Feasibility Study. Neurorehabil Neural Repair 2023;37(2–3):131–41.
57. Lang C, Birkenmeier R. Upper-extremity task-specific training after stroke or disability. Bethesda, MD: AOTA Press; 2013.
58. Takahashi CD, Der-Yeghiaian L, Le V, et al. Robot-based hand motor therapy after stroke. Brain 2008;131(Pt 2):425–37.
59. Burke Quinlan E, Dodakian L, See J, et al. Neural function, injury, and stroke subtype predict treatment gains after stroke. Ann Neurol 2015;77(1):132–45.
60. Lewthwaite R, Wulf G. Optimizing motivation and attention for motor performance and learning. Curr Opin Psychol 2017;16:38–42.
61. Available at: https://www.physio-pedia.com/The_OPTIMAL_Theory. Accessed May 8, 2023.
62. Battaglia-Mayer A, Caminiti R. Corticocortical Systems Underlying High-Order Motor Control. J Neurosci 2019;39(23):4404–21.
63. Sidarta A, Vahdat S, Bernardi NF, et al. Somatic and Reinforcement-Based Plasticity in the Initial Stages of Human Motor Learning. J Neurosci 2016;36(46):11682–92.
64. Milot MH, Marchal-Crespo L, Beaulieu LD, et al. Neural circuits activated by error amplification and haptic guidance training techniques during performance of a timing-based motor task by healthy individuals. Exp Brain Res 2018;236(11):3085–99.
65. de Havenon A, Tirschwell D, Heitsch L, et al. Variability of the Modified Rankin Scale Score Between Day 90 and 1 Year after Ischemic Stroke. Neurology Clinical Practice 2021;11(3):e239–44.
66. Cramer SC, Le V, Saver JL, et al. Intense Arm Rehabilitation Therapy Improves the Modified Rankin Scale Score: Association Between Gains in Impairment and Function. Neurology 2021;96(14):e1812–22.
67. Cramer SC, Dodakian L, Le V, et al. A Feasibility Study of Expanded Home-Based Telerehabilitation After Stroke. Front Neurol 2020;11:611453.
68. Paik SM, Cramer SC. Predicting motor gains with home-based telerehabilitation after stroke. J Telemed Telecare 2021. https://doi.org/10.1177/1357633X211023353. 1357633X211023353.
69. Podury A, Raefsky SM, Dodakian L, et al. Social Network Structure Is Related to Functional Improvement From Home-Based Telerehabilitation After Stroke. Front Neurol 2021;12:603767.
70. Chen Y, Chen Y, Zheng K, et al. A qualitative study on user acceptance of a home-based stroke telerehabilitation system. Top Stroke Rehabil 2020;27(2):81–92.

Remote Ischemic Conditioning in Stroke Recovery

Chih-Hao Chen, MD, PhD[a,b], Aravind Ganesh, MD, DPhil(Oxon) FRCPC[a,*]

KEYWORDS

- Remote ischemic conditioning • Stroke • Acute ischemic stroke • Rehabilitation

KEY POINTS

- Remote ischemic conditioning (RIC) is a noninvasive, relatively low-cost therapy that could enhance current standard treatment regimens of stroke.
- The protocol of RIC varies in terms of the target limb, repeat cycle and length, initiation timing, and treatment duration.
- Current clinical evidence suggests that applying RIC in acute stroke patients is feasible, with signals of benefit on functional outcome in patients with ischemic stroke.
- Chronic RIC may prevent recurrent stroke in patients with symptomatic intracranial atherosclerosis.
- RIC is generally safe; however, strategies to improve long-term compliance are warranted.

INTRODUCTION

Globally, stroke is the second leading cause of death and third leading cause of disability.[1] Although timely reperfusion could largely improve the functional outcome of acute ischemic stroke (AIS), only selected patients can receive these therapies,[2] and futile reperfusion may still occur.[3] During the process of AIS, brain tissues distal to the occluded vessel are hypoperfused and hypoxemic, which lead to ischemic injury. Even when reperfusion occurs, reactive oxygen species may further damage local tissues resulting in reperfusion injury.[4] Hemorrhagic stroke can also result in severe disability, yet effective therapeutic options are limited.[5] Furthermore, patients who suffer from stroke are at higher risk of recurrent stroke, which leads to worse disability. Therefore, novel approaches are being investigated to mitigate the

[a] Department of Clinical Neurosciences, University of Calgary, HMRB Room 103, 3280 Hospital Drive, NW Calgary, Alberta, Canada T2N 4Z6; [b] Department of Neurology, National Taiwan University Hospital, No.1, Changde Street, Zhongzheng District, Taipei City 100229, Taiwan (R. O.C.)
* Corresponding author.
E-mail address: aganesh@ucalgary.ca

Phys Med Rehabil Clin N Am 35 (2024) 319–338
https://doi.org/10.1016/j.pmr.2023.06.006
1047-9651/24/© 2023 Elsevier Inc. All rights reserved.

ischemic-reperfusion injury, to enhance neuroprotection that allows brain tissues to endure and recover from stroke, while protecting from recurrent stroke, thereby promoting patient recovery.

Remote ischemic conditioning (RIC) refers to a process of intermittent cycles of brief, focal ischemia and reperfusion that confers a systemic protection against further ischemic injuries in remote organs such as brain. Preclinical and clinical studies have provided evidence of benefits when applying RIC in the stroke field.[6] Therefore, RIC represents a noninvasive, relatively low-cost therapeutic strategy that can be additive to current standard treatments of stroke. This narrative review focuses on how RIC may help in stroke prevention and recovery from a clinician's perspective. This review will cover the mechanism and practical considerations of RIC, summarize clinical evidence on the safety and efficacy of RIC with a focus on stroke recovery, and discuss about unsolved questions and future study directions.

THE MECHANISM OF REMOTE ISCHEMIC CONDITIONING

The concept of RIC was first described in an animal study which found that brief (5 minutes), repetitive (4 times) cycles of occlusion and reperfusion of a coronary artery in dogs could provide protection against a subsequent experimental myocardial infarction; 25% reduction of myocardial infarct size was observed compared with controls.[7] Later it was discovered that the ischemic conditioning protocol could offer protection against ischemia in different coronary artery territories,[8] and even remote limbs or organs such as kidney or brain.[9–11] In human studies, RIC was most commonly used by applying a blood pressure cuff to a limb and inflating the pressure above certain level (ie, ~200 mm Hg), thus creating a local ischemic circumstance.

Although RIC accumulated certain evidence of benefit in preclinical and clinical studies, the mechanisms of RIC were not fully clear. It is hypothesized that the brief and repeat cycles of ischemia and reperfusion could "precondition" the target organs by introducing an endogenous protective environment that may increase organ tolerance to ischemic injury (**Fig. 1**).[12] Applying an external physical pressure to occlude blood flow to a limb can initiate remote signaling to the target organs by humoral, neurogenic, and possibly immune pathways.[13] The humoral pathway includes circulating factors such as nitrite, nitric oxide, and adenosine that could mediate vasodilatation.[14] RIC also involves activation of autonomic nervous system and peripheral sensory nerves, which are also required for the release of humoral factors.[15] Furthermore, RIC may affect immune cells and reduce the inflammatory response.[16] Pathways

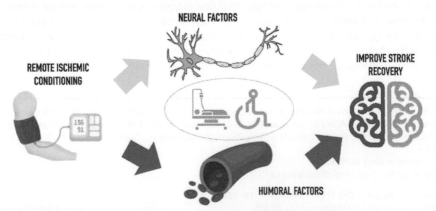

Fig. 1. Putative mechanisms of remote ischemic conditioning in stroke recovery.

triggered by RIC could ultimately improve mitochondria function against oxidative stress, modify autophagy regulation, and increase cerebral blood flow and collateral circulation.[13] The protective effect of RIC appears to occur in 2 phases: an early phase that occurs immediately and only lasts for ~2 hours, and a delayed phase that develops at 12 to 24 hours and persists for several days (the upper limit of which is unclear). Chronic, repeated cycles of RIC may induce distinct physiologic adaptations that promote stroke recovery and prevent recurrence. Although there remains a paucity of direct evidence for the repair effects of RIC in ischemic stroke, preclinical studies have suggested several potential mechanisms by which repeated RIC might promote neural repair for stroke recovery, including neurogenesis, angiogenesis, axon regeneration, synaptogenesis, and remyelination.[17]

Although the effects of RIC mainly focused on ischemic vascular disease, intracerebral hemorrhage (ICH) shares similar pathophysiologic responses such as endothelial dysfunction, impaired cerebral autoregulation, mitochondrial dysfunction, or proinflammatory state.[18] Therefore, the therapeutic benefits of RIC on ischemic stroke may also be applied in hemorrhagic stroke.

Remote Ischemic Conditioning and Exercise

Exercise, like RIC, is beneficial in cardiac and cerebrovascular protection.[13] Brief exercise-induced ischemia has been reported to reduce subsequent angina in patients with coronary artery disease, the so-called warm-up angina phenomenon.[19] Consistent evidences suggest exercise can reduce stroke risk and its severity, and provide secondary prevention of stroke.[20] In fact, there were shared biologic mechanisms of the effects of exercise and RIC, including common humoral mediators, enhanced antioxidant activity, increased endothelial function and nitric oxide signaling, and modulating immune and inflammatory responses.[21,22] Therefore, RIC can be considered as an alternative long-term treatment option to exercise, especially in stroke patients who are unable to perform post-stroke exercise due to physical limitation, fatigue, or other barriers. This can have important potential implications for the use of RIC as an adjunctive or adjuvant therapy as part of stroke rehabilitation and recovery.

HOW TO PERFORM REMOTE ISCHEMIC CONDITIONING? PRACTICAL CONSIDERATIONS

There are 3 variants of RIC, depending on the temporal relationship with stroke: before (RIPreC), during (RIPerC), and after (RIPostC).[6,13] In clinical contexts, RIPreC is usually applied in planned procedures that carry high risk of ischemic events such as cardiac surgery, carotid artery stenting, or endovascular treatment for intracranial aneurysm. RIPerC or early RIPostC are used in many clinical trials as an adjunctive strategy to the standard stroke care. Chronic RIC may include patients with previous stroke (ie, RIPostC) or at high risk of stroke (ie, RIPreC), such as symptomatic intracranial atherosclerosis or cerebral small vessel disease. The objectives for chronic RIC may involve reducing stroke recurrence, enhancement of functional recovery, or even prevention of cognitive decline.

There exists significant heterogeneity regarding the method of delivery of RIC. The protocol of RIC used can be classified according to the following aspects (also see **Table 1**):

1. Target limb: while the upper limb is more commonly used because of its feasibility, lower limb RIC has also been applied.[23] There is no direct evidence comparing the response between upper and lower limb RIC.
2. Unilateral versus bilateral limbs: during RIPerC, some studies may consider applying RIC only on the non-paretic limb.[23–26] However, safety data on bilateral

Table 1
Summary of the published studies of RIC in the stroke field

Study	Year and Country	Patients	Randomized Groups	RIC Protocol	Start Timing	Frequency and Duration	Main Outcome	Side Effects
RIPreC								
Zhao et al.[43]	2017, China	Severe carotid stenosis for carotid stenting	RIC (n = 63), sham (n = 63), control (n = 63)	Both arms, 200 mm Hg, 5 × 5 min	2 wk before stenting	Twice daily for 2 wk	↓ New DWI lesions	9.5% petechiae
RIPerC and acute RIPostC								
Hougarrd et al.[30]	2014, Denmark	AIS + IVT within 4.5 h	RIC (n = 247), control (n = 196)	Arm, 200 mm Hg, 4 × 5 min	Prehospital (before thrombolysis)	Once	No effect on penumbra and final infarct size	Higher recall of pain in RIC
RECAST-1, England et al.[24]	2017, UK	AIS within 24 h, no IVT, mRS 0–2	RIC (n = 13), sham (n = 13)	Non-paretic arm, 20 mm Hg above SBP, 4 × 5 min	Within 24 h of stroke onset	Once	Well tolerated; ↓ 90-d NIHSS	No procedure-related SAE
RECAST-2, England et al.[25]	2019, UK	AIS within 6 h, mRS 0–2	RIC (n = 31), sham (n = 29)	Non-paretic arm, 20 mm Hg above SBP, 4 × 5 min	Within 6 h of stroke onset	Increasing: 1 vs 2 vs 8 doses	Well tolerated; stroke recurrent or extension: ns	No procedure-related SAE
REVISE-1, Zhao et al.[32]	2018, China	AIS + EVT	RIC (n = 20)	Arm, 200 mm Hg, 4 × 5 min	Before recanalization	Before and after EVT, then once daily x 7 d	Well tolerated; 55% mRS 0–2, 5% symptomatic ICH	5% petechiae
RIC-rtPA, Che et al.[27]	2019, China	AIS + IVT, NIHSS 1–15, mRS 0–1	RIC (n = 15), control (n = 15)	Both arms, 200 mm Hg, 5 × 5 min	Within 2 h of IVT	First session, then twice daily x 6 d	Well tolerated; NIHSS, mRS: ns	60% pinpoint erythema
TRIPCAIS, An et al.[33]	2020, China	AIS + IVT, NIHSS <25, mRS 0–2	RIC (n = 34), control (n = 34)	Both arms, 180 mm Hg, 5 × 5 min	Within 3 h of IVT	Twice daily x hospitalization (mean 11 d)	↑ mRS 0–1 (72% vs 50%)	1 skin redness, 1 uncomfortable
SECRET-AIS, He et al.[31]	2020, China	AIS + IVT, NIHSS 5–24, mRS 0–1	RIC (n = 24), sham (n = 25)	Both arms, 200 mm Hg, 5 × 5 min	Within 6–24 h of IVT	Twice daily x 1 d	mRS 0–2: ns; NIHSS: ns	No procedure-related SAE
RESCUE-BRAIN, Pico et al.[23]	2020, France	AIS of carotid territory within 6 h, NIHSS 5–25	RIC (n = 93), sham (n = 95)	Non-paretic thigh, 110 mm Hg above SBP, 4 × 5 min	Within 6 h of onset	Once	MRI infarct growth: ns; NIHSS, mRS, symptomatic ICH: ns	2.1% erythema, visual analog scale 6

Study	Year, Country	Inclusion	Groups (n)	RIC protocol	Timing	Frequency	Outcomes	Safety
RICAMIS, Chen et al.[28]	2022, China	AIS within 48 h, NIHSS 6–16, mRS 0–1, no IVT or EVT	RIC (n = 863), control (n = 913)	Both arms, 200 mm Hg, 5 × 5 min	Within 48 h of onset	Twice daily × 10–14 d	↑ mRS 0–1 (E7% vs 62%); NIHSS, death, recurrent stroke: ns	0.2% petechiae, no pain reported
RICE, Tong et al.[29]	2022, China	AIS within 24 h, NIHSS 6–16, mRS 0–2	RIC + exercise (n = 20), Sham + exercise (n = 20)	Both arms, 200 mm Hg, 5 × 5 min	Within 24 h of onset	Once daily × 14 d	mRS 0–2: ns, NIHSS or Barthe's index: ns	80% petechiae, no procedure-related SAE
RICH-1, Zhao et al.[26]	2022, China	Supratentorial ICH, hematoma 10–30 mL, Glasgow Coma Scale >8	RIC (n = 20), control (n = 20)	Non-paretic arm, 200 mm Hg, 4 × 5 min	Within 24–48 h of onset	Once daily × 7 d	mRS 0–3: ns; ↓ hematoma resolution and relative perihematoma edema	No erythema, no safety issues
Chronic RIC								
Meng et al.[34]	2012, China	Age 18–80, symptomatic ICAS, NIHSS 0–15, mRS 2–4	RIC (n = 38), control (n = 30)	Both arms, 200 mm Hg, 5 × 5 min	Within 30 d of stroke or TIA	Twice daily × 300 d	↓ recurrent stroke or TIA, ↑ mRS 0–1, improve perfusion	No skin lesions
Meng et al.[35]	2015, China	Age > 80, symptomatic ICAS, NIHSS 0–15, mRS 2–4	RIC (n = 30), sham (n = 28)	Both arms, 200 mm Hg, 5 × 5 min	Within 7 d of stroke or TIA	Twice daily × 180 d	↓ recurrent stroke or TIA, ↑ mRS, improve perfusion	16.7% mild discomfort; no skin lesions
RICA, Hou et al.[36]	2022, China	Age 40–80, symptomatic ICAS	RIC (n = 1517), sham (n = 1516)	Both arms, 200 mm Hg, 5 × 5 min	Within 30 d of IS or 15 d of TIA	Once daily × 1 y; voluntarily after	↓ composite outcome; ↓ recurrent stroke in per-protocol only	6.9% petechiae
Mi et al.[37]	2016, China	Cerebral small vessel disease	RIC (n = 9), sham (n = 8)	Both arms, 200 mm Hg, 5 × 5 min	After enrollment	Twice daily × 1 y	↓ change in WMH volume, cognition: ns	Not reported
Wang et al.[38]	2017, China	Cerebral small vessel disease with mild cognitive impairment	RIC (n = 14), sham (n = 16)	Both arms, 200 mm Hg, 5 × 5 min	After enrollment	Twice daily × 1 y	↓ change in WMH volume, ↑ visuospatial and executive function	Not reported

Abbreviations: EVT, endovascular thrombectomy; ICAS, intracranial arterial stenosis; ICH, intracerebral hemorrhage; IVT, intravenous thrombolysis; MCI, mild cognitive impairment; mRS, modified Rankin Scale; NIHSS, National Institutes of Health Stroke Scale; RIC, remote ischemic conditioning; SAE, severe adverse event; TIA, transient ischemic attack; WMH, white matter hyperintensity.

limbs are reassuring.[27–29] Nevertheless, the inconvenience brought by applying RIC on both limbs, especially in a prolonged protocol, should be taken into consideration. It is unclear whether bilateral RIC can produce a larger ischemic stimulus than unilateral RIC, and whether the marginal effect may diminish when applying RIC on the same limb over time.

3. Cycle length and repeats: many clinical studies apply protocols with a cycle of 5 minutes of inflation (occlusion) and 5 minutes of deflation (reperfusion), repeated 4 to 5 times per bout, resulting in a total duration of 35 to 45 minutes.[12] However, different cycle lengths (3–10 minutes) and repeats do exist.

4. Frequency, timing, and duration: RIC protocol is usually carried out once or twice daily. For RIC used during acute stroke setting (ie, RIPerC), some studies have just performed RIC once, either during the transportation to the hospital or within 6 to 24 hours of onset.[23,30,31] Other studies have continued RIC treatment for 7 to 14 days after stroke event.[26,28,32,33] The duration of RIC in chronic stage is usually longer, up to 180 or 300 days.[34–38]

5. Machine and target pressure: most studies have adapted an electronic, automated sphygmomanometer with cuff that can inflate to a target pressure during the ischemic period. The target pressures can be a pre-defined 200 mm Hg, or certain level (20, 30, or even 110 mm Hg) above the measured systolic blood pressure (SBP). One important consideration for randomized clinical trials (RCTs) is the management of the control group. Applying the same device with sham treatment (no inflation, or up to 30 or 60 mm Hg only) on the control group may help achieve blinding, assuming the patients have not previously tried RIC.

IS REMOTE ISCHEMIC CONDITIONING EFFECTIVE IN STROKE RECOVERY?

To date, several clinical trials of RIC in the stroke field have been performed, with more being ongoing. The latest Cochrane Database Systematic Reviews on RIC for preventing and treating ischemic stroke was performed in 2018 and included 7 RCTs.[39] We will incorporate the above review and update studies that were published afterward until 2022, with a total of 16 clinical trials (see **Table 1**). We will begin with trials of RIC in acute setting (RIPerC and acute RIPostC), then discuss about trials of RIC applying RIPreC and chronic RIC.

Acute Ischemic Stroke: Remote Ischemic Per-Conditioning (RIPerC)

The first proof-of-concept study in patients with AIS was done by Hougaard and colleagues[30] in Denmark. They applied a single dose of 4 × 5 min RIC in 443 patients with AIS during their prehospital transportation, in addition to the standard intravenous thrombolysis (IVT) given within 4.5 hours. Although the primary outcomes of penumbra salvage, infarct size and infarct growth, as well as modified Rankin Scale (mRS) were no differences between RIC and control groups, RIC did reduce tissue at risk of infarct by MRI analysis. Following that, England and colleagues conducted the RECAST-1 (Remote Ischemic Conditioning After Stroke Trial) and RECAST-2 trials in the United Kingdom.[24,25] RECAST-1 enrolled 26 patients with AIS within 24 hours without IVT, and randomized them to once dose of RIC (4 × 5 minutes, within 24 hours of onset) or sham RIC.[24] It was a pilot study that demonstrated the tolerability and feasibility of RIC. Nevertheless, the 90-day National Institute of Health Stroke Scale (NIHSS) was lower in the intervention group, whereas vascular events were slightly more common in the control group. RECAST-2 aimed to test an increasing dose of RIC by randomizing 60 patients with AIS within 6 hours of onset to a single dose of RIC (4 × 5 minutes), 2 doses of RIC (baseline and 1 hour later), 8 doses of RIC (twice daily for 4 days), and sham control.[25] The primary outcome of feasibility was acceptable. However, the adherence dropped over time, falling to ~40% on day 3 in both the RIC and sham control groups. Stroke extension and recurrence were nonsignificantly higher in the control group.

The REmote iSchemic Conditioning in acUtE BRAin INfarction Study (RESCUE-BRAIN) was a multicenter study in France, and recruited 188 patients with AIS of carotid artery territory who had received MRI within 6 hours of onset.[23] Patients in the treatment group received 1 dose of RIC (110 mm Hg above SBP, 4 × 5 minutes) on the non-paretic thigh, whereas the control group received sham device without pressure inflation. The primary outcome of MRI infarct growth at 24 hours, and secondary outcomes of NIHSS change, 90-day mRS, reperfusion status, or symptomatic ICH were not different between the 2 groups.

Acute Ischemic Stroke: RIPerC and Acute Remote Ischemic Post-Conditioning (RIPostC)

Several trials have been conducted in China, and most of them using an RIC protocol that continue several days after the stroke event. The RIC-rtPA trial enrolled 30 patients with AIS who received IVT. RIC (200 mm Hg, both arms, 5 × 5 minutes) was given within 2 hours of IVT administration on the first day and twice daily for the following 6 days.[27] The study demonstrated the 97% of protocol completion with good tolerability. However, 60% of patients in the RIC group had erythema in their arms. The TRIP-CAIS (Thrombolysis and RIPC in Acute Ischemic Stroke) trial recruited 68 patients with AIS who received IVT, and RIC (180 mm Hg, both arms, 5 × 5 minutes) was applied within 3 hours of IVT administration and continued twice daily throughout the hospitalization period.[33] The primary outcome of a 90-day mRS score of 0 to 1 was achieved in 72% of the RIC group, compared to 50% in the placebo group ($P = 0.016$). Furthermore, the trial demonstrated significant lower plasma S100β and higher vascular endothelial growth factor in the RIC group, suggesting neuroprotective effects of RIC. The SECRET-AIS (Safety and Effectiveness of Remote Ischemic Conditioning Combined with Intravenous Thrombolysis in Treating Acute Ischemic Stroke) recruited 49 patients with AIS who received IVT, and RIC (200 mm Hg, both arms, 5 × 5 minutes) was administered at 6 and 18 hours after IVT.[31] The control group received sham treatment (60 mm Hg). The primary outcome of mRS at 3 months and NIHSS change were no different between RIC and sham control. In contrast, the REVISE-1 (Remote Ischemic Conditioning Paired With Endovascular Treatment for Acute Ischemic Stroke) is a single-arm study that enrolled 20 patients with AIS who received endovascular thrombectomy (EVT), and RIC (200 mm Hg, one arm, 4 × 5 minutes) was given before recanalization, immediately after recanalization, and then once daily for the subsequent 7 days.[32] The study confirmed the safety of RIC in the EVT patient group, with high rate of protocol completeness, and 5% of symptomatic ICH.

The RICAMIS (Remote Ischemic Conditioning for Acute Moderate Ischemic Stroke) trial was the largest trial of RIC to date in the AIS field.[28] Inclusion criteria were patients who had AIS within 48 hours of onset, NIHSS 6 to 16, were premorbid functional independent, and did not receive IVT or EVT. This multicenter study in China randomized 1893 patients either to RIC (200 mm Hg, both arms, 5 × 5 minutes) twice daily for 10 to 14 days or standard medical treatment. The primary outcome of mRS 0 to 1 at 90 days was significantly higher in the RIC than the control group (67% vs 62%, odds ratio 1.27, 95% CI 1.05–1.54, $P = 0.02$). The treatment effect was consistent across prespecified subgroups. Other secondary outcomes such as early neurologic deterioration, pneumonia, change of NIHSS, recurrent stroke, or death were comparable between the 2 groups. One notable thing is that all patients completed their RIC treatment during hospitalization. This study demonstrated that RIC administered at the acute stage may improve long-term functional recovery. Limitations of the study included a lack of sham control, no assessment of successful outcome blinding, and attrition bias because of the ~7% dropout rate after randomization.

Acute Ischemic Stroke: Remote Ischemic Conditioning and Exercise

As mentioned above, RIC and exercise shared several common biologic mechanisms. Whether there existed synergistic effects between RIC and exercise was unknown. RICE (Remote Ischemic Conditioning With Exercise) trial from China was a pilot study designed to test the effect of RIC followed by exercise in AIS.[29] The study recruited 40 patients with AIS within 24 hours of onset and NIHSS 6 to 16. The intervention group received RIC (200 mm Hg, both arms, 5 × 5 minutes) once daily for 14 days, whereas both groups started exercise on day 4, twice daily, until day 14. The exercise program consisted of out-of-bed training such as sitting, standing, and walking for 30 minutes. For the primary outcome of safety, there was no serious adverse events occurred. Favorable functional outcome (90-day mRS 0–2) was numerically higher in the intervention group (55% vs 40%, $P = 0.34$) but the study was not powered to determine the efficacy of RIC and exercise. More studies are needed to test the combination effects of RIC and exercise, or, alternatively to compare between RIC and exercise and to see if RIC can be "exercise equivalent" in stroke prevention.

Hemorrhagic Stroke: RIPerC

The only published study of RIC in hemorrhagic stroke was the RICH-1 (Remote Ischemic Conditioning for Intracerebral Hemorrhage) trial done in China.[26] This proof-of-concept study enrolled 40 patients with supratentorial ICH, hematoma size 10 to 30 mL, and Glasgow Coma Scale greater than 8. The intervention group received RIC (200 mm Hg, non-paretic arm, 4 × 5 minutes) once daily for 7 days, whereas the control group received standard medical treatment. There was no neurologic deterioration or mortality during the study period in both groups. The proportion of 90-day mRS 0 to 3 were also comparable between the 2 groups (65% vs 60%, $P = 0.74$). Interestingly, the hematoma resolution rate was higher in the RIC group ($P = 0.015$), and the relative perihematomal edema at day 7 was also lower in the RIC group ($P = 0.023$), suggesting a beneficial signal of RIC on the radiological improvement of ICH. However, lack of sham device control should be acknowledged in this trial. There are studies using RIC in aneurysmal subarachnoid hemorrhage patients but they are beyond the scope of this review.[40–42]

Preprocedural Treatment: RIPreC

Procedures such as carotid artery stenting or endovascular treatment for unruptured cerebral aneurysm are known to carry high risk of ischemic event, where preprocedural RIC (RIPreC) may be effective in reducing risk of ischemia by mechanisms mentioned above. One study in China enrolled 189 patients with severe internal carotid artery stenosis (≥70%) who are eligible for carotid artery stenting, and randomized them in a 1:1:1 ratio into 3 groups: RIC, sham RIC, and control.[43] The RIC treatment started 2 weeks before stenting, and consisted of blood target of 200 mm Hg blood pressure target on both arms, 5 × 5 minutes, twice daily in the active RIC group, and 60 mm Hg in the sham RIC group. There was no severe adverse event attributed to the RIC procedure. The primary outcome of new diffusion-weighted lesions after stenting presented in 16% in the active RIC group, 37% in the sham RIC group, and 41% in the control group ($P < 0.01$), and the volume of lesions were also significantly smaller in the active RIC group. The clinical events of recurrent stroke were nonsignificant different between the 3 groups. This study demonstrated the efficacy of RIPreC in reducing possible procedural-related ischemic brain injury in the context of carotid artery stenting.

Intracranial Artery Stenosis: Chronic Remote Ischemic Conditioning

Intracranial arterial stenosis (ICAS) attributed to atherosclerosis is a major cause of stroke especially in the Asian population, and its annual recurrent stroke rate can be up to 15% even under aggressive medical treatment.[44] Since RIC may improve collateral blood flow, stabilize atherosclerotic plaque, and reduce artery-to-artery embolism, several studies tried to apply RIC in symptomatic ICAS population.

The earliest study was done by Meng and colleagues in China, in which they recruited 68 patients with symptomatic ICAS aged 18 to 80 years with stroke or transient ischemic attack (TIA) within 30 days and divided into RIC (200 mm Hg, both arms, 5 × 5 minutes) twice daily for 300 days, and sham controls.[34] The RIC group showed a significant reduction on the primary outcome of recurrent stroke (8% vs 27% at 300 days, $P < 0.01$). Besides, RIC also increased the rate of functional recovery to mRS 0 to 1 at 90 days (65.8% vs 13.3%, $P < 0.01$). Following the success of this study, the same group performed another study with similar design, but only recruited patients older than 80 years (n = 58).[35] The intervention group received RIC (200 mm Hg, both arms, 5 × 5 minutes) twice daily for 180 days only, whereas the control group received sham RIC (30 mm Hg, both arms, 5 × 5 minutes). The efficacy of RIC in the octo- and nonagenarians stroke patients was demonstrated, as the rate of recurrent stroke and TIA (13% vs 36%, $P = 0.004$), NIHSS score (3 vs 5), and mRS score (1.4 vs 2.3) were significantly lower in the RIC group.

The RICA study was a large multicenter trial in China evaluating the effect of chronic RIC in 3033 patients with symptomatic ICAS (50%–99% stenosis).[36] Patients with stroke or TIA attributed to ICAS were randomized within 30 days of stroke or 15 days of TIA to either RIC (200 mm Hg, both arms, 5 × 5 minutes) once daily for 12 months, or sham RIC (60 mm Hg). RIC did not significantly reduce recurrent ischemic stroke (17% vs 19%, hazard ratio 0.87, 95% CI 0.74–1.03, $P = 0.12$), but did reduce the secondary outcome of composite events of ischemic stroke, TIA, or myocardial infarction (21% vs 25%, HR 0.82, 95% CI 0.71–0.95, $P = 0.0089$). Of note, only 46.5% of patients reached good compliance (ie, >50% of scheduled RIC performed). Within this per protocol population, the recurrent ischemic stroke was lower in the RIC group (15% vs 19%, HR 0.76, 95% CI 0.56–0.99 $P = 0.038$). This study suggested that RIC may be beneficial in patients with symptomatic ICAS if the treatment is appropriately carried out, but such a protocol involving both arms for 1 year may not be practical given the low compliance rate shown in the study.

Cerebral Small Vessel Disease: Chronic Remote Ischemic Conditioning

Cerebral small vessel disease (cSVD) is another major cause of stroke, and may cause both lacunar type of ischemic stroke and intracerebral hemorrhage.[45] Beyond acute stroke presentation, cSVD may also manifest with neurodegeneration features such as cognitive impairment, gait disturbance, parkinsonism, or global functional decline.[46] However, there are no effective treatment for cSVD so far, and RIC has also been tested in this field. Of note, changes of neuroimaging marker, rather than incident stroke, requires fewer sample size and is considered a more practical surrogate endpoint in clinical trials of cSVD.[47]

Two RCTs in China investigated the effects of RIC on patients with cSVD. Mi and colleagues[37] recruited 17 patients with cSVD, whereas Wang and colleagues[38] recruited 30 patients with cSVD with mild cognitive impairment. Both trials used the same treatment RIC protocol (200 mm Hg, both arms, 5×5 minutes twice daily in the RIC group; 50 mm Hg in the sham controls) for 1 year. Both trials reached primary endpoint of reduced post-treatment white matter hyperintensities volume on MRI. Number of lacunes and global cognitive function were not different between the RIC and sham control groups. However, the study by Wang and colleagues[38] observed significantly improved visuospatial and executive function in those who received RIC. The results from these pilot studies require further validation in studies with larger sample size, especially with target population of vascular cognitive impairment.

Summary of the Clinical Efficacy of Remote Ischemic Conditioning

The overall evidence from published RCTs suggests that RIC was either neutral or had marginal benefit on stroke, depending on the trials' primary outcomes. RIPreC for 2 weeks before carotid artery stenting can reduce the burden of new ischemic brain lesions.[43] Administering RIPerC once on the first day of ischemic stroke did not significantly reduce infarct burden, and was neutral on the clinical outcome.[23–25,30] However, one large sample size study found that acute RIPostC for 10 to 14 days in patients with moderate severity of ischemic stroke improved their 3 month functional outcome on the mRS.[28] Applying RIC in patients with AIS along with IVT or EVT, or even in patients with ICH seems feasible.[26,27,31,32] Chronic RIC may be more promising in patients with symptomatic ICAS, as 3 trials showed signals of reducing recurrent stroke.[34–36]

When interpreting the results from the above trials, readers should be aware of the risk of bias as assessed by previous reviews.[6,39] One source of bias may arise from potential conflict of interests between some of the investigators and the production of automated RIC device, particularly when there is no sham control. Besides, several studies showing positive effects of study outcomes only had relatively small sample size, which raises the risk of spurious results.[24,34,35,37,38]

IS REMOTE ISCHEMIC CONDITIONING SAFE?

All trials mentioned above did not report severe adverse effect attributed to RIC, either active RIC or sham RIC, suggesting the overall reassurance on the safety aspect. No limb ischemia or injury was reported. Common procedure-related side effects included skin petechiae on the treatment limbs, occurring from less than 1% to 10%.[28,36,43,48] One study reported a high incidence (60% of 20 participants) of pinpoint erythema on the treatment arms, without other discomforts nor increased plasma myoglobin.[27] Most of the local skin responses were self-limited and resolved by time without treatment. Regarding pain in the arms, the RESCUE-BRAIN study that applied one treatment session of 110 mm Hg above SBP on one thigh reported that 53% of intervention group had pain during the procedure, and the median visual analog scale was 6.[23] In contrast, the RICAMIS study, which applied RIC at 200 mm Hg on both arms twice daily for 2 weeks, did not have any pain reported from the 863 participants.[28] This discrepancy may be caused by the effects of various protocols, and may also reflect the diverse threshold of pain and willingness to report symptoms in different populations. Further studies should address this subjective issue by systematic and objective methods. Overall, RIC appears to be safe in stroke populations.

CAN REMOTE ISCHEMIC CONDITIONING BE COMBINED WITH OTHER STROKE RECOVERY STRATEGIES?

As mentioned above, RIC shares similar physiologic mechanisms with exercise. In fact, exercise and RIC can protect the brain tissue from injury through preventing apoptosis, regulating neuroplasticity, and enhancing angiogenesis.[49] Although subacute to chronic exercise rehabilitation could improve motor function and neurologic prognosis after ischemic stroke,[50] a clinical trial of very early mobilization and exercise within 24 hours of stroke onset resulted in a worse functional outcome at 3 months.[51] One possible explanation is that exercise would induce hemodynamic changes of the body due to greater demands of skeletal muscle blood flow, whereas patients in the acute phase of stroke are unable to regulate the cerebral blood flow because of impaired autoregulation; hence, the cerebral blood flow may be compromised by very early mobilization.[49] Furthermore, exercise is difficult to implement in patients with acute stroke because of the superimposed impairments, underlying comorbidities, and hemodynamic instabilities. Meanwhile, applying RIC in acute phase of stroke does not appear to induce significant changes in the body hemodynamics.[32] Stable cerebral perfusion can be an important advantage of RIC over exercise. The results from clinical trials showing the safety and possible benefit of RIC in acute stroke are also reassuring.[23–28,30–32] Therefore, RIC can be viewed as an adjunctive or alternative therapy to exercise in stroke rehabilitation during the acute phase. In the subacute to chronic phase after stroke, if the patient's condition still does not allow active exercise, RIC can still be applied as long as the patient could tolerate the protocol.

It is worth noting the similarity of RIC to blood flow restriction (BFR) training. BFR is a novel exercise modality that involves applying a cuff around a limb to partially occlude blood flow during low-intensity resistance training, and has been shown to increase muscle strength in healthy individuals and some clinical populations such as patients with musculoskeletal disorders.[52–54] Similar to RIC, BFR training may have potential benefits for stroke rehabilitation, as it could improve muscle function, hemodynamics, and even neuroplasticity in the affected limb. This treatment is being studied in an ongoing trial, BFR-Stroke RESILIENCE (The Effects of Blood Flow Restriction With Low-intensity Resistance Training Versus Traditional Resistance Exercise on Lower Limb Strength, Walking Capacity, and Balance in Patients With Ischemic Stroke; ClinicalTrials.gov Identifier: NCT05281679). More research is needed to determine the optimal parameters, safety, and effectiveness of BFR training in stroke patients, and whether this can be applied either in place of, or in conjunction with RIC.

Besides exercise, physical, occupational, and speech therapies are the cornerstone of stroke rehabilitation. The combination of RIC and these therapies also worth further investigation. In healthy participants, RIC has been shown to enhance motor learning task and improve muscle strength.[55,56] Therefore, applying RIC with pre-existing physical, occupational, and speech therapies seems feasible and may have additive effects. Furthermore, noninvasive brain stimulation such as transcranial direct current or magnetic stimulation has been applied in the stroke rehabilitation, although the optimal dose and target location are still yet to be defined.[57,58] Combining RIC together with noninvasive brain stimulation could enhance stroke recovery though different physiologic mechanisms. However, the financial and time cost of these therapies may hinder the wide applications. Finally, telerehabilitation has been increasingly emphasized, especially in remote geographic areas with limited resources.[59] RIC that requires minimal technical expertise can be an ideal home-based therapy to be implemented along with telerehabilitation in such areas.

UNSOLVED QUESTIONS AND FUTURE DIRECTIONS

Although RIC has been widely investigated in the stroke field, many unsolved questions existed. These included the optimal length, frequency, and duration of RIC, the technical considerations to improve the compliance and tolerability, and the most relevant outcomes. Several ongoing trials may help answer some of these questions (**Table 2**).

Table 2
Summary of the ongoing trials of RIC in stroke prevention and recovery

Title	ClinicalTrials.gov Identifier	Conditions	Interventions	Primary Outcomes	Country
Effects of Remote Ischemic Conditioning on Dynamic Cerebral Autoregulation, Blood Pressure and Heart Rate Variability in Patients With Cerebral Small Vessel Disease (ESCAPE-SVD)	NCT05225948	CSVD	RIC vs Sham RIC	Phase difference (cerebral autoregulation), blood pressure, and heart rate variability within 7 d	China
Remote Ischemic Conditioning for Motor Recovery After Acute Ischemic Stroke	NCT05263531	Ischemic Stroke	RIC	Changes in Fugl-Meyer score at 3 mo	China
Clinical Trial on Remote Ischemic Conditioning in Acute Ischemic Stroke Within 9 Hours of Onset in Patients Ineligible to Recanalization Therapies (TRICS-9)	NCT04400981	Ischemic Stroke	RIC vs standard medical therapy	Early neurologic improvement (NIHSS % change) at 72 h	Italy
Remote Ischemic Conditioning With Novel Optical Sensor Feedback Device in Acute Ischemic Stroke	NCT05408130	Acute Ischemic Stroke, CSVD	RIC vs Sham RIC (both groups: novel optical sensor feedback device)	Safety and feasibility (Likert scale for discomfort; any pain or persistent bruises) at 7 d	Canada
Safety and Efficacy of Remote Ischemic Conditioning for Acute Ischemic Stroke	NCT04980651	Acute Ischemic Stroke	RIC vs Sham RIC	mRS 0–2 at 3 mo	China

Title	NCT number	Condition	Intervention	Primary outcome	Country
Safety and Efficacy of Remote Ischemic Conditioning Combined With Intravenous Thrombolysis for Acute Ischemic Stroke	NCT04980625	Acute Ischemic Stroke with IV-thrombolysis	RIC vs Sham RIC	mRS 0–1 at 3 mo	China
Safety and Efficacy Study of Remote Ischemic Conditioning Combined With Endovascular Thrombectomy for Acute Ischemic Stroke Due to Large Vessel Occlusion of Anterior Circulation	NCT04977869	Acute Ischemic Stroke with endovascular thrombectomy	RIC vs Sham RIC	mRS 0–2 at 3 mo	China
Effect of Serial Remote Ischemic Conditioning on Dynamic Cerebral Autoregulation in Patients With Intravenous Thrombolysis (SRICDCA-IVT)	NCT05550103	Acute Ischemic Stroke with IV-thrombolysis	RIC vs Sham RIC	Dynamic cerebral autoregulation parameters in first 7 d	China
Remote Ischemic Conditioning in Patients With Acute Stroke (RESIST)	NCT03481777	Acute stroke (ischemic or ICH)	RIC vs Sham RIC	mRS at 3 mo	Denmark
Remote Ischemic Conditioning and Dynamic Cerebral Autoregulation in Patients With Intracranial and Extracranial Arteriosclerosis	NCT05599009	Intracranial and extracranial atherosclerosis	RIC vs Sham RIC	Dynamic cerebral autoregulation parameters in first 6 h	China
Remote Ischemic Conditioning for the Treatment of Intracerebral Hemorrhage	NCT04657133	Supratentorial ICH (10–30 mL)	RIC vs Sham RIC	mRS 0–2 at 3 mo	China
Trial of Remote Ischemic Pre-conditioning in Vascular Cognitive Impairment (TRIC-VCI)	NCT04109963	CSVD	RIC	Proportion completing 80% or more sessions	Canada

(continued on next page)

Table 2
(continued)

Title	ClinicalTrials.gov Identifier	Conditions	Interventions	Primary Outcomes	Country
REMOTE Ischemic Perconditioning Among Acute Ischemic Stroke Patients (REMOTE-CAT)	NCT03375762	Acute ischemic stroke	RIC vs Sham RIC	mRS <3 at 3 mo	Spain
Ischemic Conditioning During Air tRansport Save penUmbral Tissue (ICARUS)	NCT03481205	Acute ischemic stroke	RIC	Feasibility of RIC	United States
Remote Ischemic Conditioning for Cerebral Amyloid Angiopathy-related Intracerebral Hemorrhage (RIC-CAAH)	NCT04757597	Lobar ICH, possible or probable CAA	RIC	Safety of RIC at 3 mo	China
Safety and Efficacy of Remote Ischemic Conditioning on Cerebral Amyloid Angiopathy (RIC-CAA)	NCT05207475	Probable CAA	RIC	Changes of volume of WMHs at 6 mo and 1 y	China

Last search was done on March 19, 2023.

Abbreviations: CAA, cerebral amyloid angiopathy; CSVD, cerebral small vessel disease; ICH, intracerebral hemorrhage; RIC, remote ischemic conditioning; WMH, white matter hyperintensity.

Optimal Cycle Length, Frequency, and Duration

The most common protocols used in the published trials were 4×5 min or 5×5 min, which were adopted from the cardiology field. Whether the efficacy of RIC differ between the coronary and cerebrovascular diseases remain unknown. Only the RECAST-2 study applied a dose-escalating design; however, the trial itself was not power enough to detect differences between the RIC dose group.[25] More translational studies are required to explore the optimal number of cycles and duration of treatment, whereas clinical trials with larger sample size should also investigate any potential dose responsiveness.

As mentioned in the earlier section, the physiologic adaptative mechanisms brought by RIC may include an early and a late phase.[13] However, the effects of late phase only persisted for ~3 days. Applying RIC only once (like in the RESCUE-BRAIN or RECAST trials[23,24]) or within a brief session is theoretically insufficient to acquire meaningful long-term outcome such as enhancing stroke recovery or preventing recurrent stroke. Although there remains much uncertainty about the optimal dose and duration of therapy, it seems plausible that these variables would be influenced by the specific indication and goal of therapy. For example, a high intensity of RIC (eg, continuous cycling) over several hours may be required for acute neuroprotection in ischemic stroke while awaiting definitive reperfusion with thrombolysis or thrombectomy, whereas repeated sessions over several days may be required for ongoing neuroprotection in patients with incomplete reperfusion (or no reperfusion therapy), who might otherwise continue to have infarct progression. On the other hand, several weeks of treatment may be required to enhance stroke rehabilitation and recovery, while months of chronic RIC may be required when seeking to prevent recurrent stroke. Whether there exists a ceiling effect for chronic repeat RIC is currently unknown. Validated biomarkers on the efficacy of vascular protection of RIC can help in guiding the dose and duration of RIC protocol for these various indications, and in identifying the ideal patients who may benefit from the treatment.

Improving the Compliance and Tolerability

A prolonged course of daily RIC can be inconvenience for the participants, since they have to sit for 45 to 50 minutes per day with their arms confined to the device. Furthermore, protocols that apply RIC on both arms will cause more uneasiness. Besides, a long-term daily RIC treatment can be cumbersome for the participants. In the largest chronic RIC study, the RICA trial, good compliance was only achieved in 46.5% of patients in the first 12 months, and further decreased to 21.0% after 12 months.[36] The RICA trial also showed that the efficacy of RIC was only demonstrated in the first 12 months, but not afterward, so the benefits of RIC may be diluted over time in addition to the low compliance rate. The trial team plans to examine a newer design of a portable device that might make the intervention more practical and improve compliance. If translational studies can identify the best treatment duration, and if biomarkers can monitor the treatment response, periodic RIC, rather than chronic daily RIC, may be more acceptable to patients. That being said, even when considering daily RIC, newer RIC devices may help provide technological solutions for improving compliance, such as remote monitoring of treatment session adherence and provision of reminders.

Choosing the Most Relevant Outcomes

In the published trials, many were proof-of-concept studies, and the primary outcomes were the safety and feasibility. Choosing relevant outcomes is essential for future trial design to optimize the required sample size and study duration. For studies using only short period of RIC in the acute setting, it is reasonable to choose radiological outcomes (such as infarct growth or ischemic penumbra salvageability in AIS, or hematoma expansion in ICH) or acute clinical outcomes (such as change of NIHSS or stroke-in-evolution). Some may also consider noninvasive measurement of the cerebral blood flow such as transcranial Doppler or arterial spin labeling on MRI as surrogate outcomes,[32,34,35] as they can be used to monitor the individual participant's response of RIC.

For studies targeting on stroke recovery, mRS at 90 days is still the most pragmatic outcome assessment. The RICAMIS trial has demonstrated the benefit of RIC on mRS, although studies replicating this finding are still warranted.[28] On the basis of rehabilitation, other outcomes such as Barthel Index, instrumental activity of daily living, Fugl-Meyer Assessment of motor recovery after stroke,[60] or gait assessment can also be considered.

For studies involving secondary or even primary prevention of stroke, recurrent stroke is a straightforward outcome. However, based on trials of antiplatelets or statins, it may either require large sample size or long-term follow-up to demonstrate the efficacy.[61-63] Selecting a target population that are at higher risk of recurrent stroke, instead of all comers of stroke, may result in a more efficient trial design. This may explain the positive findings in trials that included patients with symptomatic ICAS.[34-36] However, studies are needed to expand the indication of RIC to other challenging stroke etiologies such as small-vessel disease.

Because RIC may improve cerebral blood flow and prevent recurrent stroke, this makes RIC a promising candidate in the field of vascular cognitive impairment—a disabling complication of major and cumulative minor/silent strokes.[64] Currently, only 2 studies examined the cognitive outcomes in patients with cSVD treated with chronic RIC.[37,38] However, as stated above, radiologic outcomes are more sensitive markers in the progression of cSVD, and these radiological outcomes usually parallel with cognitive decline.[65] Using advanced neuroimaging assessment such as calculating white matter hyperintensities volume or connectivity on the diffusion tensor imaging can be surrogate markers that require fewer sample size, compared to cognitive outcomes.[65]

Finally, the cost-effectiveness of RIC in stroke deserves more recognition. Although RIC has been considered as a low-cost and noninvasive treatment, it will be important to demonstrate that treatment-associated costs are accompanied by clinically meaningful benefits.

SUMMARY

In conclusion, current data suggest that RIC is a promising intervention in stroke with acceptable safety profile and potential clinical efficacy. It is intuitive, of low cost, easy to implement, and has minimal risk. The optimal treatment protocols in different stroke scenarios such as in the acute, subacute, or chronic phase, are yet to be defined. Additional high-quality studies with sham control and strategies to improve compliance are warranted before RIC can be incorporated into routine practice for improving stroke recovery.

CLINICS CARE POINTS

- RIC can be started during, after, or before stroke onset. Chronic RIC may provide benefit in stroke recovery or even prevention.

- RIC is usually done on one or both arms, applied once to twice a day, with a duration of 35 to 45 minutes per treatment. Single arm, once daily treatment is likely to be better tolerated for long-term treatment.
- RIC is generally safe, with possible side effects of self-limited skin petechiae.
- The long-term compliance of RIC is suboptimal; further studies to improve the compliance are of top priority.

DISCLOSURE

C-H. Chen has nothing to declare.

FUNDING

A. Ganesh discloses research support from the Canadian Institutes of Health Research, Alberta Innovates, Brain Canada, Campus Alberta Neuroscience, and the Heart and Stroke Foundation of Canada relevant to the published work; grant funding from the Canadian Cardiovascular Society, Government of Canada INOVAIT program, and the Alzheimer Society of Canada outside this work; consultation fees from Figure 1, MD Analytics, CTC Communications Corp, MyMedicalPanel, and Atheneum; stock options from SnapDx Inc and LetsGetProof; and a patent application (US 17/317,771) for a system for delivery of remote ischemic conditioning or other cuff-based therapies.

REFERENCES

1. Feigin VL, Stark BA, Johnson CO, et al. Global, regional, and national burden of stroke and its risk factors, 1990-2019: a systematic analysis for the Global Burden of Disease Study 2019. Lancet Neurol 2021;20(10):795–820.
2. Powers WJ, Rabinstein AA, Ackerson T, et al. Guidelines for the Early Management of Patients With Acute Ischemic Stroke: 2019 Update to the 2018 Guidelines for the Early Management of Acute Ischemic Stroke: A Guideline for Healthcare Professionals From the American Heart Association/American Stroke Association. Stroke 2019;50(12):e344–418.
3. Molina CA. Futile recanalization in mechanical embolectomy trials: a call to improve selection of patients for revascularization. Stroke 2010;41(5):842–3.
4. Lin L, Wang X, Yu Z. Ischemia-reperfusion Injury in the Brain: Mechanisms and Potential Therapeutic Strategies. Biochem Pharmacol 2016;5(4):213–29.
5. Sheth KN. Spontaneous Intracerebral Hemorrhage. N Engl J Med 2022;387(17):1589–96.
6. Landman TRJ, Schoon Y, Warle MC, et al. Remote Ischemic Conditioning as an Additional Treatment for Acute Ischemic Stroke. Stroke 2019;50(7):1934–9.
7. Murry CE, Jennings RB, Reimer KA. Preconditioning with ischemia: a delay of lethal cell injury in ischemic myocardium. Circulation 1986;74(5):1124–36.
8. Przyklenk K, Bauer B, Ovize M, et al. Regional ischemic 'preconditioning' protects remote virgin myocardium from subsequent sustained coronary occlusion. Circulation 1993;87(3):893–9.
9. Gho BC, Schoemaker RG, van den Doel MA, et al. Myocardial protection by brief ischemia in noncardiac tissue. Circulation 1996;94(9):2193–200.
10. Candilio L, Malik A, Hausenloy DJ. Protection of organs other than the heart by remote ischemic conditioning. J Cardiovasc Med 2013;14(3):193–205.

11. Jensen HA, Loukogeorgakis S, Yannopoulos F, et al. Remote ischemic preconditioning protects the brain against injury after hypothermic circulatory arrest. Circulation 2011;123(7):714–21.
12. Baig S, Moyle B, Nair KPS, et al. Remote ischaemic conditioning for stroke: unanswered questions and future directions. Stroke Vasc Neurol 2021;6(2):298–309.
13. Hess DC, Blauenfeldt RA, Andersen G, et al. Remote ischaemic conditioning-a new paradigm of self-protection in the brain. Nat Rev Neurol 2015;11(12):698–710.
14. Hess DC, Hoda MN, Khan MB. Humoral Mediators of Remote Ischemic Conditioning: Important Role of eNOS/NO/Nitrite. Acta Neurochir Suppl 2016;121:45–8.
15. Jensen RV, Støttrup NB, Kristiansen SB, et al. Release of a humoral circulating cardioprotective factor by remote ischemic preconditioning is dependent on preserved neural pathways in diabetic patients. Basic Res Cardiol 2012;107(5):285.
16. Konstantinov IE, Arab S, Kharbanda RK, et al. The remote ischemic preconditioning stimulus modifies inflammatory gene expression in humans. Physiol Genomics 2004;19(1):143–50.
17. Yu W, Ren C, Ji X. A review of remote ischemic conditioning as a potential strategy for neural repair poststroke. CNS Neurosci Ther 2023;29(2):516–24.
18. Aronowski J, Zhao X. Molecular pathophysiology of cerebral hemorrhage: secondary brain injury. Stroke 2011;42(6):1781–6.
19. Williams RP, Manou-Stathopoulou V, Redwood SR, et al. 'Warm-up Angina': harnessing the benefits of exercise and myocardial ischaemia. Heart 2014;100(2):106–14.
20. Prior PL, Suskin N. Exercise for stroke prevention. Stroke Vasc Neurol 2018;3(2):59–68.
21. Michelsen MM, Stottrup NB, Schmidt MR, et al. Exercise-induced cardioprotection is mediated by a bloodborne, transferable factor. Basic Res Cardiol 2012;107(3):260.
22. Zhao W, Li S, Ren C, et al. Chronic Remote Ischemic Conditioning May Mimic Regular Exercise:Perspective from Clinical Studies. Aging Dis 2018;9(1):165–71.
23. Pico F, Lapergue B, Ferrigno M, et al. Effect of In-Hospital Remote Ischemic Perconditioning on Brain Infarction Growth and Clinical Outcomes in Patients With Acute Ischemic Stroke: The RESCUE BRAIN Randomized Clinical Trial. JAMA Neurol 2020;77(6):725–34.
24. England TJ, Hedstrom A, O'Sullivan S, et al. RECAST (Remote Ischemic Conditioning After Stroke Trial): A Pilot Randomized Placebo Controlled Phase II Trial in Acute Ischemic Stroke. Stroke 2017;48(5):1412–5.
25. England TJ, Hedstrom A, O'Sullivan SE, et al. Remote Ischemic Conditioning After Stroke Trial 2: A Phase IIb Randomized Controlled Trial in Hyperacute Stroke. J Am Heart Assoc 2019;8(23):e013572.
26. Zhao W, Jiang F, Li S, et al. Safety and efficacy of remote ischemic conditioning for the treatment of intracerebral hemorrhage: A proof-of-concept randomized controlled trial. Int J Stroke 2022;17(4):425–33.
27. Che R, Zhao W, Ma Q, et al. rt-PA with remote ischemic postconditioning for acute ischemic stroke. Ann Clin Transl Neurol 2019;6(2):364–72.
28. Chen HS, Cui Y, Li XQ, et al. Effect of Remote Ischemic Conditioning vs Usual Care on Neurologic Function in Patients With Acute Moderate Ischemic Stroke: The RICAMIS Randomized Clinical Trial. JAMA 2022;328(7):627–36.
29. Tong Y, Lee H, Kohls W, et al. Remote ischemic conditioning (RIC) with exercise (RICE) is safe and feasible for acute ischemic stroke (AIS) patients. Front Neurol 2022;13:981498.

30. Hougaard KD, Hjort N, Zeidler D, et al. Remote ischemic perconditioning as an adjunct therapy to thrombolysis in patients with acute ischemic stroke: a randomized trial. Stroke 2014;45(1):159–67.
31. He YD, Guo ZN, Qin C, et al. Remote ischemic conditioning combined with intravenous thrombolysis for acute ischemic stroke. Ann Clin Transl Neurol 2020;7(6): 972–9.
32. Zhao W, Che R, Li S, et al. Remote ischemic conditioning for acute stroke patients treated with thrombectomy. Ann Clin Transl Neurol 2018;5(7):850–6.
33. An JQ, Cheng YW, Guo YC, et al. Safety and efficacy of remote ischemic postconditioning after thrombolysis in patients with stroke. Neurology 2020;95(24): e3355–63.
34. Meng R, Asmaro K, Meng L, et al. Upper limb ischemic preconditioning prevents recurrent stroke in intracranial arterial stenosis. Neurology 2012;79(18):1853–61.
35. Meng R, Ding Y, Asmaro K, et al. Ischemic Conditioning Is Safe and Effective for Octo- and Nonagenarians in Stroke Prevention and Treatment. Neurotherapeutics 2015;12(3):667–77.
36. Hou C, Lan J, Lin Y, et al. Chronic remote ischaemic conditioning in patients with symptomatic intracranial atherosclerotic stenosis (the RICA trial): a multicentre, randomised, double-blind sham-controlled trial in China. Lancet Neurol 2022; 21(12):1089–98.
37. Mi T, Yu F, Ji X, et al. The Interventional Effect of Remote Ischemic Preconditioning on Cerebral Small Vessel Disease: A Pilot Randomized Clinical Trial. Eur Neurol 2016;76(1–2):28–34.
38. Wang Y, Meng R, Song H, et al. Remote Ischemic Conditioning May Improve Outcomes of Patients With Cerebral Small-Vessel Disease. Stroke 2017;48(11): 3064–72.
39. Zhao W, Zhang J, Sadowsky MG, et al. Remote ischaemic conditioning for preventing and treating ischaemic stroke. Cochrane Database Syst Rev 2018;7(7): CD012503.
40. Gonzalez NR, Connolly M, Dusick JR, et al. Phase I clinical trial for the feasibility and safety of remote ischemic conditioning for aneurysmal subarachnoid hemorrhage. Neurosurgery 2014;75(5):590–8 [discussion: 598].
41. Koch S, Katsnelson M, Dong C, et al. Remote ischemic limb preconditioning after subarachnoid hemorrhage: a phase Ib study of safety and feasibility. Stroke 2011;42(5):1387–91.
42. Laiwalla AN, Ooi YC, Liou R, et al. Matched Cohort Analysis of the Effects of Limb Remote Ischemic Conditioning in Patients with Aneurysmal Subarachnoid Hemorrhage. Transl Stroke Res 2016;7(1):42–8.
43. Zhao W, Meng R, Ma C, et al. Safety and Efficacy of Remote Ischemic Preconditioning in Patients With Severe Carotid Artery Stenosis Before Carotid Artery Stenting: A Proof-of-Concept, Randomized Controlled Trial. Circulation 2017; 135(14):1325–35.
44. Gutierrez J, Turan TN, Hoh BL, et al. Intracranial atherosclerotic stenosis: risk factors, diagnosis, and treatment. Lancet Neurol 2022;21(4):355–68.
45. Pasi M, Cordonnier C. Clinical Relevance of Cerebral Small Vessel Diseases. Stroke 2020;51(1):47–53.
46. Gurol ME, Sacco RL, McCullough LD. Multiple Faces of Cerebral Small Vessel Diseases. Stroke 2020;51(1):9–11.
47. Benjamin P, Zeestraten E, Lambert C, et al. Progression of MRI markers in cerebral small vessel disease: Sample size considerations for clinical trials. J Cereb Blood Flow Metab 2016;36(1):228–40.

48. Zhao W, Li S, Ren C, et al. Remote ischemic conditioning for stroke: clinical data, challenges, and future directions. Ann Clin Transl Neurol 2019;6(1):186–96.
49. Lee H, Yun HJ, Ding Y. Timing is everything: Exercise therapy and remote ischemic conditioning for acute ischemic stroke patients. Brain Circ 2021;7(3): 178–86.
50. Pin-Barre C, Laurin J. Physical Exercise as a Diagnostic, Rehabilitation, and Preventive Tool: Influence on Neuroplasticity and Motor Recovery after Stroke. Neural Plast 2015;2015:608581.
51. group ATC. Efficacy and safety of very early mobilisation within 24 h of stroke onset (AVERT): a randomised controlled trial. Lancet 2015;386(9988):46–55.
52. Neto GR, Novaes JS, Dias I, et al. Effects of resistance training with blood flow restriction on haemodynamics: a systematic review. Clin Physiol Funct Imaging 2017;37(6):567–74.
53. Poton R, Polito MD. Hemodynamic responses during lower-limb resistance exercise with blood flow restriction in healthy subjects. J Sports Med Phys Fitness 2015;55(12):1571–7.
54. Vinolo-Gil MJ, Rodríguez-Huguet M, Martin-Vega FJ, et al. Effectiveness of Blood Flow Restriction in Neurological Disorders: A Systematic Review. Healthcare (Basel) 2022;10(12).
55. Cherry-Allen KM, Gidday JM, Lee JM, et al. Remote limb ischemic conditioning enhances motor learning in healthy humans. J Neurophysiol 2015;113(10): 3708–19.
56. Surkar SM, Bland MD, Mattlage AE, et al. Effects of remote limb ischemic conditioning on muscle strength in healthy young adults: A randomized controlled trial. PLoS One 2020;15(2):e0227263.
57. Smith MC, Stinear CM. Transcranial magnetic stimulation (TMS) in stroke: Ready for clinical practice? J Clin Neurosci 2016;31:10–4.
58. Schlaug G, Renga V, Nair D. Transcranial direct current stimulation in stroke recovery. Arch Neurol 2008;65(12):1571–6.
59. Salbach NM, Mountain A, Lindsay MP, et al. Canadian Stroke Best Practice Recommendations: Virtual Stroke Rehabilitation Interim Consensus Statement 2022. Am J Phys Med Rehabil 2022;101(11):1076–82.
60. Gladstone DJ, Danells CJ, Black SE. The fugl-meyer assessment of motor recovery after stroke: a critical review of its measurement properties. Neurorehabil Neural Repair 2002;16(3):232–40.
61. Chen ZM, Hui JM, Liu LS, et al. CAST: Randomised placebo-controlled trial of early aspirin use in 20,000 patients with acute ischaemic stroke. Lancet 1997; 349(9066):1641–9.
62. Wang Y, Wang Y, Zhao X, et al. Clopidogrel with aspirin in acute minor stroke or transient ischemic attack. N Engl J Med 2013;369(1):11–9.
63. Amarenco P, Kim JS, Labreuche J, et al. A Comparison of Two LDL Cholesterol Targets after Ischemic Stroke. N Engl J Med 2020;382(1):9.
64. Ganesh A, Barber P, Black SE, et al. Trial of remote ischaemic preconditioning in vascular cognitive impairment (TRIC-VCI): protocol. BMJ Open 2020;10(10): e040466.
65. Markus HS, van Der Flier WM, Smith EE, et al. Framework for Clinical Trials in Cerebral Small Vessel Disease (FINESSE): A Review. JAMA Neurol 2022;79(11): 1187–98.

Post Stroke Exercise Training
Intensity, Dosage, and Timing of Therapy

Robert Teasell, MD, FRCPC[a,b,c],*, Jamie L. Fleet, MD, FRCPC[a,b,c],
Amber Harnett, RN, MSc[d]

KEYWORDS

- Stroke • Rehabilitation • Exercise • Intensity • Dose • Timing • Therapy • Recovery

KEY POINTS

- Greater intensity/dosage of therapy results in improved motor outcome.
- There are practical challenges to deliver therapy at optimal intensities, including adequate resources, limited rehabilitation stays, feasibility especially with elderly patients, and uncertainty over ideal dosing.
- There are new opportunities arising through innovative approaches, including new technologies, group-based therapies, and telerehabilitation.
- As time post stroke increases, the dose of therapy required to improve motor outcomes increases.
- Intensive therapy very early on, particularly within the first 24 hours, is best avoided.

INTRODUCTION

Stroke is a leading cause of disability among the adult population.[1] Hemiparesis is an iconic feature of stroke that manifests itself in difficulties with gait, coordination, balance, and increased tone. Exercise in task-specific activities under the supervision of physiotherapists and occupational therapists is critical to maximizing motor recovery and improving functional outcomes.

Stroke rehabilitation, more than any other area of neurorehabilitation, has well-developed clinical practice guidelines aimed at standardizing best practices for patient care.[2] This initially focused on a specialized interdisciplinary rehabilitation approach (stroke rehabilitation units) and evolved to include important elements of care on those units, particularly therapy intensity, timing of rehabilitation, and a greater

[a] Parkwood Institute Research, Parkwood Institute, D4-101A, 550 Wellington Road, London, Canada; [b] St. Joseph's Health Care London, London, Canada; [c] Physical Medicine and Rehabilitation, Schulich School of Medicine and Dentistry, University of Western Ontario, London, Canada; [d] Parkwood Institute Research, Parkwood Institute, B3-123, 550 Wellington Road, London, Ontario N6C 0A7, Canada
* Corresponding author. Parkwood Institute Research, Parkwood Institute, D4-101A, 550 Wellington Road, London, Canada.
E-mail address: Robert.Teasell@sjhc.london.on.ca

Phys Med Rehabil Clin N Am 35 (2024) 339–351
https://doi.org/10.1016/j.pmr.2023.06.025
1047-9651/24/© 2023 Elsevier Inc. All rights reserved.

focus on task-specific therapy. Intensity, dosing, and timing of rehabilitation are arguably becoming one of the biggest contributors to improved rehabilitation outcomes for individuals post stroke.

INTENSITY OF THERAPY POST STROKE
Definition

The definition of *intensity* varies across studies as it relates to rehabilitation. For example, "time spent in therapy" is commonly used to describe the amount of therapy received in observational studies.[3–5] It is also defined as "augmented therapy time," which describes the extra time an experimental group spends in therapy compared with conventional care.[6,7] Other definitions include the number of repetitions, or measures of how hard a person is working. The latter can be described in a variety of ways, including heart rate or perceived level of exertion. Therefore, the definition of intensity terms is often context dependent and may not reflect the same process.

VARIABILITY IN TREATMENT PROTOCOLS

Determining the effects of intensity of therapy on functional outcomes is challenging due to variability in treatment protocols. This is complicated by differences in the type of treatments provided, timing and duration of their delivery, and the outcomes assessed. Additionally, documentation of time spent in therapy and patient engagement in rehabilitation activities differs considerably across studies, units, institutions, and countries, making it difficult to compare studies or generalize results. Variations in outcomes have also been attributed to time spent in bed, sitting out of bed, or in standing/walking activities.[8]

IMPORTANCE OF INTENSITY OF THERAPY POST STROKE

Increased therapy intensity, however defined, has been shown to improve the recovery of motor deficits following stroke.[6,7] A meta-analysis of 34 randomized controlled trial (RCTs) found that increasing time spent in therapy (57 hours in the treatment groups vs 24 hours in the control groups) strongly predicted overall functional improvement.[9] Kalra was one of the first to show that more intensive therapy, delivered on a stroke rehabilitation unit, significantly improved outcomes (Barthel Index) and reduced hospital length of stay.[10] In this study, the same amount of therapy delivered over a shorter period of time on inpatient rehabilitation resulted in significantly different outcomes (improved Barthel Index and shorter lengths of stay).[10] Given the limitations of health care systems on hospital length of stay, therapy intensity may simply reflect how much therapy is received while in hospital. In a meta-analysis, Kwakkel and colleagues[6] found that increased intensity of physical therapy, at least 16 hours of additional therapy in the first 6 months, was associated with significant improvements in activities of daily living and walking speed.

THERAPEUTIC OPTIONS
Repetitive Task-Specific Training

Repetitive task-specific training involves performing repetitions of active motor sequences within a single training session, with the goal of improving specific functions.[11] It combines elements of intensity and task specificity, and is used for both upper and lower extremity training.[11] In a systematic review, repetitive task training of sit-to-stand exercises was found to be beneficial for mobility when compared with conventional therapy.[11] Repetitive task-specific training of the upper extremity was found to be similarly beneficial in a systematic review.[12] With respect to upper limb function, increasing repetitions during rehabilitation are effective in improving functional recovery.[13–15]

High Intensity Exercise

Stroke survivors with hemiparesis require twice the energy for ambulation[16] and have half the cardiorespiratory capacity[17] compared with healthy individuals. This contributes to inactivity and deconditioning.[18,19] In turn, deconditioning limits the ability of stroke survivors to take advantage of rehabilitation therapies and achieve their full motor recovery.[20]

High intensity interval training (HIIT) involves intermittent bursts of effort separated by periods of recovery.[19,21] HIIT has been shown to be more effective in improving aerobic capacity[22–24] more quickly and efficiently through greater neuromuscular recruitment.[21] Wiener and colleagues[19] conducted a systematic review and found that HIIT using a treadmill or stationary bike resulted in significant improvements in walking speed and endurance as well as balance. Adverse effects were minor and not common. HIIT sessions were short lasting 20 to 30 minutes, 2 to 5 times a week, for 2 to 8 weeks and still resulted in improved functional outcomes.[19]

Other trials evaluating HIIT on treadmills for motor recovery post stroke revealed significant lower limb improvements in walking speed and motor evoked potentials.[25,26] Body weight supported treadmill training at faster walking speeds resulted in greater paretic limb support and peak muscle activation relative to exercise at lower walking speeds.[27] Additionally, high-intensity resistance training using training machines was shown to be more effective at improving paretic leg strength compared with lower intensity rehabilitation.[28] In this case multiple series of 8 repetitions at maximal loading was performed 3 times a week for 12 weeks with the loading progressively increased every 2 weeks. Forced exercise was also more effective improving functional movement compared with voluntary exercise.[29]

PRACTICAL CHALLENGES WITH THERAPY INTENSITY

Providing intensive rehabilitation has many practical challenges that often center around resources, or lack thereof. In many countries, there are limits to hospital length of stay; therefore, therapy intensity may simply reflect how long a person is in hospital. Another dilemma is the feasibility of high-repetition, task-specific training. Research suggests that hundreds of repetitions in task-specific practice may be required to optimize function post stroke.[13] Currently, the number of repetitions provided during post-stroke rehabilitation is a small fraction of what is optimal.[30] As an example, Lang and colleagues[30] in an observational trial found only half of upper extremity rehabilitation sessions practiced task-specific, functional upper extremity movements and in those, the average number of repetitions per session was 32. Lastly, there is a significant amount of downtime for patients undergoing rehabilitation. De Wit and colleagues[4] observed that patients spent 72% of their time in nontherapeutic activities on average. Further, an Australian study by Simpson and colleagues[31] found that patients spent more time upright and walking during the first week at home compared with their last week of rehabilitation. This suggests that stroke patients may be discouraged from achieving their full activity potential while on an organized stroke rehabilitation unit. Reasons for this may be safety concerns, lack of opportunity to be up and about, etc.

Another challenge is that the benefit of increasing therapy intensity is inconsistent across studies. In the VECTORS trial of upper extremity recovery, they found that increasing therapy intensity did not result in better outcomes.[32] Fang and colleagues[33] suggested that a physiotherapy program of greater intensity may simply enable patients to achieve independence in activities of daily living faster through compensation of the nonparetic limb rather than actual neurologic recovery. Intensity of treatment also depends on the willingness of the patient to participate in therapy, and it can hinder progress when it becomes too intense.[34] This is especially true for patients who are frail, elderly, or have significant comorbidities.

All together, these issues limit the generalizability of findings, making it difficult to draw conclusions on the overall effectiveness of higher intensity programs. Although it is recognized that greater therapy intensity improves rehabilitation outcomes, there is some uncertainty as to what the ideal dose should be. Gimigliano commenting[35] on a Cochrane review by Clark and colleagues[36] concluded, *"It seems that functioning may improve when the increase in time spent in rehabilitation exceeds a threshold; however, there is currently insufficient evidence to recommend a minimum beneficial daily dose of rehabilitation."*[35]

Guidelines

The ideal amount of therapy has never been well defined and guidelines from different countries differ regarding therapy time recommendations (**Table 1**).[3] The Canadian Best Practice Guidelines[2] recommend 3 hours of direct task-specific therapy 5 days per week, though previous work has shown few patients receive this amount.[37] This recommendation in Canada was based largely on experiences in the United States. There, this *"3 hour rule"* was legislated and shown to be feasible for many stroke patients with significantly improved outcomes[38,39] when compared with less than 3 hours a day, and when compared with Canadian results.[40] In the Ontario Stroke Rehab Audit the median amount of inpatient therapy in 2019/2020 of direct physiotherapy/occupational therapy (PT/OT) and speech language pathology (SLP) was 69 minutes per day or 60% below target.[37] This situation is not unique to Ontario and Canada, with various countries around the world reporting similar issues.[41]

Table 1
Different guidelines for inpatient rehabilitation[3]

Guideline	Recommendation
AHA/ASA 2005	"…as much therapy as needed to adapt, recover and/or establish … optimal level of functional independence."
European Stroke Organization	"Increase the duration and intensity of rehabilitation"
Intercollegiate Stroke Working Party 2008	A minimum of 45 min daily of each therapy required in the early stages of stroke
SIGN 118	Increased intensity of therapy to improve gait should be pursued Increased intensity of therapy for improving upper limb function is not recommended
National Stroke Foundation, Australia 2010	Minimum of 1 h of occupational and physiotherapy 5 d per week
Canadian Best Practice Recommendations 2010	Minimum of 1 h per day, 5 d a week of each of the relevant core therapies (PT, OT, SLP)

From Foley et al. 2012.

Increasing Intensity of Therapy Through Innovative Practices

Because of the apparent benefit, there is a desire to increase therapy time within the fiscal restraints facing most health care systems. Donnellan-Fernandez et al[42] recommended several ways to increase the intensity of therapy including constraint-induced movement therapy, robotics, circuit therapy, gaming technologies, HIIT, goal-oriented instructions, and cardiovascular exercises. Some more innovative approaches include group-based therapy, including dance therapy or playing card games,[43] and greater use of weekend therapy, though evidence these are more effective remains uncertain.[44] Newer technologies, including nonimmersive virtual reality and technology assisted devices that deliver repetitive therapy, have been shown to improve outcomes.[45,46] Telerehabilitation, with use increasing throughout the COVID-19 pandemic, may be one means to deliver increased therapy more efficiently.[47]

CLINICAL PEARLS FOR INTENSITY

- Intensity of therapy is defined in different ways, making comparisons between studies challenging.
- Increased therapy intensity has been shown to improve motor recovery when compared with less intensive therapy. This benefit is greatest when it involves repetitive task-specific training.
- HIIT offers one method of increasing intensity without increasing additional therapist time.
- There are practical challenges to implementing more intensive therapy programs which include insufficient therapy staff or inefficient practices, inability or unwillingness of patient to participate, getting in enough repetitions to further enhance recovery, insurance-related limitations on therapy frequency allowed and the demotivating nature of institutional/hospital stays.
- There are a number of innovative approaches to improving therapy intensity including greater use of technologies, telerehabilitation, additional weekend and/or group therapies, and more intensive therapy approaches such as HIIT or circuit therapy.

TIMING OF THERAPY

Timing of therapy refers to time post stroke onset. Timing of therapy impacts patient outcomes and is often studied in relation to intensity. Although many studies have examined this topic, there is no clear consensus as to the optimal time to initiate rehabilitation after stroke.

PRE-CLINICAL STUDIES

Animal studies have shown the brain demonstrates maximal response to therapies when initiated early after a stroke, and if not, delays may worsen clinical outcomes.[48–51] The precise timing of what constitutes early to achieve the window of heightened neuroplasticity has not been fully determined,[42] but delays of more than a few days appear to be detrimental.

CLINICAL ASSOCIATION BETWEEN EARLY ADMISSION TO REHABILITATION UNITS AND IMPROVED FUNCTIONAL OUTCOMES

Clinically, comparative studies have shown a strong association between early admission to rehabilitation and improved functional outcomes, as well as decreased length of stay.[52–60] For example, the Post-Stroke Rehabilitation Outcome Project (PSROP) was a prospective multisite observational study of 1291 patients from 6 inpatient facilities in the United States. They found that a longer period between stroke onset to admission to stroke rehabilitation was associated with an increased length of stay and lower Functional Independence Measure (FIM) scores at discharge,[61] particularly for individuals with moderate and severe strokes. It is possible, however, that some patients were admitted later due to a greater number of comorbidities, less medical stability, and more severe strokes, which confounds the findings. That said, other observational studies that have accounted for severity and comorbidities have found there is an association between earlier admission to rehabilitation and better recovery.[57] Delaying neurorehabilitation by a single day is associated with significant decreases in functional independence (0.3 FIM points/d) and significantly increased rates of institutionalization following discharge.[62]

MORE INTENSIVE THERAPY IN THE ACUTE PHASE

Given the importance of early transfer to rehabilitation post stroke, there has been increasing interest in the concept of very early mobilization (VEM). VEM is defined as an intervention designed to reduce the time from stroke onset to first mobilization and increasing the amount of out-of-bed physical activity shortly after stroke.[8,63] VEM occurs within 24 to 48 hours following stroke onset, generally while in acute care.

Early mobilization was studied in the Very Early Rehabilitation or Intensive Telemetry After Stroke (VERITAS) trial, an observer blinded RCT, where early mobilization was compared with standard care.[64] Mobilization activity, defined as the mean time spent upright per working day, was 61 minutes in the early mobilization group compared with 42 minutes in the standard care group. By day 5, 74% of patients in the early mobilization group were independently walking, compared with 44% of patients undergoing standard care. Patients in the very early mobilization group also experienced fewer medical complications and there was a trend toward less disability (defined as modified Rankin Scale [mRS] score of 0–2) at 3 months.

Other studies found similar results. Liu and colleagues[65] found that earlier rehabilitation (within 48 hours) was associated with greater independence at 6 months compared with later rehabilitation (after 7 days). Bai and colleagues[52,53] conducted 2 RCTs, one published in 2012 with 364 subjects and another in 2014 with 165 subjects, which evaluated a rehabilitation program provided within 24 hours of stroke onset and compared it to standard care. The very early rehabilitation programs were associated with greater improvements in impairment (Fugl-Meyer scores), independence (modified Barthel Index),[52] and spasticity (modified Ashworth Score).[53] Chippala and Sharma[66] performed an RCT of 86 subjects and showed patients who received mobilization within 24 hours had greater levels of independence based on the Barthel Index at discharge and at 3 months compared with patients receiving standard care. Morreale and colleagues[67] enrolled 340 stroke subjects into early (<24 hours post stroke) and late (>4 days) therapy involving Proprioceptive Neuromuscular Facilitation and Cognitive Therapeutic Exercise. They found with early intervention there were significant improvements in activities of daily living (Barthel Index), ambulation, and strength (Motricity Index), but not in general disability (mRS).

One of the largest studies assessing very early rehabilitation post stroke was the A Very Early Rehabilitation Trial (AVERT). This was a large, 8-year, multicenter, 3-phase trial of 2104 patients.[68] In contrast to the studies described above, AVERT found that patients receiving standard care were less likely to die or have expansion of stroke volume compared with those receiving VEM.[68] This discrepancy may be attributable to the use of different tools to assess clinical outcomes: AVERT used the mRS, whereas the other trials measured improvements using the Barthel Index. Luft and colleagues[69] argued these findings should not prolong inactivity of stroke patients early after the stroke. Paradoxically, subsequent analysis of AVERT results found that shorter and more frequent early mobilization improved chances of regaining independence, whereas higher doses of early long-term mobilization worsened outcomes.[70] This may be due to compromised reperfusion of the at-risk penumbral area with higher intensity exercise. These results suggest that intensity may be an important mediator of recovery during rehabilitation when applied very early after stroke.

Rethnam and colleagues[71] in a review of 6 studies found significantly more favorable outcomes for patients in the early mobilization compared with the usual care control group (Modified Rankin), with no difference in mortality or activities of daily living (Barthel Index). Langhorne and colleagues[11] conducted a Cochrane review and found that early mobilization was comparable to usual care, with no significant differences in mortality or functional outcomes.

Overall, it appears that most studies find early rehabilitation is important to maximize stroke recovery and function, while very early aggressive therapy in the first 24 hours after stroke may be detrimental to recovery, or at best neutral.

INTENSIVE THERAPY IN THE SUBACUTE PHASE

The above has focused on early transfer to rehabilitation and early therapy, generally within the first few days, post stroke. But what about later? Dromerick and colleagues[72] in the Critical Period After Stroke Study (CPASS) examined the optimal time for motor recovery. Twenty extra hours of self-selected task-specific motor therapy were provided to 3 different groups each at different time intervals post stroke: (1) acute ($\leq$30 days); (2) subacute (2–3 months); and (3) chronic ($\geq$6 months). Each group was compared to each other and a control group receiving standard motor rehabilitation. On the ARAT, the greatest difference when compared with the control group was in the subacute phase, there was a significant but smaller difference in the acute phase, and a non-significant improvement in the chronic phase post stroke. This may indicate that increased therapy had the greatest impact in the subacute phase to improve upper extremity function.

Several other studies have also focused on increasing therapy in the subacute phase. Kwakkel and colleagues performed a meta-analysis and found that during the first 6 months post stroke, a 16 hour increase in therapy time over standard care was associated with a favorable outcome.[6] Van Peppen and colleagues[73] noted an additional therapy time of 17 hours over 10 weeks is necessary to see significant positive effects; this was affirmed by Verbeek and colleagues[74]

The Determining Optimal Post-Stroke Exercise (DOSE) RCT was designed to study the effect of higher exercise doses on walking for rehabilitation patients 1 to 4 weeks post stroke.[75] The study consisted of 3 groups: a control group receiving standard physiotherapy for 1 hour per day, 5 days a week for 4 weeks, DOSE 1 receiving 1 hour of more intensive physiotherapy during the same period, and DOSE 2 who received 2 hours of more intensive PT per day 5 days a week for 4 weeks. Both DOSE groups showed greater walking endurance at 4 weeks and at 1 year follow-up compared with controls.

INTENSIVE THERAPY IN THE CHRONIC PHASE

Although the greatest gains in post stroke recovery occur within the first 6 months, benefits still exist for rehabilitation in the chronic phase, though literature is more conflicting. The ICARE (Interdisciplinary Comprehensive Arm Rehab Evaluation) trial, a multisite RCT, compared outpatients who received 30 hours of a structured, task-specific upper extremity exercise program over 10 weeks and found no significant difference in outcomes when compared with those receiving usual care.[76] Lang and colleagues[13] conducted a similar study and found a total of 32 hours of therapy in the chronic phase of stroke did not improve upper extremity function.

These results can be compared with 2 studies that provided much higher doses therapy.[77,78] McCabe et al[77] in a single-blind interventional study looking at upper extremity recovery found that chronic stroke patients provided 300 hours of activity-based technology assisted therapy (5 hours per day 5 days a week x 12 weeks) showed a substantial improvement of the Upper Extremity Fugl-Meyer Assessment score above the minimum clinically important difference. A retrospective review was conducted by Ward and colleagues[79] whereby 224 patients with a median of 18 months post stroke were treated with a high intensity rehabilitation program, 90 hours of therapy delivered for 6 hours a day, 5 days per week, for 3 weeks and compared it to 2 lower intensity therapy groups. The high intensity rehabilitation program resulted in significant improvement in a number of arm motor outcome measures, including the ARAT and the Upper Extremity Fugl Meyer Assessment.

Finally, a systematic review in this area conducted by Lohse and colleagues[9] examined the relationship between the amount of time spent in therapy and motor function. They found that in 34 RCTs of 1750 chronic stroke patients, those who receive more therapy as part of the intervention (on average, control was only 40% of that in the intervention group) were found to have greater improvement.

CLINICAL PEARLS FOR TIMING

- Earlier admission to a stroke rehabilitation unit/program has been associated with improved functional outcomes.
- Very early mobilization, especially if done in the first 24 hours, may be harmful and should be avoided.
- Early mobilization after the first 24 hours (with perhaps the exception of more severe stroke patients) is beneficial in improving recovery.
- Improved functional outcomes can be achieved with a more rigorous exercise program during usual planned therapy sessions at 1 to 4 weeks.
- Augmented therapy of about 20 hours in total is enough to improve motor outcomes in the subacute phase.
- Augmenting therapy in the chronic phase of stroke requires up to 90 hours of additional therapy to improve motor recovery outcomes.

SUMMARY

Although the exact intensity and timing of rehabilitation post stroke varies from study to study, in general, more intense, earlier rehabilitation results in improve motor outcomes. This is consistent with our understanding of the influence of repetitive task-specific exercises on neuroplasticity. There are pragmatic difficulties implementing more intense and earlier rehabilitation, but there are also innovative approaches including new technologies. As time goes by post stroke, the dosage of therapy required to result in improved outcomes increases. Very early rehabilitation exercises therefore offer the greatest opportunity, although rehabilitation should be carefully limited for the first 24 hours and longer for more severe strokes. Some recent data have shown that augmented rehabilitation in the subacute phase results in greater recovery in the upper extremity, when compared with recovery in the chronic phase, with a suggestion it may be as good or perhaps better than the same augmented therapy delivered in the acute phase. Therapy in the form of task-specific exercises in the chronic phase requires higher doses to produce improved motor outcomes.

CLINICS CARE POINTS

- Clinical judgement is important in determining when therapy should be implemented early post stroke onset.
- Delays in therapy, including exercise and mobilization, are common, and run the risk of not acheiving maximal potential recovery.
- Intensity of therapy is often not optimized because of a lack of or failure to maximize therapy resources.
- The impact of therapy delivered early and of appropriate intensity should not be underestimated.
- Therapy resources applied in the acute/subacute phase will result in greater improvement in motor outcomes than similar resources applied in the chronic phase.
- Therapy provided in the chronic phase can improve motor recovery outcomes.

DISCLOSURE

All authors declare that they have no commercial or financial conflicts of interest.

FUNDING

This work was supported by a grant from the Heart and Stroke Foundation of Canada and financial support from the St. Joseph's Health Centre Foundation (London, Ontario, Canada).

REFERENCES

1. Mozaffarian D, Benjamin EJ, Go AS, et al. Heart disease and stroke statistics— 2015 update: a report from the American Heart Association. Circulation 2015; 131(4):e29–322.
2. Teasell R, Salbach NM, Foley N, et al. Canadian stroke best practice recommendations: rehabilitation, recovery, and community participation following stroke. Part one: rehabilitation and recovery following stroke; update 2019. Int J Stroke 2020;15(7):763–88.
3. Foley N, Pereira S, Salter K, et al. Are recommendations regarding inpatient therapy intensity following acute stroke really evidence-based? Top Stroke Rehabil 2012;19(2):96–103.
4. De Wit L, Putman K, Dejaeger E, et al. Use of time by stroke patients: a comparison of four European rehabilitation centers. Stroke 2005;36(9):1977–83.
5. De Wit L, Putman K, Schuback B, et al. Motor and functional recovery after stroke: a comparison of 4 European rehabilitation centers. Stroke 2007;38(7):2101–7.
6. Kwakkel G, van Peppen R, Wagenaar RC, et al. Effects of augmented exercise therapy time after stroke: a meta-analysis. Stroke 2004;35(11):2529–39.
7. Veerbeek JM, Koolstra M, Ket JC, et al. Effects of augmented exercise therapy on outcome of gait and gait-related activities in the first 6 months after stroke: a meta-analysis. Stroke 2011;42(11):3311–5.

8. van Wijk R, Cumming T, Churilov L, et al. An early mobilization protocol success-fully delivers more and earlier therapy to acute stroke patients: further results from phase II of AVERT. Neurorehabilitation Neural Repair 2012;26(1):20–6.
9. Lohse KR, Lang CE, Boyd LA. Is more better? Using metadata to explore dose–response relationships in stroke rehabilitation. Stroke 2014;45(7):2053–8.
10. Kalra L. The influence of stroke unit rehabilitation on functional recovery from stroke. Stroke 1994;25(4):821–5.
11. Langhorne P, Coupar F, Pollock A. Motor recovery after stroke: a systematic re-view. Lancet Neurol 2009;8(8):741–54.
12. Pollock A, Farmer SE, Brady MC, et al. Interventions for improving upper limb function after stroke. Cochrane Database Syst Rev 2014;(11).
13. Lang CE, Strube MJ, Bland MD, et al. Dose response of task-specific upper limb training in people at least 6 months poststroke: a phase II, single-blind, random-ized, controlled trial. Ann Neurol 2016;80(3):342–54.
14. Park H, Kim S, Winstein CJ, et al. Short-duration and intensive training improves long-term reaching performance in individuals with chronic stroke. Neurorehabi-litation Neural Repair 2016;30(6):551–61.
15. Wu X, Guarino P, Lo AC, et al. Long-term effectiveness of intensive therapy in chronic stroke. Neurorehabilitation Neural Repair 2016;30(6):583–90.
16. Gerston J. External work of walking in hemiaffected patients. Scand J Rehabil Med 1971;3:85–8.
17. MacKay-Lyons MJ, Makrides L. Exercise capacity early after stroke. Archives of physical medicine and rehabilitation 2002;83(12):1697–702.
18. Billinger SA, Coughenour E, MacKay-Lyons MJ, et al. Reduced cardiorespiratory fitness after stroke: biological consequences and exercise-induced adaptations. Stroke Res Treat 2012;2012:959120.
19. Wiener J, McIntyre A, Janssen S, et al. Effectiveness of high-intensity interval training for fitness and mobility post stroke: A systematic review. PM&R 2019; 11(8):868–78.
20. Ivey FM, Hafer-Macko CE, Macko RF. Task-oriented treadmill exercise training in chronic hemiparetic stroke. J Rehabil Res Dev 2008;45(2):249.
21. Gibala MJ. High-intensity interval training: a time-efficient strategy for health pro-motion? Curr Sports Med Rep 2007;6(4):211–3.
22. Milanović Z, Sporiš G, Weston M. Effectiveness of high-intensity interval training (HIT) and continuous endurance training for VO 2max improvements: a system-atic review and meta-analysis of controlled trials. Sports Med 2015;45:1469–81.
23. Weston M, Taylor KL, Batterham AM, et al. Effects of low-volume high-intensity in-terval training (HIT) on fitness in adults: a meta-analysis of controlled and non-controlled trials. Sports Med 2014;44:1005–17.
24. Gist NH, Fedewa MV, Dishman RK, et al. Sprint interval training effects on aerobic capacity: a systematic review and meta-analysis. Sports Med 2014;44:269–79.
25. Boyne P, Dunning K, Carl D, et al. High-intensity interval training and moderate-intensity continuous training in ambulatory chronic stroke: feasibility study. Phys Ther 2016;96(10):1533–44.
26. Madhavan S, Stinear JW, Kanekar N. Effects of a single session of high intensity interval treadmill training on corticomotor excitability following stroke: implications for therapy. Neural Plast 2016;2016.
27. Burnfield JM, Buster TW, Goldman AJ, et al. Partial body weight support treadmill training speed influences paretic and non-paretic leg muscle activation, stride characteristics, and ratings of perceived exertion during acute stroke rehabilita-tion. Hum Mov Sci 2016;47:16–28.

28. Severinsen K, Jakobsen JK, Pedersen AR, et al. Effects of resistance training and aerobic training on ambulation in chronic stroke. Am J Phys Med Rehabil 2014; 93(1):29–42.
29. Linder SM, Rosenfeldt AB, Dey T, et al. Forced aerobic exercise preceding task practice improves motor recovery poststroke. Am J Occup Ther 2017;71(2). 7102290020p7102290021-7102290020p7102290029.
30. Lang CE, MacDonald JR, Reisman DS, et al. Observation of amounts of movement practice provided during stroke rehabilitation. Archives of physical medicine and rehabilitation 2009;90(10):1692–8.
31. Simpson DB, Breslin M, Cumming T, et al. Go home, sit less: the impact of home versus hospital rehabilitation environment on activity levels of stroke survivors. Archives of physical medicine and rehabilitation 2018;99(11):2216–21, e2211.
32. Dromerick A, Lang C, Birkenmeier R, et al. Very early constraint-induced movement during stroke rehabilitation (VECTORS): a single-center RCT. Neurology 2009;73(3):195–201.
33. Fang Y, Chen X, Li H, et al. A study on additional early physiotherapy after stroke and factors affecting functional recovery. Clin Rehabil 2003;17(6):608–17.
34. Belagaje SR. Stroke rehabilitation. CONTINUUM: Lifelong Learning in Neurology 2017;23(1):238–53.
35. Gimigliano F. Does time spent in rehabilitation makes a difference on activity limitation and impairment in people with stroke?-A Cochrane Review summary with commentary. J Rehabil Med 2022;54:jrm00315.
36. Clark B, Whitall J, Kwakkel G, et al. The effect of time spent in rehabilitation on activity limitation and impairment after stroke. Cochrane Database Syst Rev 2021;(10).
37. Ontario OAGo. Value for Money Audit Cardiac Disease and Stroke Treatment. 2021:1-81.
38. Wang H, Camicia M, Terdiman J, et al. Daily treatment time and functional gains of stroke patients during inpatient rehabilitation. PM&R 2013;5(2):122–8.
39. Prusynski RA, Gustavson AM, Shrivastav SR, et al. Rehabilitation intensity and patient outcomes in skilled nursing facilities in the United States: a systematic review. Phys Ther 2021;101(3):pzaa230.
40. Teasell R, Meyer MJ, Foley N, et al. Stroke rehabilitation in Canada: a work in progress. Top Stroke Rehabil 2009;16(1):11–9.
41. Bonifacio GB, Ward NS, Emsley HC, et al. Optimising rehabilitation and recovery after a stroke. Practical Neurol 2022;22(6):478–85.
42. Donnellan-Fernandez K, Ioakim A, Hordacre B. Revisiting dose and intensity of training: Opportunities to enhance recovery following stroke. J Stroke Cerebrovasc Dis 2022;31(11):106789.
43. Renner CI, Outermans J, Ludwig R, et al. Group therapy task training versus individual task training during inpatient stroke rehabilitation: a randomised controlled trial. Clin Rehabil 2016;30(7):637–48.
44. English C, Bernhardt J, Crotty M, et al. Circuit class therapy or seven-day week therapy for increasing rehabilitation intensity of therapy after stroke (CIRCIT): a randomized controlled trial. Int J Stroke 2015;10(4):594–602.
45. Saposnik G, Cohen LG, Mamdani M, et al. Efficacy and safety of non-immersive virtual reality exercising in stroke rehabilitation (EVREST): a randomised, multi-centre, single-blind, controlled trial. Lancet Neurol 2016;15(10):1019–27.
46. Lo HS, Xie SQ. Exoskeleton robots for upper-limb rehabilitation: State of the art and future prospects. Med Eng Phys 2012;34(3):261–8.

47. Dodakian L, McKenzie AL, Le V, et al. A home-based telerehabilitation program for patients with stroke. Neurorehabilitation Neural Repair 2017;31(10–11): 923–33.

48. Biernaskie J, Chernenko G, Corbett D. Efficacy of rehabilitative experience declines with time after focal ischemic brain injury. J Neurosci 2004;24(5):1245–54.

49. Tian S, Zhang Y, Tian S, et al. Early exercise training improves ischemic outcome in rats by cerebral hemodynamics. Brain Res 2013;1533:114–21.

50. Park J-W, Bang M-S, Kwon B-S, et al. Early treadmill training promotes motor function after hemorrhagic stroke in rats. Neurosci Lett 2010;471(2):104–8.

51. Hordacre B, Austin D, Brown KE, et al. Evidence for a window of enhanced plasticity in the human motor cortex following ischemic stroke. Neurorehabilitation Neural Repair 2021;35(4):307–20.

52. Bai Y, Hu Y, Wu Y, et al. A prospective, randomized, single-blinded trial on the effect of early rehabilitation on daily activities and motor function of patients with hemorrhagic stroke. J Clin Neurosci 2012;19(10):1376–9.

53. Bai Y-l, Hu Y-s, Wu Y, et al. Long-term three-stage rehabilitation intervention alleviates spasticity of the elbows, fingers, and plantar flexors and improves activities of daily living in ischemic stroke patients: a randomized, controlled trial. Neuroreport 2014;25(13):998–1005.

54. Horn SD, DeJong G, Smout RJ, et al. Stroke rehabilitation patients, practice, and outcomes: is earlier and more aggressive therapy better? Archives of physical medicine and rehabilitation 2005;86(12):101–14.

55. Hu M-H, Hsu S-S, Yip P-K, et al. Early and intensive rehabilitation predicts good functional outcomes in patients admitted to the stroke intensive care unit. Disabil Rehabil 2010;32(15):1251–9.

56. Paolucci S, Antonucci G, Grasso MG, et al. Early versus delayed inpatient stroke rehabilitation: a matched comparison conducted in Italy. Archives of physical medicine and rehabilitation 2000;81(6):695–700.

57. Jutai J, Foley NC, Bhogal SK, et al. Impact of early vs delayed admission to rehabilitation on functional outcomes in persons with stroke. J Rehabil Med 2006; 38(113117/ϸ).

58. Wang H, Camicia M, DiVita M, et al. Early inpatient rehabilitation admission and stroke patient outcomes. Am J Phys Med Rehabil 2015;94(2):85–100.

59. Wang H, Camicia M, Terdiman J, et al. Time to inpatient rehabilitation hospital admission and functional outcomes of stroke patients. Pm&r 2011;3(4):296–304.

60. Yagi M, Yasunaga H, Matsui H, et al. Impact of rehabilitation on outcomes in patients with ischemic stroke: a nationwide retrospective cohort study in Japan. Stroke 2017;48(3):740–6.

61. Maulden SA, Gassaway J, Horn SD, et al. Timing of initiation of rehabilitation after stroke. Archives of physical medicine and rehabilitation 2005;86(12):34–40.

62. Murie-Fernández M, Ortega-Cubero S, Carmona-Abellán M, et al. "Time is brain": only in the acute phase of stroke? Neurologia 2012;27(4):197–201.

63. Bernhardt J, Dewey H, Thrift A, et al. A very early rehabilitation trial for stroke (AVERT) phase II safety and feasibility. Stroke 2008;39(2):390–6.

64. Langhorne P, Stott D, Knight A, et al. Very early rehabilitation or intensive telemetry after stroke: a pilot randomised trial. Cerebrovasc Dis 2010;29(4):352–60.

65. Liu N, Cadilhac DA, Andrew NE, et al. Randomized controlled trial of early rehabilitation after intracerebral hemorrhage stroke: difference in outcomes within 6 months of stroke. Stroke 2014;45(12):3502–7.

66. Chippala P, Sharma R. Effect of very early mobilisation on functional status in patients with acute stroke: a single-blind, randomized controlled trail. Clin Rehabil 2016;30(7):669–75.
67. Morreale M, Marchione P, Pili A, et al. Early versus delayed rehabilitation treatment in hemiplegic patients with ischemic stroke: proprioceptive or cognitive approach. Eur J Phys Rehabil Med 2016;52(1):81–9.
68. Bernhardt J, Langhorne P, Lindley RI, et al. Efficacy and safety of very early mobilisation within 24 h of stroke onset (AVERT): a randomised controlled trial. Lancet 2015;386(9988):46–55.
69. Luft AR, Macko RF, Forrester LW, et al. Treadmill exercise activates subcortical neural networks and improves walking after stroke: a randomized controlled trial. Stroke 2008;39(12):3341–50.
70. Bernhardt J, Churilov L, Ellery F, et al. Prespecified dose-response analysis for a very early rehabilitation trial (AVERT). Neurology 2016;86(23):2138–45.
71. Rethnam V, Langhorne P, Churilov L, et al. Early mobilisation post-stroke: a systematic review and meta-analysis of individual participant data. Disabil Rehabil 2022;44(8):1156–63.
72. Dromerick AW, Geed S, Barth J, et al. Critical Period After Stroke Study (CPASS): A phase II clinical trial testing an optimal time for motor recovery after stroke in humans. Proc Natl Acad Sci USA 2021;118(39). e2026676118.
73. Van Peppen RP, Kwakkel G, Wood-Dauphinee S, et al. The impact of physical therapy on functional outcomes after stroke: what's the evidence? Clin Rehabil 2004;18(8):833–62.
74. Veerbeek JM, van Wegen E, van Peppen R, et al. What is the evidence for physical therapy poststroke? A systematic review and meta-analysis. PLoS One 2014; 9(2):e87987.
75. Klassen TD, Dukelow SP, Bayley MT, et al. Higher doses improve walking recovery during stroke inpatient rehabilitation. Stroke 2020;51(9):2639–48.
76. Winstein CJ, Wolf SL, Dromerick AW, et al. Interdisciplinary Comprehensive Arm Rehabilitation Evaluation (ICARE): a randomized controlled trial protocol. BMC Neurol 2013;13(1):1–19.
77. McCabe J, Monkiewicz M, Holcomb J, et al. Comparison of robotics, functional electrical stimulation, and motor learning methods for treatment of persistent upper extremity dysfunction after stroke: a randomized controlled trial. Archives of physical medicine and rehabilitation 2015;96(6):981–90.
78. Daly JJ, McCabe JP, Holcomb J, et al. Long-dose intensive therapy is necessary for strong, clinically significant, upper limb functional gains and retained gains in severe/moderate chronic stroke. Neurorehabilitation Neural Repair 2019;33(7): 523–37.
79. Ward NS, Brander F, Kelly K. Intensive upper limb neurorehabilitation in chronic stroke: outcomes from the Queen Square programme. J Neurol Neurosurg Psychiatr 2019;90(5):498–506.

Integrating Cardiac Rehabilitation in Stroke Recovery

Sara J. Cuccurullo, MD*, Talya K. Fleming, MD,
Hayk Petrosyan, PhD

KEYWORDS

- Stroke • Cerebrovascular accident • Stroke rehabilitation • Cardiac rehabilitation
- Exercise • Physical activity

KEY POINTS

- After a stroke, individuals significantly reduce physical activity and spend most of their time in sedentary activities.
- It has been formally recommended to incorporate aerobic exercise as part of stroke management; however, its implementation has proven to be challenging.
- Cardiac rehabilitation (CR) programs have a well-established structure that offers patients physical activity, cardiovascular exercise, risk factor education, and behavior change.
- Numerous studies have demonstrated the safety and effectiveness of programs modeled after CR for stroke patients.

INTRODUCTION

Stroke is a devastating condition with more than 795,000 people affected annually only in the United States.[1] Despite modern multidisciplinary team efforts and advances in stroke care, approximately a third of stroke survivors remain dependent following their stroke event, greatly impacting their daily life.[2]

Motor impairments of stroke survivors enable inactive lifestyles resulting in spending approximately ~80% of their time in sedentary behaviors.[3,4] Significantly decreased physical activity results in further deconditioning in this patient population, thus increasing the risk of cardiovascular events and recurrent stroke who are already at significant risk for cardiovascular disease.

Current rehabilitation strategies start early poststroke and aim to address the disability and needs with balance, limited mobility, and daily activities.[5] Numerous

Department of Physical Medicine and Rehabilitation, JFK Johnson Rehabilitation Institute at Hackensack Meridian Health, 65 James Street, Edison, NJ, USA
* Corresponding author.
E-mail address: Sara.Cuccurullo@hmhn.org

Phys Med Rehabil Clin N Am 35 (2024) 353–368
https://doi.org/10.1016/j.pmr.2023.06.007

innovations incorporating technological advancements, virtual reality/gaming, and electrical stimulation modalities are being used in rehabilitation programs and are successful in accelerating the recovery of function.[6-8] Nonetheless, existing rehabilitation programs are mostly aimed to address mobility deficits and confront functional limitations with daily activities, that is, upper extremity function, devoting other concomitant functional deficits little attention.

In addition to motor impairments, stroke survivors have a significant decline in cardiovascular capacity with stroke patients exhibiting approximately 60% of the normative values for healthy sedentary individuals.[9] These detrimental numbers are comparable to patients after myocardial infarction[9] demonstrating the necessity to address this critical problem in this patient population.

Cardiovascular disease poststroke is a significant challenge and one of the major factors obstructing the successful adaptation of poststroke rehabilitation.[10-12] Stroke survivors exhibit reduced oxygen uptake and a significant decrease in endurance for exercise.[9,13,14] Neuromuscular impairments and decreased cardiovascular capacity together lead to limited activity in stroke survivors, which is heightened by the high metabolic demand and as much as three times greater energy cost of walking for stroke survivors compared with individuals without neurologic impairments.[9,15]

The development of rehabilitative services that incorporate cardiovascular exercise into poststroke rehabilitation is critical for achieving effective recovery of function and lowering the risk for recurrent stroke. National and international clinical practice guidelines and recommendations promote strategies to incorporate aerobic exercise in rehabilitation for stroke survivors.[16-18]

The American Heart Association (AHA) and American Stroke Association (ASA) recommend moderate-intensity aerobic exercise, lasting 20 to 60 minutes, performed three to five times a week as part of management for stroke survivors.[17,18] In the past decade, more studies have incorporated aerobic exercise into poststroke rehabilitation demonstrating significant benefits and increasing awareness among clinicians and researchers.[19-24]

Aerobic exercise is an essential part of the cardiac rehabilitation (CR) program, a proven model that significantly improved the health of cardiac patients.[25,26] Studies incorporating aerobic exercise for stroke patients and modeled after a CR program have demonstrated significant effects on recovery of function as well as hospital readmission and mortality for stroke survivors.[20,22,27-29]

This review aims to synthesize available evidence to inform clinicians and researchers regarding the benefits of aerobic exercise and programs modeled after CR for stroke survivors and relevant challenges.

Benefits of Aerobic Exercise After Stroke

There are several approaches that are used during stroke rehabilitation to improve health and function after stroke. Although stroke rehabilitation strategies emphasize various types of physical activity (eg, anaerobic exercise, resistance/strength training, gait training, and coordination/balance training),[17,30] this review focuses on the evidence of the specific principles and benefits of aerobic exercise after cerebrovascular disease. The Centers for Disease Control and Prevention defines aerobic exercise as "a type of physical activity that involves planned, structured, and repetitive bodily movement done to maintain or improve one or more components of physical fitness."[31] Unfortunately, traditional stroke rehabilitation and physical activity recommendations provide a mean of only 3 minutes of low-intensity aerobic training ($\geq$40% of heart rate reserve) per session and therefore do not adequately substitute the specific benefits achieved by a structured aerobic exercise program.[17] With global rates of stroke at more than 13 million cases, and approximately 25% of these strokes classified as recurrent strokes, there is emerging clinical evidence supporting supervised progressive aerobic exercise along with risk factor modification delivered by CR programs for the stroke population.[32]

Favorable physiologic adaptations to the cardiovascular system are associated with moderate-vigorous exercise training. Aerobic exercise interventions have consistently shown improvements in exercise capacity measured as peak oxygen consumption (Vo$_2$ peak)[27,33–35] and the 6-minute walk test (6MWT) in survivors of chronic stroke.[24,27,28,36] Exercise performance is often measured in metabolic equivalents (METs; 1 MET = 3.5 mL O$_2$/kg per min = approximate resting O$_2$ consumption[37] and MET-minutes [METs multiplied by exercise minutes[38]]) providing a convenient method to describe functional capacity or exercise tolerance. When comparing the start to completion of aerobic exercise programs, a significant increase of 2.04 METs (31.4%) in mean aerobic capacity[37] and 78% of MET-minutes[20] has also been shown post-36 sessions of a modified CR. Importantly, the AHA acknowledged in their 2014 Scientific Statement that aerobic exercise in subacute stroke survivors facilitated improvements in cardiorespiratory and vascular health.[17]

Exercise and risk factor modification programs are associated with improved cardiovascular disease risk factors, reduced 3-year risk for recurrent stroke, vascular death, myocardial infarction, and reduced all-cause mortality.[32] A modified CR program demonstrated a reduction in 1-year all-cause mortality[20] and a reduction in 1-year all-cause hospital readmission rate.[29] In addition, aerobic exercise promotes improvements in multiple aspects of the cardiometabolic profile after stroke. The benefits of regular exercise in the general population include improved exercise tolerance, lowered blood pressure, and increased insulin sensitivity.[39] In subacute stroke survivors, aerobic exercise improves the stroke vascular risk factor profile and cardiovascular fitness.[17,32] Poststroke aerobic exercise has been demonstrated to significantly lower serum levels of total cholesterol (TC) (6.8%), TC/high-density lipoprotein (TC/HDL) (11.6%), triglycerides (16.5%), waist circumference (2.4%), body mass index (1.8%), and body weight (1.7%)[37] with a protocol of 20 to 60 minute sessions, two to four times per week for 50 sessions. Furthermore, the decrease in low-density lipoprotein (LDL) (10.3%), systolic blood pressure (2.4%), and diastolic blood pressure (3.0%) as well as the increase in HDL (4.4%) approached statistical significance.[37]

Evolving research proposes that aerobic exercise after stroke bestows clinically meaningful health benefits in several physical and psychosocial domains that extend beyond the bounds of the cardiovascular system. Exercise is an effective and feasible strategy for improving motor and cognitive recovery following ischemic stroke through the facilitation of neuroplasticity.[40] Chronic aerobic exercise induces greater levels of circulating brain-derived neurotrophic factor, insulin-like growth factor, and vascular endothelial growth factor, thereby promoting gliogenesis, neurogenesis, synaptogenesis, and angiogenesis.[41,42] Increases in gray matter volume, white matter volume, and neural activity are associated with improvements in motor and cognitive function.[41] The 2016 AHA/ASA guidelines for adult stroke rehabilitation and recovery reported that as a degree of impairment, exercise positively affects bone health, fatigue, executive functioning and memory, emotional well-being, and depression symptoms.[18,32] A Cochrane review summarized that "there is clear evidence that cardiorespiratory training improves measures of walking performance (walking speed and walking capacity)."[15] Functional progress was also noted in upper extremity muscle strength and walking ability (endurance more than speed).[18,29] Among stroke survivors, there is also evidence demonstrating improved cognition after exercise.[17,20,24,32] Moreover, evidence indicates an association between exercise training after stroke and social participation as well as return to work.[18] As a common goal for many stroke survivors, a meta-analysis reported that exercise interventions significantly benefit health-related quality of life.[18]

More recently, exercise recommendations have evolved to include more specific guideline recommendations as a standard of care after stroke.

- In 2014, the AHA/ASA guidelines for physical activity and exercise recommendations for stroke survivors describe that "where appropriate, aerobic exercise with the goals/objectives including to: increase walking speed and efficiency, improve exercise tolerance (functional capacity), increase independence in activities of daily living, reduce motor impairment and improve cognition, improve vascular health and induce other cardioprotective benefits (eg, vasomotor reactivity, decrease risk factors)."[17]
- In 2019, the Aerobic Exercise Recommendations to Optimize Best Practices in Care After Stroke: AEROBICS 2019 Update includes 20 recommendations and specifically states that "Aerobic training should be incorporated into a comprehensive, interprofessional program of stroke rehabilitation, vascular risk reduction, and secondary stroke prevention."[43]
- In 2021, the AHA/ASA guideline for the prevention of stroke in patients with stroke and transient ischemic attack states that "patients with stroke or TIA who are capable of physical activity, engaging in at least moderate-intensity aerobic activity for a minimum of 10 minutes 4 times a week or vigorous-intensity aerobic activity for a minimum of 20 minutes twice a week is indicated to lower the risk of recurrent stroke and the composite cardiovascular end point of recurrent stroke, MI, or vascular death"(Class 1, Level C-LD).[44]
- In 2021, the AHA/ASA guideline for the prevention of stroke in patients with stroke and transient ischemic attack reports that "in patients with deficits after a stroke that impair their ability to exercise, supervision of an exercise program by a health care professional such as a physical therapist or cardiac rehabilitation professional, in addition to routine rehabilitation, can be beneficial for secondary stroke prevention" (Class 2a, Level C-EO).[44]

Although these recommendations are clinically important and relevant, incorporation of these recommendations into a structured, medically supervised program continues to be a challenge in the administration of traditional stroke rehabilitation.

What Is Cardiac Rehabilitation?

The American Association of Cardiovascular and Pulmonary Rehabilitation (AACVPR) defines CR as the provision of comprehensive long-term services involving medical evaluation, prescriptive exercise, cardiac risk factor modification, education, counseling, and behavioral interventions.[45] CR has a class 1 indication (ie, strong recommendation) after heart surgery, myocardial infarction, or coronary intervention, and for stable angina or peripheral artery disease.[45] It has a class 2a indication (ie, moderate recommendation) for stable systolic heart failure.[45] CR guidelines endorse a multidisciplinary team providing skilled delivery of evidence-based components of secondary prevention of vascular disease.[46]

Most CR programs include medically supervised progressive aerobic exercise combined with cardiac risk factor modification including education and behavioral intervention addressing specific secondary prevention for cardiac disease (eg, optimization of blood pressure, blood glucose control, lipid management, body mass index, nutrition, smoking cessation, and physical activity). In addition, behavioral management including medication adherence, nutritional counseling, exercise training, and psychosocial education is included as a part of the program. Medical and functional outcomes such as weight, blood pressure, serum lipid level, serum glucose level, and functional capacity are assessed at the beginning and end of the CR program for comparison.[47] Risk factors are targeted to reduce the rates of morbidity and mortality, improve functional capacity, and alleviate activity-related symptoms.[45] The AHA and the AACVPR encourage all CR/secondary prevention programs to meet the standards for AACVPR program certification, including the core components of CR/secondary prevention programs: (1) blood pressure management, (2) lipid management, (3) diabetes management, (4) tobacco cessation, (5) psychosocial management, (6) physical activity counseling, and (7) exercise training. Evaluation, interventions, and expected outcomes are recorded for each area.[48]

CR has several documented benefits in the treatment of cardiac disease after an acute cardiovascular incident. Persons participating in CR have a dose-dependent reduced rate of cardiovascular mortality (relative risk 0.74), and fewer hospital readmissions (relative risk 0.82).[45] Medicare beneficiaries who participated in CR found that those who attended more sessions had a lower rate of morbidity and death at 4 years, particularly if they participated in more than 11 sessions. Those who attended the full 36 sessions had a mortality rate 47% lower than those who attended a single session.[45] In addition to cardiovascular health, the benefits of CR include improved functional capacity, greater ease with activities of daily living, and improved quality of life.[45] CR programs are recommended as a standard of care by major clinical guidelines.[49]

Owing to the benefits demonstrated by CR, there has been increasingly more attention focused on expanding CR-like programs for patients with stroke[20,28,32] and other vascular diseases such as peripheral artery disease.[50] Additional evidence-based medicine from rigorous clinical research will provide further information about the effects of CR interventions in various populations.

Clinical Similarities Between Patients with Stroke and Cardiovascular Disease

While often overlooked, the pathophysiology driving cardiovascular disease and cerebrovascular disease/stroke has many clinical similarities. Both ischemic stroke and myocardial infarction are disease states that are a consequence of derangements to the vascular system resulting in a lack of blood flow to the end organ, namely the brain and heart, respectively. Stroke and myocardial infarction share common pathologic mechanisms and clinical risk factors.[51] Moreover, coronary artery disease is an important cause of death in patients with cerebrovascular disease,[51] highlighting a common clinical pathway caused by systemic vascular disease (**Fig. 1**).

The concept of cardiovascular health was recently expanded to not only apply to cardiovascular disease risk factors but also to promote the health of the individual and the population as a whole.[52] The AHAs presidential advisory recently redefined an enhanced approach to assessing cardiovascular health, termed Life's Essential 8. The components of Life's Essential 8 include the management of blood pressure, blood glucose, blood lipids, body mass index, diet, physical activity, nicotine exposure, and sleep health.[52] These eight areas are the key to achieving optimal cardiovascular health for both stroke and cardiovascular disease. Mechanisms by which higher cardiovascular health is associated with lower cardiovascular disease risk have identified several potential pathways involving inflammation, endothelial function, atherosclerosis, cardiac stress and remodeling, hemostatic factors, and epigenetics, among others.[52]

Secondary prevention strategies for stroke, as well as cardiovascular disease, have typically incorporated models of behavioral interventions to address lifestyle

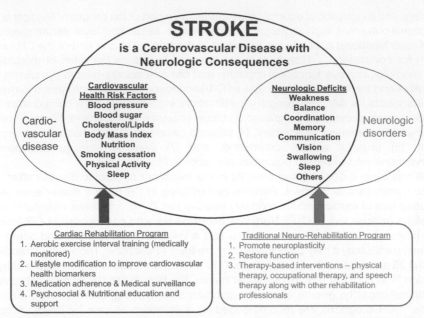

Fig. 1. Stroke as a vascular and neurologic disease and the benefits of cardiac rehabilitation in combination with neuro-rehabilitation.

management and exercise intervention to address underlying risk factors promoting cardiovascular health. People with stroke, especially those with atherosclerotic risk factors and subclinical cardiac disease detected by testing, should incorporate comprehensive and aggressive risk factor reduction.[51]

Aerobic Exercise and Cardiac Rehabilitation Available for Stroke Patients: Programs and Research

Numerous studies have investigated the efficacy of aerobic exercise or implemented programs modeled after CR for stroke patients. The available literature includes large cohort studies, randomized controlled trials, feasibility, and pilot studies that incorporated patients with both ischemic and hemorrhagic stroke, with a spectrum of deficits, ranging from minor strokes to moderate impairments. They have demonstrated the feasibility and practicality of adaptation of aerobic exercise and programs modeled after CR for these patients.[20–24,27,53]

The studies were conducted across several countries, including the United States, Canada, Europe, and Australia (**Table 1**). The exercise programs varied in both frequency and duration. Most of the studies involved patients engaging in facility-based aerobic exercise two to three times a week,[20,21,34,37,57] whereas others had a combination of facility-based exercise performed once a week and have patients continue the program four times a week at home.[36] The length of the exercise programs also differed, ranging from 4 weeks to 6 months, with the majority lasting around 12 weeks. Most exercise sessions were 30 minutes in duration. However, in studies conducted in Canada, where stroke patients participated in a traditional CR program with cardiac patients, sessions had 60 and 90 minutes duration incorporating additional activities besides aerobic exercise.[19,54] The programs included various types of aerobic exercise, including total body recumbent stepper, cycle ergometer,

Table 1
Summary of studies and their outcomes incorporating cardiac rehabilitation programs or aerobic exercise for stroke patients

Reference	Country	Type of the Study/Setting	Stroke Type	Sample Size	Concurrent to Neurorehabilitation	Description of Intervention	Initiation Poststroke	Frequency (per Week)	Session and Program Duration (Total Number of Sessions)	Intensity	Risk Factor Education	Improved Clinical Outcomes	Improved Functional and Psychosocial Outcomes
Billinger et al,[27] 2012	USA	Cohort; feasibility /research laboratory	NR	10	NR	Total body recumbent stepper	<6 mo; (15–123 d) average 68 d	3x	20–40 min sessions over 8 wk (total 24 sessions)	50%–59% of HR for 4 wk then 60%–69% HR; Moderate-to-high intensity	No	Brachial artery diameter; flow-mediated dilation; SBP	6MWT; VO2 peak; Watts
Calmels et al,[37] 2011	France	Cohort; feasibility /outpatient PM&R clinic	Ischemic or hemorrhagic	14	NR	Adapted cycle ergometer	>3 mo, <2 y; average 12 mo	3x	30 min sessions over 2 mo (total sessions NR)	60 rpm	No	NR	6MWT; VO2 peak; Muscle strength; watts
Clague-Baker et al,[21] 2022	United Kingdom	Mixed-methods feasibility/ CR clinic	Ischemic or hemorrhagic; mild-to moderate	32	NR	Adapted traditional CR program (bike, treadmill, side steps, back steps)	Greater than 1 wk, <6 mo; average 88 d	2x	55 min sessions over 6 wk (total sessions NR)	50%–70% of max HR	Yes	NR	ISWT
Cuccurullo et al,[20] 2022	USA	Prospective cohort/ outpatient PM&R clinic	Ischemic or hemorrhagic	449	Yes	Modified CR program	<45 d	2x–3x	30 min sessions over 3–4 mo (total 36 sessions)	Low-to-moderate level	Yes	1-y all-cause mortality	AM-PAC-basic mobility, daily activity, applied cognitive; MET-min
MacKay-Lyons et al,[54] 2022	Canada	RCT/PT supervised	TIA and NDS	184	NR	Treadmill, cycling stepping	<3 mo	2x	60 min sessions over 12 wk (total sessions NR)	60%–80% of VO2 peak	Yes	DBP LDL-C	NR
Kirk et al,[53] 2014	United Kingdom	RCT/CR clinic	Minor stroke or TIA	24	Yes	Traditional CR program	NR (acute poststroke)	NR	Phase 3: 60 min sessions over 6 wk (total sessions NR) Phase 4: (total 12 sessions)	50%–70% max HR	Yes	CVD risk score	SF-36 physical and mental health domain

(continued on next page)

Table 1
(continued)

Reference	Country	Type of the Study/Setting	Stroke Type	Sample Size	Concurrent to Neurorehabilitation	Description of Intervention	Initiation Poststroke	Frequency (per Week)	Session and Program Duration (Total Number of Sessions)	Intensity	Risk Factor Education	Improved Clinical Outcomes	Improved Functional and Psychosocial Outcomes
Orme et al,[55] 2020	United Kingdom	Prospective before after/ CR clinic	Mild-to-moderate stroke	24	NR	Adapted traditional CR program	>1 wk, <6 mo	2x	30 min over 6 wk (total sessions NR)	50%–70% max HR	Yes	NR	Daily steps; moderate-vigorous physical activity
Lennon et al,[22] 2020	Ireland	Matched group analysis with CR patients/CR clinic	TIA and NDS	94	NR	Traditional CR program	NR. (acute poststroke)	2x	Session duration NR over 8 wk (total 16 sessions)	NR	Yes	SBP LDL TC Triglycerides	METs
Prior et al,[38] 2011	Canada	Cohort/CR clinic	TIA and NDS	100	Yes	Traditional CR program	<1 y	2x	20–60 min sessions, program duration 6 mo (50-session option)	40%–70% HR reserve	Yes	TC TC/HDL Triglycerides FBG-nondiabetic Waist circumference BMI Body weight	METs
Reynolds et al,[23] 2021	Australia	Pilot RCT/ outpatient PT gym	Ischemic or hemorrhagic	20	Yes	Cycle ergometer, recumbent bike, treadmill, upper extremity ergometer, stepper	>6 wk, <1 y; (72–175 d) average 109 d	2x	30 min sessions over 12 wk (total sessions NR)	40%–59% HR reserve; moderate intensity	No	NR	VO2peak
Sandberg et al,[56] 2016	Sweden	RCT/PT monitored clinic at the hospital	Ischemic or hemorrhagic; mild stroke	56	No (mild strokes did not get any neuro-rehab therapy according to standard of care)	Cycle ergometer, walking, standing	Greater than 3 d; average 22 d	2x	60 min sessions over 12 wk (total sessions NR)	60%–80% of max HR	No	Peak work rate (Watts)	6MWT 10MWT TUG SLS EQ-5D VAS SIS recovery

Study	Country	Design/Setting	Stroke type	N		Modality	Time since stroke	Frequency	Session	Intensity				
Tang et al,[34] 2009	Canada	Matched control/IRF	Ischemic or hemorrhagic; mild stroke	57	Yes	Cycle ergometer	<3 mo; (6–62 d) average 17 d	3x	30 min sessions over 4 wk (up to 10 sessions, depending on duration of IRF stay)	4–6 RPE 50%–75% of work rate (Watts)	No	Positive trend (NSS)	Positive trend (NSS)	
Vanroy et al,[57] 2017	Belgium	RCT/IRF Or home	Ischemic or hemorrhagic	59	Yes	Seated cycling program, MOTOmed leg trainer	>3 wk; <10 wk	3x	30 min sessions over 3 mo (total sessions NR)	[HRpeak – HRrest]x [60% to 75%] +HRrest	Yes	Watt peak	Positive trend (NSS)	
Regan et al,[24] 2021	USA	Pre-post mixed methods/CR clinic	Ischemic or hemorrhagic	29	No	Traditional CR program	>3 mo (average 2.4 y)	3x	31–50 min sessions over 12 wk (total 36 sessions)	11–14 RPE	Yes	NR	6MWT; SIS-mobility; METs; FTSS; SIS-ADL; SIS-memory; SIS-participation	
Marzolini et al,[19] 2016	Canada	Pro-retrospective/ CR clinic	Ischemic or hemorrhagic/ TIA	85	NR	Traditional CR program	Average 14 mo	1x	90 min sessions over 6 mo (total sessions NR)	60%–80% VO₂ peak	Yes	BMI	VO₂ peak; CES-D	
Tang et al,[36] 2010	Canada	Prospective cohort/ outpatient CR program	Ischemic or hemorrhagic; mild-to moderate stroke	41	NR	Overground walking, semi-recumbent cycle ergometer	>3 mo; (3–113 mo) average 30 mo	1x in the facility 4x at home	30–60 min sessions over 6 mo (total sessions NR)	60%–80% HR reserve	Yes	VO₂ peak Labs-positive trend (NSS)	Positive trend (NSS)	

Abbreviations: 10MWT, 10-minute walk test; ADL, activities of daily living; BMI, body mass index; CES-D, center for epidemiologic studies depression; CR, cardiac rehabilitation; CVD, cardiovascular disease; D, days; DBP, diastolic blood pressure; EQ5D, EuroQol 5 dimension; FBG, fasting blood glucose; FTSS, five times sit to stand test; HDL, high-density lipoprotein; HR, heart rate; IRF, inpatient rehabilitation facility; ISWT, incremental shuttle walk test; LDL, low-density lipoprotein; LDL-C, low-density lipoprotein cholesterol; MET, metabolic equivalent; MET-min, metabolic equivalent minutes; MIN, minutes; NDS, non-disabling stroke; NR, not reported; NSS, non-statistically significant; PM&R, physical medicine and rehabilitation; PT, physical therapy; RCT, randomized clinical trial; RPE, rating of perceived exertion; RPM, revolutions per minute; SBP, systolic blood pressure; SF, short form health survey; SIS, stroke impact scale; SLS, single leg stance; TC, total cholesterol; TIA, transient ischemic attack; TUG, timed up and go; VAS, visual analog scale; VO₂ peak, peak oxygen uptake.

treadmill walking, and cycling, among others.[35,36,54,56,58] Some studies also incorporated resistance training exercises and activities designed to enhance balance and mobility.[21,56] The intensity of the exercise program was also varied, with the majority of them being in the mild-to-moderate level. The studies reviewed included stroke patients at various stages of their recovery, including the early subacute phase[20,21,27,34,54,56] and the chronic phase.[19,24,36] This indicates that aerobic exercise and CR programs can be implemented at different stages of recovery with no significant risks for patients.

Importantly, many studies included stroke patients into the existing traditional CR programs, making necessary modifications and adaptations to suit the unique needs of stroke patients. Some studies conducted in Europe, Canada, and the United States had stroke patients participate in the traditional center-based CR program and exercised alongside cardiac patients with no modifications.[19,22,24,37] The ability of stroke patients to perform diverse forms of exercise and the successful adaptation of existing programs to include stroke patients suggests the feasibility of this approach.

The current results demonstrate significant effects of aerobic exercise and CR programs on various health outcomes of stroke survivors, such as improvements in cardiovascular health (eg, V_{O_2} peak, blood pressure, serum biomarkers),[22,27,37,38,54] physical function (eg, walking distance, muscle strength, MET-minutes, balance, and endurance),[20,37,55,56] cognitive function, memory, quality of life, and mood.[20,24,53,56] In addition, some studies showed significant effects on major clinical outcomes, such as rehospitalization rates and mortality of stroke patients.[20]

In summary, the studies reviewed provide compelling evidence supporting the feasibility and effectiveness of aerobic exercise and CR programs for stroke patients. The inclusion of stroke patients at various stages of recovery and with diverse deficits underscores the potential of these programs to improve various aspects of physical and cognitive function, quality of life, and overall health outcomes in the stroke population.

DISCUSSION

A large body of data available in the literature provides strong evidence regarding the positive impact of aerobic exercise on health improvements for stroke survivors. These studies highlight the importance of implementing aerobic exercise in poststroke rehabilitation. Aerobic exercise training is a safe and effective intervention for stroke survivors across various stages of recovery that leads to improved cardiovascular function, cardiovascular capacity, peak oxygen uptake, walking distance, and physical and cognitive function. According to a recent systematic review and meta-analysis, stroke survivors improve their aerobic capacity by participating in aerobic exercise programs that match the dosage of US CR programs, regardless of the specific type of aerobic activity undertaken.[28] Improving cardiovascular function can enable patients to increase their participation in neurorehabilitation potentially leading to better recovery outcomes. It is important to emphasize that with aerobic exercise, as with any exercise regimen, risk assessment, adapted approach, and oversight by qualified health care providers are necessary to guarantee the safety and efficacy of the program for every patient.

Aerobic exercise is the main component of the well-established traditional medically supervised CR program. CR is a comprehensive structured program that includes risk factor education and counseling in addition to exercise training to improve cardiovascular health. Risk factor education and counseling on nutrition, stress management, smoking cessation, and other lifestyle factors play a significant role in improving health outcomes. The multifaceted approach of CR has been shown to reduce hospital readmissions, secondary events (cardiac events, reinfarction), and mortality of patients with cardiovascular diseases.[25,26,57] Current evidence demonstrates that programs modeled after CR can also provide significant benefits for patients with stroke or transient ischemic attack at all stages of recovery, from subacute to chronic stages.[19-21,24,59] Implementation of these programs can help to improve cardiovascular function, enhance the overall quality of life, and reduce the risk of future cardiovascular events, rehospitalizations, and mortality of stroke patients.[20,32] In addition, these programs can also improve other aspects of physical and mental health, such as mobility, balance, mood, and cognitive function.[20,24,53,56] Thus, CR-based programs are an effective approach to stroke recovery, offering a range of benefits that extend beyond cardiovascular health.

Even though aerobic exercise provides strong benefits to stroke patients, it cannot be regarded as a replacement for conventional neurorehabilitation programs or their medical treatments but rather serve as an addition. Similarly, stroke survivors require customized neurorehabilitation that specifically addresses their individual functional needs. For stroke survivors to achieve their highest level of recovery, it is necessary to provide them with programs that focus on their functional needs and that improve their cardiovascular function. Several studies have demonstrated that the incorporation of cardiovascular exercise in addition to standard-of-care therapies for stroke patients is feasible, safe, and results in significant health benefits.[20,23,33,37,55]

Adaptation of existing CR programs for stroke survivors can be a cost-effective way to provide a proven rehabilitation model that has already been shown to provide significant health benefits in patients with cardiac disease. By using existing infrastructure and resources, such as exercise equipment and trained personnel, rehabilitation programs for stroke survivors can be implemented nationally relatively easily and more cost-effectively.

Currently, various obstacles prevent stroke patients from participating in CR programs. These barriers may include physical limitations, difficulties with cognitive functioning, and existing comorbidities. Functional challenges can be a significant barrier for stroke patients seeking to participate in traditional CR programs. For example, they may have difficulty with mobility, balance, and coordination, which can make it challenging to perform certain exercises or activities. Modifications to the exercise program may be necessary to accommodate these challenges. Another barrier currently existing is the lack of clinicians' confidence and comfort level in prescribing safe and effective aerobic exercise for stroke patients.[32,53,60] The existing neurorehabilitation programs do not address the cardiovascular health of stroke patients. Addressing these barriers is essential for promoting successful rehabilitation outcomes for stroke patients. Providing support and resources can help ensure that stroke survivors receive the care they need to fully recover and regain their independence.

Most importantly lack of funding is a significant barrier for stroke patients to participate in CR programs in the United States. In Canada and Australia, most traditional CR programs currently accept patients with stroke.[61,62] The results of implementing CR programs for stroke survivors demonstrate significant improvements in various health parameters, such as cardiovascular health, muscular strength, and mobility. Overall, the successful implementation of CR programs in Canada for stroke survivors, traditional CR programs, or adapted programs for patients with functional limitations emphasizes the importance of individualized rehabilitation programs that cater to the unique needs of each patient in achieving positive health outcomes.

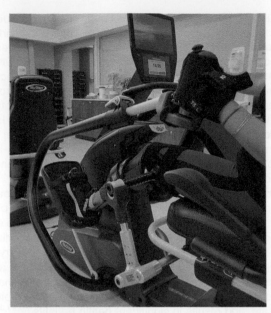

Fig. 2. A patient on the recumbent exercise bike with hand and leg accommodations.

Several studies have demonstrated the successful adaptation of CR programs for stroke patients. These adaptations may include the use of recumbent cross-trainer bikes with a thigh cuff and foot plate strap to support leg weakness and a hand mitt to support arm weakness, a chair with seatbelt support if necessary, and assistance with transfers on and off the machines (**Fig. 2**). During the sessions, patients can remain on the recumbent cross-trainer bike for at least 31 minutes, alternating between using both arms and legs, only the arms, and only the legs. This approach eliminates the need to transfer the patients to multiple pieces of equipment during the rehabilitation sessions.

Although there is abundant evidence demonstrating the benefits of aerobic exercise and programs modeled after CR for stroke survivors during their recovery, it is unfortunate that Medicare reimbursement for CR programs is not currently available to stroke patients. Research studies examining the efficacy and cost-effectiveness of adding stroke to the list of compliant CR diagnoses are vital to fill this gap. The future direction of research needs to focus on generating data-driven evidence to support policy change, which will add stroke to the list of compliant diagnoses for CR programs funded by the Centers for Medicare and Medicaid Services. This policy change would enable stroke patients to access the same beneficial program that is currently available to patients with other cardiovascular conditions.

SUMMARY

Implementation of a CR program for stroke survivors can potentially make a substantial impact on public health at a national level. Adapting a rehabilitation program modeled after CR to meet the needs of stroke survivors can be an effective approach to enhance recovery outcomes for stroke survivors, reduce the risk of future cardiovascular and cerebrovascular events, and decrease the economical strain that stroke places on society.

CLINICS CARE POINTS

- The incorporation of aerobic exercise in poststroke rehabilitation significantly improves cardiovascular fitness, strength, balance, and overall functional ability in stroke survivors.

- It is well-known that cardiac patients benefit greatly from a structured cardiac rehabilitation program. Patients with stroke have similar risk factors as cardiac disease and therefore will benefit similarly from having this comprehensive program in addition to neurorehabilitation.

- The implementation of strategies modeled after cardiac rehabilitation for stroke survivors has the potential to make a significant national impact on public health by improving outcomes for people with stroke and reducing the economical burden of stroke on society.

DISCLOSURE

The authors have no disclosures related to this work.

REFERENCES

1. Tsao CW, Aday AW, Almarzooq ZI, et al. Heart Disease and Stroke Statistics—2022 Update: A Report From the American Heart Association. Circulation 2022; 145(8). https://doi.org/10.1161/CIR.0000000000001052.
2. James SL, Abate D, Abate KH, et al. Global, regional, and national incidence, prevalence, and years lived with disability for 354 diseases and injuries for 195 countries and territories, 1990–2017: a systematic analysis for the Global Burden of Disease Study 2017. Lancet 2018;392(10159):1789–858.
3. Tieges Z, Mead G, Allerhand M, et al. Sedentary Behavior in the First Year After Stroke: A Longitudinal Cohort Study With Objective Measures. Arch Phys Med Rehabil 2015;96(1):15–23.
4. Fini NA, Bernhardt J, Said CM, et al. How to Address Physical Activity Participation After Stroke in Research and Clinical Practice. Stroke 2021;52(6). https://doi.org/10.1161/STROKEAHA.121.034557.
5. Stinear CM, Lang CE, Zeiler S, et al. Advances and challenges in stroke rehabilitation. Lancet Neurol 2020;19(4):348–60.
6. Chen Y, Abel KT, Janecek JT, et al. Home-based technologies for stroke rehabilitation: A systematic review. Int J Med Inf 2019;123:11–22.
7. Di Pino G, Pellegrino G, Assenza G, et al. Modulation of brain plasticity in stroke: a novel model for neurorehabilitation. Nat Rev Neurol 2014;10(10):597–608.
8. Silva GS, Schwamm LH. Advances in Stroke: Digital Health. Stroke 2022;53(3): 1004–7.
9. MacKay-Lyons MJ, Makrides L. Exercise capacity early after stroke. Arch Phys Med Rehabil 2002;83(12):1697–702.
10. Virani SS, Alonso A, Aparicio HJ, et al. Heart Disease and Stroke Statistics—2021 Update: A Report From the American Heart Association. Circulation 2021; 143(8). https://doi.org/10.1161/CIR.0000000000000950.
11. Scheitz JF, Sposato LA, Schulz-Menger J, et al. Stroke–Heart Syndrome: Recent Advances and Challenges. J Am Heart Assoc 2022;11(17):e026528.
12. Buckley BJR, Harrison SL, Hill A, et al. Stroke-Heart Syndrome: Incidence and Clinical Outcomes of Cardiac Complications Following Stroke. Stroke 2022;53(5):1759–63.
13. Tang A, Sibley KM, Thomas SG, et al. Maximal Exercise Test Results in Subacute Stroke. Arch Phys Med Rehabil 2006;87(8):1100–5.

14. Baert I, Daly D, Dejaeger E, et al. Evolution of Cardiorespiratory Fitness After Stroke: A 1-Year Follow-Up Study. Influence of Prestroke Patients' Characteristics and Stroke-Related Factors. Arch Phys Med Rehabil 2012;93(4):669–76.

15. Saunders DH, Sanderson M, Hayes S, et al. Physical fitness training for stroke patients. Cochrane Stroke Group. Cochrane Database Syst Rev 2016. https://doi.org/10.1002/14651858.CD003316.pub6.

16. Pang MYC, Charlesworth SA, Lau RWK, et al. Using Aerobic Exercise to Improve Health Outcomes and Quality of Life in Stroke: Evidence-Based Exercise Prescription Recommendations. Cerebrovasc Dis 2013;35(1):7–22.

17. Billinger SA, Arena R, Bernhardt J, et al. Physical Activity and Exercise Recommendations for Stroke Survivors: A Statement for Healthcare Professionals From the American Heart Association/American Stroke Association. Stroke 2014;45(8):2532–53.

18. Winstein CJ, Stein J, Arena R, et al. Guidelines for Adult Stroke Rehabilitation and Recovery: A Guideline for Healthcare Professionals From the American Heart Association/American Stroke Association. Stroke 2016;47(6). https://doi.org/10.1161/STR.0000000000000098.

19. Marzolini S, Danells C, Oh PI, et al. Feasibility and Effects of Cardiac Rehabilitation for Individuals after Transient Ischemic Attack. J Stroke Cerebrovasc Dis 2016;25(10):2453–63.

20. Cuccurullo SJ, Fleming TK, Zinonos S, et al. Stroke Recovery Program with Modified Cardiac Rehabilitation Improves Mortality, Functional & Cardiovascular Performance. J Stroke Cerebrovasc Dis Off J Natl Stroke Assoc 2022;31(5):106322.

21. Clague-Baker N, Robinson T, Gillies CL, et al. Adapted cardiac rehabilitation for people with sub-acute, mild-to-moderate stroke: a mixed methods feasibility study. Physiotherapy 2022;115:93–101.

22. Lennon O, Gallagher A, Cooney H, et al. A COMPARISON OF CARDIAC REHABILITATION FOR NON-DISABLING STROKE AND CARDIAC CONDITIONS: OUTCOMES AND HEALTHCARE PROFESSIONALS' PERCEPTIONS. EMJ Interv Cardiol. Published online November 2020;17:26–38.

23. Reynolds H, Steinfort S, Tillyard J, et al. Feasibility and adherence to moderate intensity cardiovascular fitness training following stroke: a pilot randomized controlled trial. BMC Neurol 2021;21(1):132.

24. Regan EW, Handlery R, Stewart JC, et al. Integrating Survivors of Stroke Into Exercise-Based Cardiac Rehabilitation Improves Endurance and Functional Strength. J Am Heart Assoc 2021;10(3):e017907.

25. Lawler PR, Filion KB, Eisenberg MJ. Efficacy of exercise-based cardiac rehabilitation post–myocardial infarction: A systematic review and meta-analysis of randomized controlled trials. Am Heart J 2011;162(4):571–84.e2.

26. Anderson L, Oldridge N, Thompson DR, et al. Exercise-Based Cardiac Rehabilitation for Coronary Heart Disease. J Am Coll Cardiol 2016;67(1):1–12.

27. Billinger SA, Mattlage AE, Ashenden AL, et al. Aerobic Exercise in Subacute Stroke Improves Cardiovascular Health and Physical Performance. J Neurol Phys Ther 2012;36(4):159–65.

28. Regan EW, Handlery R, Beets MW, et al. Are Aerobic Programs Similar in Design to Cardiac Rehabilitation Beneficial for Survivors of Stroke? A Systematic Review and Meta-Analysis. J Am Heart Assoc 2019;8(16):e012761.

29. Cuccurullo SJ, Fleming TK, Kostis JB, et al. Impact of Modified Cardiac Rehabilitation Within a Stroke Recovery Program on All-Cause Hospital Readmissions. Am J Phys Med Rehabil 2022;101(1):40–7.

30. Cuccurullo SJ, Fleming TK, Kostis WJ, et al. Impact of a Stroke Recovery Program Integrating Modified Cardiac Rehabilitation on All-Cause Mortality, Cardiovascular Performance and Functional Performance. Am J Phys Med Rehabil 2019;98(11):953–63.

31. CDC. Published April 27, 2023. https://www.cdc.gov/nchs/nhis/physical_activity/pa_glossary.htm.

32. Marzolini S. Including Patients With Stroke in Cardiac Rehabilitation: BARRIERS AND FACILITATORS. J Cardiopulm Rehabil Prev 2020;40(5):294–301.

33. Tang A, Sibley KM, Thomas SG, et al. Effects of an Aerobic Exercise Program on Aerobic Capacity, Spatiotemporal Gait Parameters, and Functional Capacity in Subacute Stroke. Neurorehabil Neural Repair 2009;23(4):398–406.

34. Saunders DH, Sanderson M, Hayes S, et al. Physical Fitness Training for Patients With Stroke. Stroke 2020;51(11). https://doi.org/10.1161/STROKEAHA.120.030826.

35. Tang A, Marzolini S, Oh P, et al. Feasibility and effects of adapted cardiac rehabilitation after stroke: a prospective trial. BMC Neurol 2010;10:40.

36. Calmels P, Degache F, Courbon A, et al. The faisability and the effects of cyclo-ergometer interval-training on aerobic capacity and walking performance after stroke. Preliminary study. Ann Phys Rehabil Med 2011;54(1):3–15.

37. Prior PL, Hachinski V, Unsworth K, et al. Comprehensive Cardiac Rehabilitation for Secondary Prevention After Transient Ischemic Attack or Mild Stroke: I: Feasibility and Risk Factors. Stroke 2011;42(11):3207–13.

38. Garber CE, Blissmer B, Deschenes MR, et al. Quantity and Quality of Exercise for Developing and Maintaining Cardiorespiratory, Musculoskeletal, and Neuromotor Fitness in Apparently Healthy Adults: Guidance for Prescribing Exercise. Med Sci Sports Exerc 2011;43(7):1334–59.

39. Myers J. Exercise and Cardiovascular Health. Circulation 2003;107(1). https://doi.org/10.1161/01.CIR.0000048890.59383.8D.

40. Xing Y, Bai Y. A Review of Exercise-Induced Neuroplasticity in Ischemic Stroke: Pathology and Mechanisms. Mol Neurobiol 2020;57(10):4218–31.

41. El-Sayes J, Harasym D, Turco CV, et al. Exercise-Induced Neuroplasticity: A Mechanistic Model and Prospects for Promoting Plasticity. Neuroscientist 2019; 25(1):65–85.

42. Cramer SC, Sur M, Dobkin BH, et al. Harnessing neuroplasticity for clinical applications. Brain 2011;134(6):1591–609.

43. MacKay-Lyons M, Billinger SA, Eng JJ, et al. Aerobic Exercise Recommendations to Optimize Best Practices in Care After Stroke: AEROBICS 2019 Update. Phys Ther 2020;100(1):149–56.

44. Kleindorfer DO, Towfighi A, Chaturvedi S, et al. 2021 Guideline for the Prevention of Stroke in Patients With Stroke and Transient Ischemic Attack: A Guideline From the American Heart Association/American Stroke Association. Stroke 2021;52(7). https://doi.org/10.1161/STR.0000000000000375.

45. Simon M, Korn K, Cho L, et al. Cardiac rehabilitation: A class 1 recommendation. Cleve Clin J Med 2018;85(7):551–8.

46. Supervia M, Turk-Adawi K, Lopez-Jimenez F, et al. Nature of Cardiac Rehabilitation Around the Globe. EClinicalMedicine 2019;13:46–56.

47. American Association of Cardiovascular & Pulmonary Rehabilitation. In: Guidelines for cardiac rehabilitation programs. 6th edition. Champaign: Human Kinetics; 2021.

48. Balady GJ, Williams MA, Ades PA, et al. Core Components of Cardiac Rehabilitation/Secondary Prevention Programs: 2007 Update: A Scientific Statement From the American Heart Association Exercise, Cardiac Rehabilitation, and

Prevention Committee, the Council on Clinical Cardiology; the Councils on Cardiovascular Nursing, Epidemiology and Prevention, and Nutrition, Physical Activity, and Metabolism; and the American Association of Cardiovascular and Pulmonary Rehabilitation. Circulation 2007;115(20):2675–82.

49. Bellmann B, Lin T, Greissinger K, et al. The Beneficial Effects of Cardiac Rehabilitation. Cardiol Ther 2020;9(1):35–44.

50. Supervised Exercise Therapy (SET) for Symptomatic Peripheral Artery Disease (PAD). https://www.cms.gov/medicare-coverage-database/view/ncacal-decision-memo.aspx?proposed=N&NCAId=287.

51. Adams RJ, Chimowitz MI, Alpert JS, et al. Coronary risk evaluation in patients with transient ischemic attack and ischemic stroke: a scientific statement for healthcare professionals from the Stroke Council and the Council on Clinical Cardiology of the American Heart Association/American Stroke Association. Stroke 2003; 34(9):2310–22.

52. Lloyd-Jones DM, Allen NB, Anderson CAM, et al. Life's Essential 8: Updating and Enhancing the American Heart Association's Construct of Cardiovascular Health: A Presidential Advisory From the American Heart Association. Circulation 2022; 146(5):e18–43.

53. Boyne P, Billinger S, MacKay-Lyons M, et al. Aerobic Exercise Prescription in Stroke Rehabilitation: A Web-Based Survey of US Physical Therapists. J Neurol Phys Ther JNPT 2017;41(2):119–28.

54. Sandberg K, Kleist M, Falk L, et al. Effects of Twice-Weekly Intense Aerobic Exercise in Early Subacute Stroke: A Randomized Controlled Trial. Arch Phys Med Rehabil 2016;97(8):1244–53.

55. Kirk H, Kersten P, Crawford P, et al. The cardiac model of rehabilitation for reducing cardiovascular risk factors post transient ischaemic attack and stroke: a randomized controlled trial. Clin Rehabil 2014;28(4):339–49.

56. Vanroy C, Feys H, Swinnen A, et al. Effectiveness of Active Cycling in Subacute Stroke Rehabilitation: A Randomized Controlled Trial. Arch Phys Med Rehabil 2017;98(8):1576–85.e5.

57. Long L, Mordi IR, Bridges C, et al. Exercise-based cardiac rehabilitation for adults with heart failure. Cochrane Heart Group. Cochrane Database Syst Rev 2019;2019(1). https://doi.org/10.1002/14651858.CD003331.pub5.

58. MacKay-Lyons M, Gubitz G, Phillips S, et al. Program of Rehabilitative Exercise and Education to Avert Vascular Events After Non-Disabling Stroke or Transient Ischemic Attack (PREVENT Trial): A Randomized Controlled Trial. Neurorehabil Neural Repair 2022;36(2):119–30.

59. Orme MW, Clague-Baker NJ, Richardson M, et al. Does cardiac rehabilitation for people with stroke in the sub-acute phase of recovery lead to physical behaviour change? Results from compositional analysis of accelerometry-derived data. Physiotherapy 2020;107:234–42.

60. Bayley MT, Hurdowar A, Richards CL, et al. Barriers to implementation of stroke rehabilitation evidence: findings from a multi-site pilot project. Disabil Rehabil 2012;34(19):1633–8.

61. Howes T, Mahenderan N, Freene N. Cardiac Rehabilitation: Are People With Stroke or Transient Ischaemic Attack Being Included? A Cross-Sectional Survey. Heart Lung Circ 2020;29(3):483–90.

62. Toma J, Hammond B, Chan V, et al. Inclusion of People Poststroke in Cardiac Rehabilitation Programs in Canada: A Missed Opportunity for Referral. CJC Open 2020;2(4):195–206.

Neurostimulation After Stroke

Hala Osman, PhD[a,b,1], Ricardo Siu, PhD[a,c,1],
Nathan S. Makowski, PhD[a,b,c], Jayme S. Knutson, PhD[a,c,d],
David A. Cunningham, PhD[a,c,d],*

KEYWORDS

- Transcranial direct current stimulation • Repetitive transcranial magnetic stimulation
- Functional electrical stimulation • Vagus nerve stimulation • Motor impairment
- Stroke rehabilitation

KEY POINTS

- Neural stimulation has been commonly applied with stroke survivors both as a therapeutic tool and as an assistive device.
- Targeted neural stimulation to promote neuroplasticity can benefit recovery and help the nervous system relearn abilities that have been lost after stroke.
- Neural stimulation technology is used to allow stroke survivors to participate in functional task practice, despite poor functional motor abilities.

INTRODUCTION

Fifty percent of stroke survivors are reported to have motor and functional limitations.[1] Although some motor function recovery usually occurs, full recovery is rare. The most rapid recovery occurs within the first month, and by 3- to 6-month poststroke, progress, typically plateaus and disabilities, remains a life-long issue. Targeted rehabilitation, including task-specific repetitive training based on the principles of motor learning and neuroplasticity, can benefit recovery and help the nervous system relearn abilities that have been lost after stroke.[2] Therefore, it is important for motor recovery rehabilitation to facilitate neuroplasticity to improve functional capacity. However, these therapies may take a long time to show progress, and some patients may have physical limitations that prevent them from participating fully in the therapy.

[a] MetroHealth Center for Rehabilitation Research, 4229 Pearl Dr, Cleveland, OH 44109, USA; [b] APT Center, 10701 East Boulevard, Cleveland, OH 44106, USA; [c] Department of Physical Medicine and Rehabilitation, Case Western Reserve University, 9501 Euclid Avenue, Cleveland, OH 44106, USA; [d] Cleveland FES Center, 10701 East Boulevard, Cleveland, OH 44106, USA
[1] These authors contributed equally.
* Corresponding author. 4229 Pearl Road, Cleveland, OH 44109.
E-mail address: Dxc536@case.edu

Phys Med Rehabil Clin N Am 35 (2024) 369–382
https://doi.org/10.1016/j.pmr.2023.06.008
1047-9651/24/© 2023 Elsevier Inc. All rights reserved.

pmr.theclinics.com

To address these challenges, researchers are exploring strategies that target the central nervous system (CNS) to augment the neuroplastic potential of occupational and physical therapeutic strategies. By facilitating the brain's ability to reorganize and form new connections, these strategies aim to improve functional recovery. In addition, neural stimulation technology is being developed as a supportive technology to allow stroke survivors to participate in functional task practice, despite poor functional motor abilities.

In this article, the authors first discuss neural stimulation targeting the CNS via noninvasive brain stimulation (NIBS) techniques, repetitive transcranial magnetic stimulation (rTMS), and transcranial direct current stimulation (tDCS) as well as with vagus nerve stimulation (VNS). The authors then discuss neural stimulation targeting the peripheral nervous system. The authors explore the application of peripheral neuromuscular electrical stimulation as a technology for both therapeutic and assistive purposes. Here, the authors review three applications that exemplify these principles: functional electrical stimulation (FES), neuromuscular electrical stimulation (NMES), and transcutaneous electrical nerve stimulation (TENS).

Throughout this article, the authors review the mechanisms of action for each technology, efficacy and safety, and Food and Drug Administration (FDA) status when applicable. The authors also highlight how these approaches can improve recovery and their limitations.

NONINVASIVE BRAIN STIMULATION

NIBS technologies aim to modulate cortical firing rate by directly generating an electric field or by indirectly doing so through a magnetic field which produces an electric field at the level of the cortex without the need for surgery. NIBS modulates the target's spontaneous firing rate to decrease or increase neural excitability. Studies suggest that NIBS approaches to treat poststroke impairments increase brain circuitry's neuroplastic capabilities, restoring and/or building new connections that supplement or replace those lost due to the vascular injury. Because NIBS increases potential for plasticity rather than driving the plastic changes themselves, it must be paired with adjunctive rehabilitation approaches to generate positive functional changes.[3]

The application of NIBS is largely based on conceptual models of adaptive and maladaptive neuroplasticity after stroke, with the most common approach being the interhemispheric competition model.[4] This model suggests that increased activation of the non-lesioned hemisphere leads to excessive inhibition of the primary motor cortex of the lesioned hemisphere. Therefore, the model suggests that paresis arises due to the diminished corticospinal output to the weakened limb and is exacerbated by interhemispheric imbalances between the two hemispheres. To enhance rehabilitative outcomes, NIBS methods have primarily focused on increasing excitability in the affected hemisphere while reducing excitability in the unaffected hemisphere either during or before physical/occupational therapy. However, recent evidence indicates that two important factors need to be considered.[5] First, the interhemispheric competition model seems to be applicable specifically during the chronic phase of stroke, that is, greater than 6-month poststroke. Second, the interhemispheric imbalances might actually reflect the brain's recovery progress and/or result from reduced utilization of the paretic limb, rather than directly impacting motor function. Consequently, there is now growing uncertainty whether these imbalances should be targeted as a therapeutic intervention for all patients.

Newer poststroke models, such as the bimodal balance recovery model, provide different patient-specific NIBS approaches.[6,7] The bimodal balance-recovery model links reorganization patterns following stroke to the extent of damage to the lesioned hemisphere and pathways. When damage is mild, the lesioned hemisphere mainly contributes to recovery, and the non-lesioned hemisphere contributes to upper limb paresis. Conversely, if the damage is severe, the non-lesioned hemisphere may take the primary role in the recovery of paretic upper limb function via uncrossed ipsilateral pathways. Several groups have tested the efficacy of facilitating the non-lesioned hemisphere based on this model for patients with more severe motor impairments.[7–10] The following sections introduce rTMS and tDCS and provide a broad overview of their clinical applications, safety, and current regulatory status.

Repetitive Transcranial Magnetic Stimulation

rTMS is a noninvasive technique that uses an electromagnetic coil placed above the scalp (**Fig. 1**A), through which a brief alternating current is passed.[11] This generates a rapidly pulsed magnetic field that passes through the skull and into the brain, inducing current within the targeted area and electrically stimulating neural tissue up to approximately 1.5 cm deep into the brain. The extent of the stimulated region varies with the shape of the coil.[12] In stroke rehabilitation research, rTMS is usually set up to target the primary motor cortex, although studies targeting other cortical regions, such as the premotor cortex[8,13,14] and prefrontal cortex,[15] are ongoing or have been investigated. Typically, rTMS is applied for 10 to 30 minutes before a rehabilitation session at subthreshold intensities in an attempt to increase susceptibility to plasticity from training.[11] Depending on the frequency of the pulses being delivered, it is possible to either increase or decrease corticospinal excitability. At stimulation frequencies above 5 Hz, corticospinal excitability is increased, likely due to an increase in synaptic strength of the target area. However, frequencies at approximately 1 Hz tend to have an inhibitory effect, likely due to a decrease in synaptic strength.[3] rTMS has also been delivered to match theta rhythms in the brain, known as theta burst stimulation (TBS). There are two primary patterns of TBS: continuous TBS (cTBS) and intermittent TBS (iTBS). iTBS is applied in bursts of three at a frequency of 50 Hz for a total of 2 seconds, where there are 10-second intervals between each set of stimulation. cTBS is similar except the bursts of stimulation are applied continuously without the 10-second intervals. iTBS is considered to have an excitatory effect, and cTBS is considered to have an inhibitory effect.[16]

Clinical applications

Poststroke rTMS studies have primarily focused on upper limb motor recovery along with adjunctive therapies such as physical and occupational therapies. Two recent meta-analyses have concluded a general positive effect of rTMS on motor recovery. He and colleagues[16] included 20 randomized controlled trials (RCTs) with a total

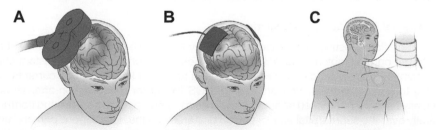

Fig. 1. Neural stimulation targeting the corticomotor system. (*A*) Repetitive transcranial magnetic stimulation, (*B*) transcranial direct current stimulation, and (*C*) implanted vagus nerve stimulation. (Illustration by Emily Imka. © 2023 Cleveland FES Center, Cleveland, OH.)

841 stroke participants and concluded that inhibitory rTMS (<1 Hz) targeting the contralesional hemisphere has a positive effect on grip strength and lower limb function as assessed by the Fugl–Meyer assessment. Zhang and colleagues[17] included 34 RCTs with a total of 904 participants and concluded that rTMS is beneficial for upper limb motor function, where 11 studies (310 participants) showed a benefit long-term (assessments made at or after 1 month). Further, they report that iTBS is more beneficial than cTBS, low-frequency rTMS targeting the contralesional hemisphere is more beneficial than high-frequency rTMS targeting the ipsilesional hemisphere, and participants with subcortical lesions are more likely to benefit than other lesion sites (ie, cortical lesions). Of note, more pronounced effects were reported when rTMS was administered during the acute phase of stroke. However, it remains challenging to separate the effects of NIBS from spontaneous recovery during the early and intermediate phases following a stroke event.

Still, there are major challenges that are currently under investigation. These challenges include heterogeneity in the patient population, etiology, location, and spread of the vascular injury. In addition, more research needs to be done to optimize the delivery of rTMS with regard to adequate dosing, timing of the intervention in terms of time since injury, duration of treatment, and optimization of stimulation parameters.[18] For a full list and history of US FDA milestones for TMS devices, refer to Cohen and colleagues.[19]

Safety/FDA status

Side effects include local transient scalp pain and discomfort (39%), sleepiness, and mild headaches (28%), which tend to quickly subside after stimulation. In rare instances (<1%), seizures have occurred as a result of rTMS. To reduce the risk of seizures, the patient's history of seizures and their drug and substance use should be taken into consideration. This and many other safety guidelines have led to a decrease in onset of seizures caused by rTMS.[11,20] Absolute contraindications include metal in the head and implanted electrical devices in close contact to the discharging coil (ie, cochlear implants, internal pulse generator or medication pumps). Other contraindications to consider based on risk/benefit ratio include epilepsy or history of convulsion or a seizure, use of medications that lower the seizure threshold, history of fainting spells, severe head trauma, hearing problems or ringing in the ears, and pregnancy. rTMS is classified as a Class II device by the FDA and has been approved for the treatment of depression and obsessive compulsive disorder. In addition, single-pulse TMS (Cerena Transcranial Magnetic Stimulator) is approved for the treatment of migraine (The eNeura Therapeutics, Sunnyvale, CA). The FDA approval for use to improve hemiparesis for stroke survivors has not yet been attained. For a full list and history of US FDA milestones for TMS devices, refer to Cohen and colleagues.[19]

Transcranial Direct Current Stimulation

tDCS modulates resting membrane potentials by applying a constant direct current to the target cortical regions (**Fig. 1**B). Surface electrodes connected to a constant current stimulator are placed on the scalp and used to deliver low-amplitude currents (0–4 mA) to cortical regions. Research using tDCS for motor rehabilitation after stroke typically uses saline-soaked sponges placed on the primary motor cortex and contralaterally over the supraorbital area or placed bilaterally on the homologous primary motor cortices.[21,22] However, studies have applied tDCS to alternate regions such as the premotor cortex.[23–25] More recent research using tDCS have investigated the use of high-density electrode arrays to deliver stimulation that is believed to be more localized, better sustained, and longer-lasting.[26,27] Much like rTMS, the rehabilitative potential of tDCS seems to be greater when delivered in conjunction with other reha-bilitative training approaches.[28-30]

tDCS can have both excitable and inhibitory effects. The current delivered through tDCS is thought to change the resting membrane potentials, changing the threshold at which action potentials are evoked. The direction of the current flow determines the effect, with anodal tDCS being excitatory as it depolarizes the membrane potential and cathodal tDCS being inhibitory as it hyperpolarizes the membrane potential.[31] Preclinical research has shown that the application of tDCS in conjunction with motor learning induces long-term potentiation/depression-like plasticity, increasing the syn-aptic connections involved in that task through brain-derived neurotrophic factor (BDNF) and possibly gamma-aminobutyric acid (GABA)-related mechanisms.[32-34]

Clinical applications

There has been growing interest in the use of tDCS to help restore motor function after stroke, including upper and lower extremity motor recovery. Typically, tDCS applied during the chronic phase of stroke is most effective.[21] In regard to upper limb motor recovery, multiple studies have shown evidence that anodal (excitatory) tDCS applied to the ipsilesional motor cortex alongside motor training resulted in greater improve-ments in upper limb motor function compared with motor training alone.[22,28,35] A recent meta-analysis of eight RCTs with a total of 213 stroke subjects[21] concluded that tDCS produces superior motor recovery compared with sham stimulation and found a positive dose–response relationship, with electrode sizes and current ampli-tudes that produce higher current and charge densities being superior (ie, smaller electrode size). Also, studies that used the bihemispheric montage (anodal tDCS to the ipsilesional hemisphere + cathodal [inhibitory] tDCS to the contralesional hemi-sphere) compared with unilateral montage (anodal tDCS to the ipsilesional hemi-sphere or cathodal tDCS to the contralesional hemisphere) had the largest improvements.[22]

Although research on the use of tDCS for lower limb motor recovery after stroke is less extensive, a systematic review has shown that tDCS with physiotherapy focused on gait training leads to improvements in gait parameters, static and dynamic balance, and lower limb function,[36] whereas tDCS with gait training has shown improvements in functional metrics such as 6-minute walking test and 10-minute walking test.[36,37] Still, future research is required to determine which tDCS montage is most effective for lower limb recovery (ie, anodal tDCS to the ipsilesional hemisphere, cathodal tDCS to the contralesional hemisphere, or bihemispheric tDCS).

Despite the promising results, the same challenges that affect rTMS need to be addressed for tDCS before it can be widely used as a rehabilitative treatment for post-stroke motor impairments. These include optimizing the stimulation parameters, dosing, timing of the intervention, and patient selection based on the site and extent of the stroke lesion.

Safety/FDA status

Common side effects of tDCS include moderate fatigue (35%), transient mild head-aches (11.8%), and tingling of the scalp at the stimulation location.[38] However, unlike rTMS, there have been no reported instances of seizures when using tDCS. In 2016, a report based on 33,000 sessions of tDCS found no evidence for irreversible injury pro-duced by tDCS sessions lasting up to 40 minutes with stimulation intensities of up to 4 mA.[39] Absolute contraindications include metal in the head and implanted electrical devices in close contact to the electrodes (ie, cochlear implants, internal pulse gener-ator, or medication pumps). Other contraindications to consider based on risk/benefit ratio include epilepsy or history of convulsion or a seizure, use of medications that lower the seizure threshold, history of fainting spells, severe head trauma, hearing problems or ringing in the ears, and pregnancy. The FDA classifies tDCS as a Class II device and, as of the writing of this article, has yet to approve its use outside of an investigational setting.

Vagus Nerve Stimulation

VNS is an emerging neuromodulatory approach for poststroke upper limb motor recovery. VNS involves delivering electrical current to the vagus nerve, either invasively with the use of an implanted stimulator and cuff electrodes (**Fig. 1**C) or noninvasively using an external stimulator with surface electrodes. VNS is hypothesized to invoke neuroplasticity via cholinergic and noradrenergic modulation through afferent inputs to the nucleus tractus solitarius, which in turn project to the cholinergic neurons within the nucleus basalis and noradrenergic neurons in the locus coeruleus.[40] Both of these areas are highly networked in wide areas of the cortex, including the motor network. Similar to rTMS and tDCS, the rehabilitative potential of VNS seems to be greater when delivered in conjunction with other rehabilitative training approaches.

The investigation of optimal stimulation parameters is still ongoing. Most of the studies have used a stimulation protocol consisting of 0.8 mA, 100 μs pulse width, 20 to 30 Hz pulse frequency, and a pulse train lasting 0.5 seconds delivered every 10 seconds for 30 minutes.[40,41] However, it has been reported that the relationship between pulse frequency and neuroplasticity is an inverted-U-shaped curve. Moderate-frequency pulse trains are reported to improve cortical plasticity, whereas slower and faster pulse rates do not significantly enhance plasticity.[42]

Clinical applications

There have been several clinical studies exploring the efficacy and safety of combining VNS with rehabilitation exercise for treating upper extremity motor deficits in people with chronic stroke.[41,43] The largest trial to date involved 106 participants who were randomly assigned to either VNS treatment with rehabilitation or sham VNS plus rehabilitation. Both groups underwent 300 to 500 repetitions of progressive, functionally relevant exercises per session, three times per week, for 6 weeks followed by a home exercise program. The study found that on the first day after completing in-clinic therapy, the VNS group saw an average increase of 5.0 points in their upper extremity Fugl–Meyer assessment score (UEFM) compared with the control group's increase of 2.4 points.[44] Most recently, Gao and colleagues[43] performed a systematic review and meta-analysis on the effect of motor training with or without concurrent VNS on motor recovery after stroke. Seven RCTs involving 263 stroke patients showed a medium effect size in favor of the VNS group, with nearly half of the VNS group achieving at least an additional six points on the UEFM compared with a quarter of those who underwent training only.

Although VNS shows promise in aiding upper limb motor recovery poststroke, there are still some challenges that need to be addressed as noted by Ward.[45] The need for further research to compare implanted and external devices, determine the optimal dose and type of rehabilitation training that should be used in conjunction with VNS, and last, identify the specific patient phenotype that is most likely to benefit from VNS, including assessing the relevant anatomic pathways.

Safety/FDA status

Recent studies have tested the safety of VNS for patients with chronic stroke. The most common side effects include dysphonia, dysphagia, nausea, skin redness, dysgeusia, and pain related to device implantation.[41] As of the writing of this article, there is currently one VNS device, the ViviStim System (MircroTransponder Inc, Austin TX), which has been FDA-approved to treat moderate to severe upper extremity motor deficits associated with chronic ischemic stroke. The Vivistim System is a prescription device that may be used both in the clinical and at-home setting and is intended to be used in conjunction with rehabilitation exercises.

Peripheral Nerve Stimulation

Peripheral neural stimulation has been commonly used with stroke survivors both as a therapeutic tool and as an assistive device. Electrical currents generate action potentials along the afferent and efferent pathways to generate muscle contractions and send signals back up to the brain. Peripheral stimulation modalities have been described as FES, NMES, and TENS. Differentiating factors are the level of activation and whether stimulation is applied for functional use. FES indicates stimulation is incorporated into a functional task and usually means multiple channels are applied to generate functional movements. NMES describes stimulation that elicits muscle contractions, but is not necessarily part of a functional movement. TENS commonly describes stimulation applied at sub-motor and in some cases sub-sensory thresholds; it is commonly applied for pain, but has not been shown to be efficacious. TENS is explicitly applied through the skin, whereas FES and NMES could be applied with surface or implanted electrodes.

The stimulation devices typically consist of a control unit and at least one pair of electrodes. The control unit contains a wired power supply, a pulse generator, and controls to set stimulus parameters such as frequency, amplitude, and pulse width. The control unit connects to electrodes that are positioned near targeted nerves.[46–48] Stimulators and electrodes have been implemented transcutaneously (surface stimulation) or with implanted components. Surface stimulation systems do not require surgery and have a smaller risk profile. Implanted systems have a more reliable response, can target deeper muscles, and eliminate the need for daily donning and doffing wearable gear. Implanted electrodes also allow bypassing cutaneous sensory receptors, decreasing some discomfort elicited by stimulation.

Peripheral neural stimulation can be implemented either as a therapeutic tool where the individual uses the device as part of therapy and then retains improvements after treatment or as an assistive device or neuroprosthesis where they use the device to assist with daily tasks. It is worth noting that in some cases, there may be therapeutic or exercise benefits from using a device on a daily basis because it allows for an increase in the number of movement repetitions (ie, increase motor therapy dose). Multiple control paradigms have been implemented with stimulation. The simplest is cyclic NMES where stimulation cycles on and off based on preset timers. In addition, stimulation has been triggered by electromyography (EMG) or other sensors such as a button. In research settings, proportional control has been implemented.

Safety considerations

Commercial surface neural stimulation devices, such as NMES devices, are contraindicated for individuals with demand pacemakers, implanted defibrillators, and severely impaired cognition.[48] The concern about interaction with other implanted devices is that the stimuli could interact with other implanted devices, either damaging those devices or preventing their intended effect. This is likely out of an abundance of caution; however, future studies should determine whether this risk is real. Current-controlled surface stimulators have a risk of burns in cases where there is poor electrode contact or a damaged wire due to a high charge density. The benefit of current-controlled devices is that they deliver a consistent current, which is what activates nerves. Voltage-controlled stimulators are less likely to cause injury, but the current delivered varies based on tissue impedance. It is of particular importance that individuals with impaired sensation monitor sites to avoid potential electrical burns. Implanted devices have the same risks as other implants, such as infection. Both implanted and surface stimulation have the risk of eliciting uncomfortable sensations, but this can be mitigated by decreasing the stimulus intensity levels.

Upper Limb Clinical Applications and FDA Status

Upper limb therapy approaches have primarily focused on hand opening. Commercially available NMES devices include the Neuromove (Zynex Medical, Inc, Englewood, CO) and Bioness H200 (Bioventus). An RCT ($n = 122$) in acute stroke survivors (<6 months) found that sensory stimulation (TENS), cyclic NMES, and EMG-triggered NMES for hand opening reduced impairment and improved function, but there were no significant differences between groups.[49]

An emerging FES approach, known as contralaterally controlled FES (CCFES; **Fig 2**), has shown efficacy in recent clinical trials. CCFES uses surface electrodes over the paretic finger and thumb extensors to deliver stimulation with intensity proportional to the degree of volitional opening of the less affected contralateral hand by, traditionally, wearing an instrumented glove. Thus, volitional opening of the non-paretic hand

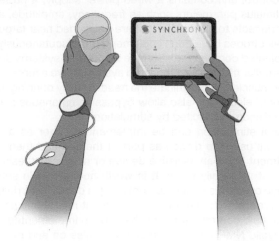

Fig. 2. Example neural stimulation for the upper limb. Contralaterally controlled functional electrical stimulation (CCFES), an innovative method of applying NMES for the upper limb for individuals poststroke. Traditionally, CCFES has consisted of a kinematic sensor glove, stimulation control unit, surface electrodes, and touchscreen interface. However, a wireless model is currently in development (Synapse Biomedical Inc) which replaces the kinematic sensor glove with an optical sensor worn on the less-affected hand (right hand). The optical sensor records movement of the digits and in turn delivers stimulations to the hemiplegic limbs (left hand) with intensity proportional to the degree of volitional opening of the less–affected hand. A touchscreen interface is used to program the stimulator. The CCFES device enables stroke survivors to practice using their paretic hand to perform tasks in therapy and to self-administer hand opening exercises. (Illustration by Emily Imka. © 2023 Cleveland FES Center, Cleveland, OH.)

produces stimulation-assisted opening of the paretic hand, which enables the patient to practice functional tasks with the paretic hand in therapy sessions. A recent meta-analysis of six RCTs with a total of 267 stroke participants concluded that CCFES produces greater improvements in upper extremity hemiplegia when compared with NMES.[50] Owing to the limited number of relevant articles, it is still unclear which stroke recovery phase would benefit the most. The largest study to date included 80 participants with chronic (>6 months) moderate to severe upper limb hemiparesis and reported that the improvements from CCFES were greatest in the subset of participants who were moderately impaired and less than 2 years post-stroke, with 57% achieving clinically relevant gains in dexterity (>8 block increase in the box and block test) compared with 14% of subjects receiving conventional electrical stimulation.[51]

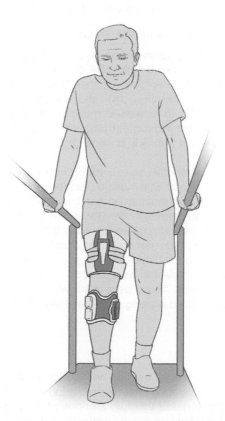

Fig. 3. Example of neural stimulation for the lower limb. The L300 Go is an FES system that incorporates 3D motion detection via an adaptive algorithm to precisely detect gait events. It consists of an ergonomic cuff, a control unit, and gait sensor. The L300 Go provides 3D motion detection of gait, multichannel stimulation and includes a mobile application to track user activity. The device delivers electrical stimulation and uses information from a three-axis gyroscope and accelerometer. Individuals' movement is monitored in all three planes and stimulation is implemented when needed during the gait cycle. The adaptive algorithm accommodates changes in gait dynamics and a high-speed processor deploys stimulation within 10 ms of detecting a valid gait event (with permission; Image courtesy of Bioventus). (Illustration by Emily Imka. © 2023 Cleveland FES Center, Cleveland, OH.)

NMES has also reduced poststroke shoulder pain compared with usual care ($n = 25$).[52] Sprint (SPR Therapeutics, Brooklyn Park, MN) has an FDA-approved percutaneous stimulator; a single electrode was placed to elicit contractions from the posterior and middle deltoid, whereas stimulation was applied for 6 hours a day for 3 weeks. A follow-up study evaluated an implanted pulse generator for individuals who had pain return.[53] Pain significantly reduced for four of the five participants 2 years post-implant.[53] There is no commercial device for this approach, but it could be implemented with a device like the Bioventus StimRouter. TENS has been evaluated for poststroke shoulder pain as well, but was found to be ineffective.[54]

Implanted approaches are also being explored under investigational device exemptions (IDEs). A pilot study ($n = 1$) demonstrated that a 12-channel FES system could generate hand opening and grasp patterns, whereas the user was relaxed, but had difficulty in the presence of simultaneous effort; incorporating nerve block approaches may make this more effective for individuals with severe hemiparesis in the future.[55]

Lower Limb Clinical Applications and FDA Status

FES has been applied to the peroneal nerve to prevent foot drop, both as a therapy and as an assistive device. There are three FDA-approved surface stimulation devices available: Walkaide (Innovative Neurotronics Inc), Odstock Dropped-Foot Stimulator (Salisbury District Hospital, Salisbury, UK), and the L300Go (Bioventus). Although there are physiologic benefits to increased muscle activation, meta-analyses show that both the therapeutic and neuroprosthetic effects are similar to an ankle foot orthosis (AFO).[56,57] It is worth noting that some individuals prefer the form factor of these devices to an AFO.

Companies and researchers have been adding channels to wearable FES systems to determine if activation of additional muscles further improves walking. The Bioness L300Go (**Fig 3**) adds a thigh cuff that can be configured to stimulate the quadriceps or hamstrings. Results ($n = 48$) demonstrate modest improvement over stimulation for dorsiflexion alone.[58] Additional companies are adding channels to surface stimulation devices for walking, but they have not demonstrated improvements over the existing systems yet. Under an IDE, a pilot study ($n = 1$) also implanted a stroke survivor with an eight-channel system with electrodes activating muscles that cross the hip, knee, and ankle on the paretic side. There were minimal therapeutic improvements, but walking with the device doubled walking speed and significantly improved endurance while using the device.[59]

SUMMARY

Neurostimulation holds promise for treating and aiding poststroke hemiplegia. Targeting the corticomotor system through neuromodulation technologies, when combined with occupational and/or physical therapy, can potentially expedite and enhance recovery. Assistive technologies also enable patients with physical limitations to participate in activities they would not otherwise be able to, augmenting the therapeutic benefits of functional task practice. However, it is important to acknowledge that the degree of benefit varies among individuals. To maximize therapeutic gains, it will be important to identify the clinical characteristics of individuals who would benefit the most. Furthermore, future research should concentrate on translating these technologies into clinical practice, as many devices discussed in this article are still in development. When evaluating the clinical impact, it is important to consider not only the technology's effectiveness but also its practical implementation within existing standards of care.

CLINICS CARE POINTS

- Fifty percent of stroke survivors are reported to have motor and functional limitations.

- Noninvasive brain stimulation technologies modulate the target's spontaneous firing rate to decrease or increase neural excitability and must be paired with adjunctive rehabilitation approaches to generate positive functional changes.

- Vagus nerve stimulation is an emerging neuromodulatory approach for poststroke upper limb motor recovery. It involves delivering electrical current to the vagus nerve, either invasively with the use of implants or noninvasively using surface electrodes.

- Functional electrical stimulation is a method used to assist with functional task practice and promote neuroplasticity following a stroke.

- Neurostimulation devices have been successfully used to treat neurologic conditions, particularly in movement disorders.

- Additional research should be directed toward translating the technology so that it is clinically available while considering its practical implementation.

DISCLOSURE

The work was supported by the National Institutes of Health and National Institute of Child Health and Human Development (NICHD) (Grant Number 1R01HD109299)

REFERENCES

1. Shumway-Cook A, Woollacott MH. Motor Control: Translating Research into Clinical Practice. 4th edition Wolters Kluwer Health/Lippincott Williams & Wilkins; 2012. http://catdir.loc.gov/catdir/enhancements/fy1211/2010029395-t.html. Accessed April 19, 2023.
2. Subramaniam S, Hui-Chan CWY, Bhatt T. Effect of dual tasking on intentional vs. reactive balance control in people with hemiparetic stroke. J Neurophysiol 2014; 112(5):1152–8.
3. Dayan E, Censor N, Buch ER, et al. Noninvasive brain stimulation: from physiology to network dynamics and back. Nat Neurosci 2013;16(7):838–44.
4. Di Pino G, Di Lazzaro V. The balance recovery bimodal model in stroke patients between evidence and speculation: Do recent studies support it? Clin Neurophysiol 2020;131(10):2488–90.
5. Xu J, Branscheidt M, Schambra H, et al. Rethinking interhemispheric imbalance as a target for stroke neurorehabilitation. Ann Neurol 2019;85(4):502–13.
6. Di Pino G, Pellegrino G, Assenza G, et al. Modulation of brain plasticity in stroke: a novel model for neurorehabilitation. Nat Rev Neurol 2014;10(10):597–608.
7. Lin YL, Potter-Baker KA, Cunningham DA, et al. Stratifying chronic stroke patients based on the influence of contralesional motor cortices: An inter-hemispheric inhibition study. Clin Neurophysiol 2020;131(10):2516–25.
8. Sankarasubramanian V, Machado AG, Conforto AB, et al. Inhibition versus facilitation of contralesional motor cortices in stroke: Deriving a model to tailor brain stimulation. Clin Neurophysiol 2017;128(6):892–902.
9. Dodd KC, Nair VA, Prabhakaran V. Role of the Contralesional vs. Ipsilesional Hemisphere in Stroke Recovery. Front Hum Neurosci 2017;11:469.
10. McCambridge AB, Stinear JW, Byblow WD. Revisiting interhemispheric imbalance in chronic stroke: A tDCS study. Clin Neurophysiol 2018;129(1):42–50.

11. Rossi S, Antal A, Bestmann S, et al. Safety and recommendations for TMS use in healthy subjects and patient populations, with updates on training, ethical and regulatory issues: Expert Guidelines. Clin Neurophysiol 2021;132(1):269–306.

12. Klomjai W, Katz R, Lackmy-Vallée A. Basic principles of transcranial magnetic stimulation (TMS) and repetitive TMS (rTMS). Annals of Physical and Rehabilitation Medicine 2015;58(4):208–13.

13. Mohapatra S, Harrington R, Chan E, et al. Role of contralesional hemisphere in paretic arm reaching in patients with severe arm paresis due to stroke: A preliminary report. Neurosci Lett 2016;617:52–8.

14. Lüdemann-Podubecká J, Bösl K, Nowak DA. Inhibition of the contralesional dorsal premotor cortex improves motor function of the affected hand following stroke. Eur J Neurol 2016;23(4):823–30.

15. Kim J, Cha B, Lee D, et al. Effect of Cognition Recovery by Repetitive Transcranial Magnetic Stimulation on Ipsilesional Dorsolateral Prefrontal Cortex in Subacute Stroke Patients. Front Neurol 2022;13. https://www.frontiersin.org/articles/10.3389/fneur.2022.823108. Accessed April 4, 2023.

16. He Y, Li K, Chen Q, et al. Repetitive Transcranial Magnetic Stimulation on Motor Recovery for Patients With Stroke: A PRISMA Compliant Systematic Review and Meta-analysis. Am J Phys Med Rehabil 2020;99(2):99–108.

17. Zhang L, Xing G, Fan Y, et al. of Repetitive Transcranial Magnetic Stimulation on Upper Limb Motor Function after Stroke: a Systematic Review and Meta-Analysis. Clin Rehabil 2017;31(9):1137–53.

18. Cunningham DA, Lin YL, Potter–Baker KA, et al. Chapter 18-efficacy of noninvasive brain stimulation for motor rehabilitation after stroke. In: Wilson R, Raghavan P, editors. Stroke rehabilitation. St. Louis, MO: Elsevier; 2019. p. 249–65.

19. Cohen SL, Bikson M, Badran BW, et al. A visual and narrative timeline of US FDA milestones for Transcranial Magnetic Stimulation (TMS) devices. Brain Stimul 2022;15(1):73–5.

20. Wassermann EM. Risk and safety of repetitive transcranial magnetic stimulation: report and suggested guidelines from the International Workshop on the Safety of Repetitive Transcranial Magnetic Stimulation, June 5–7, 1996. Electroencephalogr Clin Neurophysiol 1998;108(1):1–16.

21. Chhatbar PY, Ramakrishnan V, Kautz S, et al. Transcranial Direct Current Stimulation Post-Stroke Upper Extremity Motor Recovery Studies Exhibit a Dose–Response Relationship. Brain Stimul 2016;9(1):16–26.

22. Lindenberg R, Renga V, Zhu LL, et al. Bihemispheric brain stimulation facilitates motor recovery in chronic stroke patients. Neurology 2010;75(24):2176–84.

23. Unger RH, Lowe MJ, Beall EB, et al. Stimulation of the Premotor Cortex Enhances Interhemispheric Functional Connectivity in Association with Upper Limb Motor Recovery in Moderate-to-Severe Chronic Stroke. Brain Connect 2023. https://doi.org/10.1089/brain.2022.0064.

24. Pavlova EL, Semenov RV, Pavlova-Deb MP, et al. Transcranial direct current stimulation of the premotor cortex aimed to improve hand motor function in chronic stroke patients. Brain Res 2022;1780:147790.

25. Cunningham DA, Varnerin N, Machado A, et al. Stimulation targeting higher motor areas in stroke rehabilitation: A proof-of-concept, randomized, double-blinded placebo-controlled study of effectiveness and underlying mechanisms. Restor Neurol Neurosci 2015;33(6):911–26.

26. Parlikar R, Vanteemar SS, Shivakumar V, et al. High definition transcranial direct current stimulation (HD-tDCS): A systematic review on the treatment of neuropsychiatric disorders. Asian J Psychiatr 2021;56:102542.

27. Kuo HI, Bikson M, Datta A, et al. Comparing cortical plasticity induced by conventional and high-definition 4 × 1 ring tDCS: a neurophysiological study. Brain Stimul 2013;6(4):644–8.

28. Klomjai W, Aneksan B. A randomized sham-controlled trial on the effects of dual-tDCS "during" physical therapy on lower limb performance in sub-acute stroke and a comparison to the previous study using a "before" stimulation protocol. BMC Sports Science Medicine Rehabilitation 2022;14(1):68.

29. Middleton A, Fritz SL, Liuzzo DM, et al. Using clinical and robotic assessment tools to examine the feasibility of pairing tDCS with upper extremity physical therapy in patients with stroke and TBI: A consideration-of-concept pilot study. NeuroRehabilitation 2014;35(4):741–54.

30. Zheng X, Schlaug G. Structural white matter changes in descending motor tracts correlate with improvements in motor impairment after undergoing a treatment course of tDCS and physical therapy. Front Hum Neurosci 2015;9. https://www.frontiersin.org/articles/10.3389/fnhum.2015.00229. Accessed April 4, 2023.

31. Nitsche MA, Paulus W. Excitability changes induced in the human motor cortex by weak transcranial direct current stimulation. J Physiol 2000;527 Pt 3(Pt 3):633–9.

32. Kronberg G, Rahman A, Sharma M, et al. Direct current stimulation boosts hebbian plasticity in vitro. Brain Stimul 2020;13(2):287–301.

33. Longo V, Barbati SA, Re A, et al. Transcranial Direct Current Stimulation Enhances Neuroplasticity and Accelerates Motor Recovery in a Stroke Mouse Model. Stroke 2022;53(5):1746–58.

34. Stagg CJ, Bachtiar V, Johansen-Berg H. The role of GABA in human motor learning. Curr Biol 2011;21(6):480–4.

35. Kim DY, Lim JY, Kang EK, et al. Effect of Transcranial Direct Current Stimulation on Motor Recovery in Patients with Subacute Stroke. Am J Phys Med Rehabil 2010;89(11):879.

36. Navarro-López V, Molina-Rueda F, Jiménez-Jiménez S, et al. Effects of Transcranial Direct Current Stimulation Combined with Physiotherapy on Gait Pattern, Balance, and Functionality in Stroke Patients. A Systematic Review. Diagnostics 2021;11(4):656.

37. Mitsutake T, Imura T, Hori T, et al. Effects of Combining Online Anodal Transcranial Direct Current Stimulation and Gait Training in Stroke Patients: A Systematic Review and Meta-Analysis. Front Hum Neurosci 2021;15. https://www.frontiersin.org/articles/10.3389/fnhum.2021.782305. Accessed April 4, 2023.

38. Dhaliwal SK, Meek BP, Modirrousta MM. Non-Invasive Brain Stimulation for the Treatment of Symptoms Following Traumatic Brain Injury. Front Psychiatry 2015;6:119.

39. Bikson M, Grossman P, Thomas C, et al. Safety of Transcranial Direct Current Stimulation: Evidence Based Update 2016. Brain Stimul 2016;9(5):641–61.

40. Engineer ND, Kimberley TJ, Prudente CN, et al. Targeted Vagus Nerve Stimulation for Rehabilitation After Stroke. Front Neurosci 2019;13:280.

41. Ramos-Castaneda JA, Barreto-Cortes CF, Losada-Floriano D, et al. Efficacy and Safety of Vagus Nerve Stimulation on Upper Limb Motor Recovery After Stroke. A Systematic Review and Meta-Analysis. Front Neurol 2022;13:889953.

42. Buell EP, Loerwald KW, Engineer CT, et al. Cortical map plasticity as a function of vagus nerve stimulation rate. Brain Stimul 2018;11(6):1218–24.

43. Gao Y, Zhu Y, Lu X, et al. Vagus nerve stimulation paired with rehabilitation for motor function, mental health and activities of daily living after stroke: a systematic review and meta-analysis. J Neurol Neurosurg Psychiatry 2023;94(4):257–66.
44. Dawson J, Liu CY, Francisco GE, et al. Vagus Nerve Stimulation Paired with Rehabilitation for Upper Limb Motor Function After Ischaemic Stroke (VNS-REHAB): A Randomised, Blinded, Pivotal, Device Trial. Lancet 2021;397(10284):1545–53.
45. Ward N. The prospects for poststroke neural repair with vagal nerve stimulation. J Neurol Neurosurg Psychiatry 2023;94(4):255–6.
46. Fu MJ, Knutson JS. Chapter 14-neuromuscular electrical stimulation and stroke recovery. In: Wilson R, Raghavan P, editors. Stroke rehabilitation. St. Louis, MO: Elsevier; 2019. p. 199–213.
47. Kristensen MGH, Busk H, Wienecke T. Neuromuscular Electrical Stimulation Improves Activities of Daily Living Post Stroke: A Systematic Review and Meta-analysis. Arch Rehabil Res Clin Transl 2022;4(1):100167.
48. Chae J, Knutson J, Sheffler L. Chapter 60-stimulation for return of function after stroke. In: Krames ES, Peckham PH, Rezai AR, editors. Neuromodulation. London, UK: Academic Press; 2009. p. 743–51.
49. Wilson RD, Page SJ, Delahanty M, et al. Upper-Limb Recovery After Stroke: A Randomized Controlled Trial Comparing EMG-Triggered, Cyclic, and Sensory Electrical Stimulation. Neurorehabil Neural Repair 2016;30(10):978–87.
50. Loh MS, Kuan YC, Wu CW, et al. Upper Extremity Contralaterally Controlled Functional Electrical Stimulation Versus Neuromuscular Electrical Stimulation in Post-Stroke Individuals: A Meta-Analysis of Randomized Controlled Trials. Neurorehabil Neural Repair 2022;36(7):472–82.
51. Knutson JS, Gunzler DD, Wilson RD, et al. Contralaterally Controlled Functional Electrical Stimulation Improves Hand Dexterity in Chronic Hemiparesis: A Randomized Trial. Stroke 2016;47(10):2596–602.
52. Wilson RD, Gunzler DD, Bennett ME, et al. Peripheral nerve stimulation compared with usual care for pain relief of hemiplegic shoulder pain: a randomized controlled trial. Am J Phys Med Rehabil 2014;93(1):17–28.
53. Wilson RD, Bennett ME, Nguyen VQC, et al. Fully Implantable Peripheral Nerve Stimulation for Hemiplegic Shoulder Pain: A Multi-Site Case Series With Two-Year Follow-Up. Neuromodulation 2018;21(3):290–5.
54. Whitehair VC, Chae J, Hisel T, et al. The effect of electrical stimulation on impairment of the painful post-stroke shoulder. Top Stroke Rehabil 2019;26(7):544–7.
55. Knutson JS, Chae J, Hart RL, et al. Implanted neuroprosthesis for assisting arm and hand function after stroke: a case study. J Rehabil Res Dev 2012;49(10):1505–16.
56. Prenton S, Hollands KL, Kenney LPJ, et al. Functional electrical stimulation and ankle foot orthoses provide equivalent therapeutic effects on foot drop: A meta-analysis providing direction for future research. J Rehabil Med 2018;50(2):129–39.
57. Prenton S, Hollands KL, Kenney LPJ. Functional electrical stimulation versus ankle foot orthoses for foot-drop: A meta-analysis of orthotic effects. J Rehabil Med 2016;48(8):646–56.
58. Springer S, Vatine JJ, Lipson R, et al. Effects of dual-channel functional electrical stimulation on gait performance in patients with hemiparesis. Sci World J 2012;2012:530906.
59. Makowski NS, Kobetic R, Lombardo LM, et al. Improving Walking with an Implanted Neuroprosthesis for Hip, Knee, and Ankle Control After Stroke. Am J Phys Med Rehabil 2016;95(12):880–8.

Technological Advances in Stroke Rehabilitation
Robotics and Virtual Reality

Deepthi Rajashekar, PhD[a], Alexa Boyer, MASc[a,b],
Kelly A. Larkin-Kaiser, PhD[a,c,d],
Sean P. Dukelow, PhD, MD, FRCPC[a,c,e,*]

KEYWORDS

● Stroke ● Robotics ● Rehabilitation ● VR ● Physical therapy

KEY POINTS

- Robotics and virtual reality (VR) are widely studied in stroke rehabilitation to facilitate intensive, repetitive, and engaging therapies.
- Currently, there are some discrepancies between the findings of meta-analyses and some of the larger clinical trials in the field.
- More large, high-quality, randomized, multicenter trials are required to improve our understanding of the impact of robotics and VR on stroke recovery.
- Robotics and VR can augment and complement conventional therapy and have the potential to be used as precision rehabilitation approaches.

INTRODUCTION

Stroke is a leading cause of disability, including reduced mobility, aphasia, depression, and cognitive decline.[1] Studies have estimated that the yearly cost of post-stroke care, including rehabilitation, ranges from 40 to 60K USD per patient in high-income countries, including the United States, Canada, Western Europe, Russia, Australia, and China (as of 2020).[2] Traditional rehabilitation methods rely on multidisciplinary teams (physiotherapy, occupational, recreational therapy, etc.) that often focus efforts on frequent and intense repetition to gradually improve skilled, goal-oriented movements.[3,4] Specifically, the frequency and duration of rehabilitation appear to be

[a] Department of Clinical Neurosciences, Cumming School of Medicine, University of Calgary, Calgary, Alberta, Canada; [b] Schulich School of Engineering: Department of Biomedical Engineering, University of Calgary, Calgary, Alberta, Canada; [c] Hotchkiss Brain Institute, University of Calgary, Calgary, Alberta, Canada; [d] Ablerta Children's Hospital Research Institute, University of Calgary, Calgary, Alberta, Canada; [e] Division of Physical Medicine and Rehabilitation, Cumming School of Medicine, University of Calgary, Calgary, Alberta, Canada
* Corresponding author. Department of Clinical Neurosciences, Foothills Medical Centre, 1403 29th Street Northwest, South Tower, Calgary, Alberta T2N 2T9, Canada.
E-mail address: spdukelo@ucalgary.ca

Phys Med Rehabil Clin N Am 35 (2024) 383–398
https://doi.org/10.1016/j.pmr.2023.06.026
1047-9651/24/© 2023 Elsevier Inc. All rights reserved.

important in facilitating better outcomes. In cases where remediation is not possible, the rehabilitation focus may turn toward teaching the patient to compensate for lost function using devices (eg, gait aids, orthoses). Despite the critical role of rehabilitation after a stroke, several challenges can limit its effectiveness. Common obstacles include access to care, resource constraints, coordination of multidisciplinary teams, and insurance coverage.[5] There is an increasing need to develop effective rehabilitation interventions that help stroke survivors regain independence. Therefore, integrating appropriate technology-based therapies may allow the potential for objective, repetitive, engaging, and personalized rehabilitation to help complement and augment traditional rehabilitation approaches.

Robots for Rehabilitation

The integration of robotics in rehabilitation began in the late 1990s and has steadily gained attention from researchers studying how to optimize stroke recovery.[6] For rehabilitation purposes, robotics can be categorized into end effectors and exoskeletons (**Fig. 1**). End effectors are designed to guide the distal parts of the limb to interact with the environment and perform specific tasks, such as grasping and reaching. In contrast, exoskeletons are designed to work with torque actuators that control joint movement and therefore can augment the movements of each joint they cross.[7] These systems enable the design of specific rehabilitation tasks and provide objective feedback through visual, motor/sensory, and cognitive mechanisms. Robotic devices tend to focus on either the upper or lower extremity and are employed to target improving motor function, patterns of muscular activity, range of motion, and in some cases enhanced activity and mobility in the community.[8] Although most studies have explored the use of robots in a therapeutic nature, they can also be used as an orthosis, replacing a particular body function.[9,10] Further, robots can be used to measure the kinematics and/or kinetics of movement to track changes in impairment over time.[11,12] This information can be critical to understanding therapy-induced improvements in impairment.

Upper-limb Robotics

Early studies of robotics in the upper-limb focused on their ability to provide a rehabilitative treatment intervention.[13] However, soon after their implementation as

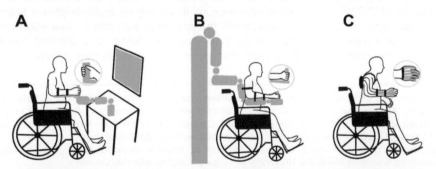

Fig. 1. Upper limb robotic solutions for stroke rehabilitation with stroke patient seated in a wheelchair (*black*) using (*A*) an end effector sometimes paired with a video screen (*green*) such as InMotion2,[20,21,23] NEREBOT,[84] Haptic Master,[85] ArmeoSpring,[86] and Bi-Manu Track[87]; (*B*) an exoskeleton (*green*) such as KINARM,[15] ARMin,[26] T-WREX,[88] and ARMOR[89]; (*C*) soft wearable hand robotic device (*green*) with a power supply backpack such as GloReha.[90] (Figure is adapted from Gassert and Dietz, with permission.[91])

rehabilitation tools, researchers and clinicians recognized their ability to act as assessment tools[14] to quantify various aspects of impairment. Conventional clinical assessments tend to be largely observer-based, ordinal scales, posing challenges related to floor and ceiling effects and reliability, robots, on the other hand, can allow for precise and accurate quantification of sensory-motor impairments,[15,16] spasticity,[17] kinaesthesia,[18,19] and proprioception.[11,12] A variety of robotic devices that have been used for assessment include the InMotion,[20–23] KINARM,[15] ARM Guide,[24] MIME,[25] and ArmIn[26] among others.

As mentioned above, a substantial focus in the early literature was the use of robots as a therapeutic tool. A 2018 Cochrane review included 45 randomized clinical trials (RCT), 9 robotic devices, and 1619 stroke patients and found high evidence supporting the use of robot-assisted arm therapy (RAAT) in improving overall arm function as measured by Upper Extremity Fugl-Meyer Assessment (UE-FM). Specifically, the author concluded that RAATs contributed to improvement in function, muscle strength, and performance of activities of daily living, with a caveat that there was high variability in training intensity (duration and frequency), the robotic device used, participant characteristics, and clinical outcomes.[27] Similarly, a network meta-analysis summarizing the effects of RAAT on motor function and activity[a] in upper-limb rehabilitation from 18 RCTs reported that the effectiveness of RAAT depended on 3 main factors: duration of intervention, level of impairment, and time since stroke.[28] Although RAAT was most effective in improving motor function as measured by UE-FM in subacute patients with severe to moderate impairments with 6 to 15 hours of intervention delivered, chronic patients with mild impairments benefited from RAAT with 15 to 30 hours of intervention delivered. However, RAAT did not result in significant improvements in activities of daily living (Barthel Index) when compared to conventional therapy. Despite these reviews suggesting chronic patients would benefit from RAAT, the largest clinical trial, the RATULS trial with 770 participants (largely chronic stroke) concluded that RAAT (delivered with the InMotion2 robot, 45 minutes session, three times a week, for 12 weeks) had no clinically meaningful functional improvements compared with conventional therapy (45 minutes a session, a minimum of 5 weeks, until rehabilitation goals were met).[29] Furthermore, another systematic review and meta-analysis of 11 RCTs in subacute stroke reported that the only requirement for effective upper-limb rehabilitation was highly intensive and repetitive movements, regardless of whether they were facilitated by robots or therapists.[30] A recommendation for future trials has been to carefully consider the optimal therapy dose and time since stroke in any ensuing RAAT studies.[31,32]

It is important to recognize that there were substantial differences in the types of robotic devices included in the above metanalyses.[27,28,30] Robots varied in their design and in what part of the upper extremity was targeted (ie, shoulder, elbow, wrist, hand, finger). A systematic review (149 participants, 5 trials) found exoskeletons to be more effective than end-effectors for finger-hand motor recovery.[33] In contrast, a larger review (2654 participants, 55 trials) compared the relative efficacy of 28 different types of robotic devices on activities of daily living, arm function, and strength and concluded that no one type of intervention (either unilateral or bilateral end-effector vs exoskeleton for distal vs proximal) was significantly better than the other.[34] Overall, there is weak evidence in the literature favoring either the exoskeletons or end effectors for improving arm function[35–37] but it is rare to see an actual head-to-head comparison of the robotic devices.

---

[a] By the International Classification of Functioning, Disability and Health (ICF) definition, activity is the execution of a task by an individual.

The integration of exoskeletons with noninvasive brain stimulation (through transcranial direct current stimulation [tDCS]), neuromuscular stimulation, and functional electrical stimulation has gained some attention in chronic stroke patient rehabilitation (368 patients, 10 trials)[38] with upper-limb impairment. Although there was some promise of functional improvements with wrist and hand components when RAAT is coupled with stimulation,[39,40] there was weak evidence to suggest that arm training is benefited by coupling RAAT with stimulation.[41] More high-quality studies are warranted to establish when to employ brain stimulation in rehabilitating upper extremities with RAAT.

In summary, although RAAT has demonstrated some promise as a tool for the assessment and treatment of the post-stroke upper extremity, there are still fundamental questions about the optimal dose and timing of administration. However, the same could be said of traditional stroke rehabilitation practice. The sheer number of devices and relative lack of comparative studies make navigating which robot might be best for a given patient challenging. Implementation into health care systems has proven challenging in some jurisdictions because of the initial expense of the device, reimbursement mechanisms for robotic therapy, and a lack of clear guidelines around best practices for integrating RAAT into clinical practice. The possibility of further augmenting RAAT with noninvasive brain stimulation or peripheral nerve stimulation remains an active area of research. Perhaps at present, RAAT is best viewed as a reasonable way to augment upper-limb therapy after stroke with much work to be done to facilitate and support clinical translation.

Lower-limb Robotics

Independent walking after a stroke is a predictor of autonomy and optimized quality-of-life outcomes.[42] Stroke-induced lower-limb impairments often involve an abnormal gait, impaired balance, asymmetric weight distribution (more weight on the unaffected side), and increased postural oscillation. Earlier studies in robot-assisted gait training (RAGT) focused largely on the use of devices that offered partial body weight support and incorporated a treadmill such as the Lokomat[43,44] or moved the patient's feet in an elliptical-like motion such as the Gait Trainer 1.[45] More recently, wearable exoskeletons (like the EksoGT,[46,47] ReWalk,[48] Indego,[49] or HAL[50]) are being clinically evaluated and adopted for stroke rehabilitation[51] (Fig. 2). RAGT devices have demonstrated the ability to allow patients to ambulate in a supported environment which might be challenging to accomplish without several human therapists assisting, particularly for those individuals with more severe lower-limb impairment. In some devices, a patient can be fully supported, and the robot can simply be used to move the limbs through a range of motion passively, while at other times the patient must initiate a movement to trigger the next step, making the rehabilitation more active in nature.

A recent meta-analysis, which included 15 studies, examined the effectiveness of using treadmill-based exoskeletons as an adjunct to conventional therapy for gait training, compared with the effectiveness of conventional therapy alone. Although the authors identified no significant differences in ambulatory function, walking speed, or walking endurance, they reported marked improvements in balance function and cadence in chronic stroke in the RAGT group.[52] Interestingly, this improvement in balance was not witnessed in studies where the robot only moved the patient's limbs passively, which suggests the importance of encouraging active movement during gait rehabilitation to maximize effectiveness.

Similar to RAAT, some authors have attempted to determine whether the type of device employed in RAGT may have an impact on outcomes. In a meta-analysis of 13

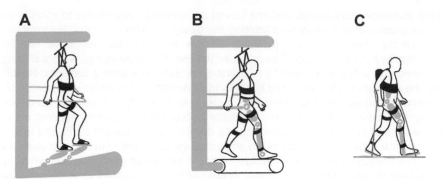

Fig. 2. Lower-limb robotics solutions for stroke rehabilitation with stroke patient walking (black): (*A*) on a gait training system (*green*) with body weight support (*black*) such as Gait Trainer 1,[45] G-EO,[92] GAR,[93] and Lexo[94]; (*B*) on a treadmill with an exoskeleton (*green*) and body weight support (*black*) such as Lokomat and LokomatPro; some commercially available devices as pictured in (*A*) and (*B*) may come with video display screens; (*C*) overground with forearm crutches (*black*) using a wearable exoskeleton (*green*) such as EksoGT,[43,44,46] ReWalk,[48] HAL,[50] Indego,[49] and SMA.[58] (Figure is adapted from Gassert and Dietz, with permission.[91])

studies, Bruni and colleagues[53] investigated the differences between exoskeletons (218 participants, 6 robots) and end effectors (469 participants, 7 robots) in RAGT across chronic (167 participants, 4 trials) and subacute (520 participants, 9 trials) stroke participants. Their observations indicate that, unlike exoskeletons, end-effector devices can independently improve walking speed in comparison to conventional therapy. However, this effect was statistically significant for subacute patients only, suggesting that non-ambulatory patients derive the most benefit from RAGT when robots support distal parts of the limb and mimic the stance and swing phases of gait within a few weeks from stroke.[53] Furthermore, exoskeletons have also been successful in reducing the perception of pain,[44,54] reducing spasticity,[55] improving muscle tone at the hip, knee, and ankle,[43,44] and maximizing the effectiveness of physiotherapists during gait training.[8]

A recent systematic review of 71 clinical trials investigated the design and clinical evaluation of nearly 25 commercially available wearable exoskeletons (as of 2021) for rehabilitating patients with either stroke, spinal cord injury, or other neurologic diseases.[56] They found that wearables can improve various aspects of lower-limb ambulation, including cadence, speed, and asymmetries in step length or stride length. RCTs comparing the SMA with functional training for stroke patients demonstrated significant increases in step length of the paretic leg,[57] endurance (6MWT),[58] balance,[58] cortical motor excitability of the paretic rectus femoris,[58] and reductions in asymmetry[57] (all cases, $P < .05$). Another RCT comparing a custom robotics-assisted ankle-foot orthosis (AFO) with a passive AFO in conventional therapy found that the robotic group showed significant improvements in vertical loading and braking forces on the affected side, as well as improved knee flexion on the unaffected side based on ground reaction data.[59] However, the adoption of wearable exoskeletons was often challenged by economic cost,[60,61] ergonomic issues,[62] and human-exoskeleton interaction based control issues.[63] The latter included the weight of the device that increased the metabolic cost of walking, the extensive time required for donning/doffing the device (up to 30 minutes), and the technical expertise required for implementing the use. The authors highlighted the lack of dynamic assist-as-needed algorithms and the use of deterministic algorithms to identify the various phases of gait as factors limiting the design of patient-centric rehabilitative interventions. These findings (both qualitative and quantitative) were recently confirmed by the ExStRA trial,[46] which used the EksoGT for stepping, weight shifting, and walking practice in a cohort of 36 first-time, subacute stroke patients. Results from the as-treated analysis of the ExStRA trial showed that patients who completed the exoskeleton regime had better gait, walking endurance, and walked more independently. However, therapists and patients also confirmed a steep learning curve, confusion, and intimidation in handling the device, lack of trained staff, and lack of therapy time outside the exoskeleton as limitations for implementing their use clinically. The therapists also acknowledged that the exoskeleton allowed early walking for individuals with severe stroke who would not be rehabilitated as early with conventional therapeutic approaches.[47]

Recently, RAGT has been coupled with noninvasive brain stimulation techniques to improve the efficacy of lower-limb rehabilitation.[38] In a randomized sample of 37 chronic stroke participants, Naro and colleagues[64] investigated the safety and efficacy of combining task-specific and repetitive RAGT through the LokomatPro with dual-site tDCS to restore interhemispheric balance. This study reported improvements in gait stability, balance, and walking endurance among patients who received brain stimulation during and after RAGT, as opposed to modulating cortical excitability before each RAGT session.[64] Another recent RCT used the Stride Management Assist (SMA) exoskeleton with 50 chronic stroke patients and concurrently manipulated the cortical motor excitability using transcranial magnetic stimulation (TMS).[58] This study concluded the SMA group had better endurance and higher absolute activity level (step count) on therapy days and observed larger changes in the corticomotor excitability of the paretic rectus femoris muscle.[58] Furthermore, by combining robotics with modulation of motor excitability, these studies have demonstrated the potential for using RAGT to target specific muscle groups (such as the hamstring, tibialis anterior, and quadriceps) to improve lower-limb strength and function.

In summary, the last few decades have produced some promising evidence for robotic therapy for lower-limb rehabilitation post-stroke, particularly for individuals with more severe gait impairments. That said, there are ongoing challenges with robot designs and control strategies in many devices that have limited uptake. Like RAAT, implementation has proven challenging in many centers because of the cost and technical training required for staff to operate the devices. Further technical optimizations, speeding up donning and doffing, and lessening the burden on clinicians trying to operate the robots may lead to more widespread adoption of these technologies into the health care system and homes.

Virtual Reality for Rehabilitation

VR is a set of computer-generated simulations that allow users to engage and interact with a simulated environment in a naturalistic fashion, resulting in a wide range of experiences from non-immersive, semi-immersive, and fully immersive[65] (**Fig. 3**). The adoption of VR to enhance the efficacy of conventional rehabilitative interventions[66] in stroke began in the 1990s,[67] with a primary focus on improving patient engagement,[68] and successful translation of the therapy from hospitals to homes.

A 2017 Cochrane review on VR for both upper- and lower-limb stroke rehabilitation included 2470 participants and 72 trials.[69] The authors suggested for the upper-limb (22 trials) that VR on its own was not superior to conventional therapy. However, when VR was used as an add-on to effectively increase the dose of therapy delivered, there were notable improvements in UE-FM scores amongst other outcomes. However, the

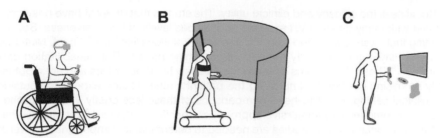

Fig. 3. VR solutions for stroke rehabilitation: (*A*) stroke patient seated in a wheelchair (*black*) with an immersive VR headset and VR controllers (*green*) such as Oculus,[95] HTC Vive[96]; (*B*) stroke patient on a treadmill with body weight support (*black*) in front of a semi-immersive VR screen (*green*) (eg, Motek GRAIL,[97] Motek CAREN,[98] Motek C-mill[99]); (*C*) stroke patient standing in front of a video screen holding a VR controller connected to non-immersive VR gaming systems (*green*) such as Xbox Kinect,[100] Playstation,[101] Nintendo Wii,[102] and Leap Motion.[103]

evidence was considered to come from low-quality studies (as ranked by GRADE). Recently, another systematic review (2271 participants, 50 trials) concluded that VR[b] was superior to conventional treatment for upper-limb impairment (UE-FM) and activities of daily living, but not for performance on Box and Block Test and Wolf Motor Function Test.[70] The consistent criticism in both these reviews was that VR trials are often low-quality studies that have a high risk of bias.

In the lower-limb literature, a large systematic review (2328 participants, 61 trials)[71] comparing VR gait training with body weight support gait training concluded that VR gait training helps improve performance on balance battery assessments and dynamic balance, but not steady-state balance. Two meta-analyses (809 participants, 32 studies[72]; 337 participants, 18 trials[73]) compared VR with treadmill-based training, or RAGT for chronic stroke patients and reported significant improvements in cadence, stride length, and gait speed in VR-based gait training. A smaller systematic review (183 participants, 11 trials, 2 RAGT trials)[74] with similar results suggested a minimum of 10 sessions are required to derive any meaningful changes in motor function, with immersive VR being more effective than semi- or non-immersive VR.

Some studies have examined the potential impact of VR on cognitive function. A large meta-analysis of 87 clinical trials involving 3540 participants examined the ability of VR to improve upper- and lower-limb function, activities of daily living, and cognition. In this analysis, Zhang and colleagues[75] found that only 7 studies reported on the Mini-Mental State Examination, which included 210 participants. Despite the low sample size and moderate heterogeneity, Mini-Mental State scores were higher in the VR groups compared with conventional therapy groups within 4 weeks of the intervention. Another smaller meta-analysis (196 patients, 8 trials)[76] that specifically investigated the effect of VR on post-stroke cognition alone found no significant differences between groups who received VR alone and those who received a combination of VR and conventional therapy.

In summary, there have been many studies examining the use of VR for stroke rehabilitation. Critics have consistently suggested higher-quality studies are needed to

---

[b] In this paper, VR, augmented reality, and mixed reality technologies were compared with conventional therapy for upper-limb. Of these, the VR technologies reviewed were largely off-the shelf solutions like the Nintendo Wii and Xbox Kinect.

better assess the efficacy and clinical utility. The studies that do exist have been conducted with many different VR systems and various levels of immersiveness. Several existing trials were conducted using off-the-shelf solutions like Xbox Kinect, Nintendo Wii, and PlayStation, to study the effects of gaming-based VR in rehabilitation programs.[77,78] These VR systems cost as little as a few hundred dollars and are a potentially promising solution for improving the patient's rehabilitation experience outside the clinical setting. Head-to-head comparisons of these less costly VR approaches and more complex, fully immersive approaches specifically designed for stroke rehabilitation are scarce. More studies are needed to determine how important the level of immersiveness is in stroke recovery.

The Potential of Combining Robotics and Virtual Reality

Given that rehabilitation is a complex, multifactorial process, Clarke and colleagues[79] investigated the efficacy of individually using robotics and VR as an adjunct to conventional therapy versus the combination of robotics and VR (Robotic Therapy [RT] + CT, VR + CT vs RT + VR + CT). The authors suggested the benefit of coupling robotics with VR was the ability to facilitate repetitive, high-intensity and task-specific interventions while also engaging patients, reducing frustration and fatigue, while providing visual and cognitive feedback in a gamified manner, thus enhancing the overall therapy experience.[79]

In a systematic review by Mubin and colleagues[80] of 30 studies that employed VR coupled with robotics (VR + RT) showed that the VR, augmented reality, or gamification technologies aided in the transition of exoskeleton-based rehabilitation from hospitals to homes. In assessing the effectiveness of VR + RT to improve health-related quality of life across different neurologic conditions (RT = 52 studies, VR + RT = 18, largely pilot studies), Zanatta and colleagues[81] found that in comparison to using robotics alone, the VR + RT significantly improved quality of life in patients with stroke, despite the shorter therapy and session duration. Most of the studies considered for this used non-immersive VR mediated through screens and monitors. As a result, it has been suggested that the combination of VR + RT has the potential to stimulate motor learning and neuroplasticity better than using either in isolation.[79]

DISCUSSION

In this review, we have described different robotic and VR applications in stroke rehabilitation and briefly reviewed the existing evidence for their use. Broadly speaking, both robotics and VR have demonstrated some level of efficacy in several studies. However, results should be interpreted with caution as much of the evidence comes from small clinical trials with significant heterogeneity in the devices used, patient characteristics, and outcome measures employed.

In examining the literature, there are frequent discrepancies between the findings of large meta-analyses and some of the larger individual clinical trials. We suspect this may be due to several factors. Smaller trials are common in the literature and impact the results of meta-analyses, despite the risk of these trials being underpowered and having a higher risk of bias. Multiple systematic reviews remarked on the lower quality ratings of the trials included, and most trials tended to employ a single device. One would suspect the type of device might impact the outcome, although some suggestions have been that this may not be the case.[34] Lastly, patient factors such as time since stroke and stroke location can drastically influence a trial outcome. In most systematic reviews and meta-analyses, but not all, different stroke subtypes and/or stroke chronicity (eg, subacute, chronic) are collapsed together despite differences in expected outcomes. Ultimately, we need to consider employing larger, high-quality, randomized, multicenter trials with appropriate control groups to fully understand the efficacy of device-specific robotic interventions tailored to specific patient cohorts.

Despite the challenges above, robotics and VR have more evidence behind them than some other common rehabilitation interventions (eg, splinting for spasticity), yet their adoption by clinicians and the healthcare system in many parts of the world is limited. To encourage easy adoption, the technical design of robotic devices needs to consider the challenges that both therapists and patients face when learning to use them. Early career therapists in Canada (n = 127) reported a lack of awareness of robotic (62.2%) and VR-based (37%) interventions as a primary reason for not adopting them in clinical practice, along with a lack of access (RT: 21.2%; VR: 44% did not have access), increased cost (RT: 11%; VR:12.6%), and lack of time (RT: 0.04%; VR: 0.1%) to use emerging technologies.[82] These challenges exist despite the emphasis on evidence-based practice in post-secondary training institutions, resulting in a drastic need for knowledge translation that can drive the implementation of technology-based solutions in the clinic. When evaluating the cost-effectiveness of VR + RT technologies, it is important to consider not only the upfront purchasing cost but also the operational cost of administering therapy. For example, although the hardware for VR solutions is affordable, ongoing expenses for software development and maintenance can be significant. Additionally, in some countries, a clear reimbursement pathway for interventions is lacking, which limits their uptake in the clinical setting.

FUTURE PROSPECTS

Although the effectiveness of robotics and VR (or a combination of both) in comparison to conventional care remains mixed, these technologies can be used to facilitate and augment early, intensive, and patient-centered therapy. Robotics has the potential to be an adjunct to one-on-one therapy, especially in clinical settings with limited availability of skilled and qualified therapists if someone has the skills to operate the robot. Furthermore, robotics can minimize the demand for therapists to facilitate repetitive movements and thereby reduce potential injuries.[83] Both VR and robotics have demonstrated their ability to safely and effectively engage patients with severe impairments earlier in therapy than is possible with conventional care alone. Furthermore, the emerging field of wearables combined with affordable VR solutions can enhance the probability of rehabilitation to extend beyond the clinical setting, allowing patients to continue their therapy comfortably at home.

The field of integrated robotics and multimodal stimulation in therapy is still in its infancy. However, with ongoing advancements in the development of more human-like movements and immersive mixed-reality headsets, the potential for adoption in stroke rehabilitation and improving activities of daily living is encouraging. As the technology continues to evolve, researchers and clinicians must work together across multiple centers to gather high-quality evidence to support and optimize the integration of these emerging solutions into clinical practice.

More importantly, there is also a wealth of data on the severity of impairment and patient engagement that these robotics and VR solutions capture. This creates a tremendous opportunity to better understand the impairment and recovery process following a stroke. It also allows clinicians the potential to integrate kinematic and kinetic information into clinical care and tailor therapy to the individual patient, paving the way for precision rehabilitation.

SUMMARY

This review highlights the existing evidence for using robotics and VR in stroke rehabilitation. Although there are technical and cost-related challenges in the widespread adoption of robotics and VR in stroke rehabilitation, these emerging solutions offer a unique advantage by capturing a wealth of data on patient impairment, engagement, and comfort. This can aid in a precision rehabilitation approach, but it can also help address staff shortages by delivering therapy effectively in clinics where human resources may be scarce.

CLINICS CARE POINTS

- Robotic devices can be helpful in increasing repetitive training for stroke survivors retraining their upper and lower limbs. Appropriate patient and device selection would seem to be important but at present, little data exists to guide these decisions.
- VR can be helpful to supplement ongoing rehabilitation to achieve greater gains and is often combined in studies with other technology-based tools such as robotics or treadmills.
- At present, several robotic and VR devices are available, but there is little data comparing different devices.

FUNDING

DR and AB are funded by the Cumming Medical Research Fund from the University of Calgary and the Hotchkiss Brain Insitute Graduate Studentship award respectively.

DISCLOSURE

SPD: Speakers fees from Abbvie, Merz. He has been part of advisory boards for Ipsen Pharmaceuticals.Consultancy fees from Prometheus Medical.Operating grants from the University of Calgary, Canadian Institutes of Health Research, Heart and Stroke Foundation, and Brain Canada.He has collaborated with Red Iron Labs on the development of a virtual reality intervention for stroke rehabilitation. **DR and AB**: No disclosures. **KLK**: Dr. Kelly Kaiser is a founder and holds equity in HEMOtx.

REFERENCES

1. Katan M, Luft A. Global burden of stroke. Semin Neurol 2018;38(2):208–11.
2. Strilciuc S, Grad DA, Radu C, et al. The economic burden of stroke: a systematic review of cost of illness studies. J Med Life 2021;14(5):606–19.
3. Johansson BB. Current trends in stroke rehabilitation. a review with focus on brain plasticity. Acta Neurol Scand 2011;123(3):147–59.
4. Dobkin BH. Strategies for stroke rehabilitation. Lancet Neurol 2004;3(9):528–36.
5. Stinear CM, Lang CE, Zeiler S, et al. Advances and challenges in stroke rehabilitation. Lancet Neurol 2020;19(4):348–60.
6. Aisen ML, Krebs HI, Hogan N, et al. The effect of robot-assisted therapy and rehabilitative training on motor recovery following stroke. Arch Neurol 1997;54(4):443–6.
7. Chang WH, Kim YH. Robot-assisted therapy in stroke rehabilitation. J Stroke 2013;15(3):174–81.
8. Cho JE, Yoo JS, Kim KE, et al. Systematic Review of Appropriate Robotic Intervention for Gait Function in Subacute Stroke Patients. BioMed Res Int 2018; 2018:e4085298.

9. Iida S, Kawakita D, Fujita T, et al. Exercise using a robotic knee orthosis in stroke patients with hemiplegia. J Phys Ther Sci 2017;29(11):1920–4.
10. Chen A, Winterbottom L, Park S, et al. Thumb stabilization and assistance in a robotic hand orthosis for post-stroke hemiparesis. IEEE Robot Autom Lett 2022; 7(3):8276–82.
11. Scott SH, Dukelow SP. Potential of robots as next-generation technology for clinical assessment of neurological disorders and upper-limb therapy. J Rehabil Res Dev 2011;48(4):335–53.
12. Semrau JA, Herter TM, Scott SH, et al. Examining differences in patterns of sensory and motor recovery after stroke with robotics. Stroke 2015;46(12):3459–69.
13. Burgar CG, Lum PS, Shor PC, et al. Development of robots for rehabilitation therapy: the Palo Alto VA/Stanford experience. J Rehabil Res Dev 2000;37(6): 663–73.
14. Reinkensmeyer DJ, Schmit BD, Rymer WZ. Mechatronic assessment of arm impairment after chronic brain injury. Technol Health Care 1999;7(6):431–5.
15. Coderre AM, Amr AZ, Dukelow SP, et al. Assessment of upper-limb sensorimotor function of subacute stroke patients using visually guided reaching. Neurorehabilitation Neural Repair 2010;24(6):528–41.
16. Dukelow SP, Herter TM, Moore KD, et al. Quantitative assessment of limb position sense following stroke. Neurorehabilitation Neural Repair 2010;24(2): 178–87.
17. de-la-Torre R, Oña ED, Balaguer C, et al. Robot-aided systems for improving the assessment of upper limb spasticity: a systematic review. Sensors 2020;20(18): 5251.
18. Kenzie JM, Semrau JA, Findlater SE, et al. Localization of impaired kinesthetic processing post-stroke. Front Hum Neurosci 2016;10:505.
19. Semrau JA, Herter TM, Scott SH, et al. Differential loss of position sense and kinesthesia in sub-acute stroke. Cortex J Devoted Study Nerv Syst Behav 2019; 121:414–26.
20. Bosecker C, Dipietro L, Volpe B, et al. Kinematic robot-based evaluation scales and clinical counterparts to measure upper limb motor performance in patients with chronic stroke. Neurorehabilitation Neural Repair 2010;24(1):62–9.
21. Rohrer B, Fasoli S, Krebs HI, et al. Movement smoothness changes during stroke recovery. J Neurosci 2002;22(18):8297–304.
22. Dipietro L, Krebs HI, Fasoli SE, et al. Changing motor synergies in chronic stroke. J Neurophysiol 2007;98(2):757–68.
23. Palazzolo JJ, Ferraro M, Krebs HI, et al. Stochastic estimation of arm mechanical impedance during robotic stroke rehabilitation. IEEE Trans Neural Syst Rehabil Eng Publ IEEE Eng Med Biol Soc 2007;15(1):94–103.
24. Reinkensmeyer DJ, Dewald JP, Rymer WZ. Guidance-based quantification of arm impairment following brain injury: a pilot study. IEEE Trans Rehabil Eng Publ IEEE Eng Med Biol Soc 1999;7(1):1–11.
25. Lum PS, Burgar CG, Kenney DE, et al. Quantification of force abnormalities during passive and active-assisted upper-limb reaching movements in post-stroke hemiparesis. IEEE Trans Biomed Eng 1999;46(6):652–62.
26. Guidali M, Schmiedeskamp M, Klamroth V, Riener R. Assessment and training of synergies with an arm rehabilitation robot. IEEE; 2009. p. 772–6.
27. Mehrholz J, Pohl M, Platz T, et al. Electromechanical and robot-assisted arm training for improving activities of daily living, arm function, and arm muscle strength after stroke. Cochrane Database Syst Rev 2018;9. https://doi.org/10. 1002/14651858.CD006876.pub5.

28. Everard G, Declerck L, Detrembleur C, et al. New technologies promoting active upper limb rehabilitation after stroke: an overview and network meta-analysis. Eur J Phys Rehabil Med 2022;58(4).

29. Rodgers H, Shaw L, Bosomworth H, et al. Robot Assisted Training for the Upper Limb after Stroke (RATULS): study protocol for a randomised controlled trial. Trials 2017;18(1):340.

30. Chien WT, Chong YY, Tse MK, et al. Robot-assisted therapy for upper-limb rehabilitation in subacute stroke patients: a systematic review and meta-analysis. Brain Behav 2020;10(8):e01742.

31. Bernhardt J, Mehrholz J. Robotic-assisted training after stroke: RATULS advances science. Lancet 2019;394(10192):6–8.

32. Rodgers H, Bosomworth H, Krebs HI, et al. Robot assisted training for the upper limb after stroke (RATULS): a multicentre randomised controlled trial. Lancet 2019;394(10192):51–62.

33. Moggio L, de Sire A, Marotta N, et al. Exoskeleton versus end-effector robot-assisted therapy for finger-hand motor recovery in stroke survivors: systematic review and meta-analysis. Top Stroke Rehabil 2022;29(8):539–50.

34. Mehrholz J, Pollock A, Pohl M, et al. Systematic review with network meta-analysis of randomized controlled trials of robotic-assisted arm training for improving activities of daily living and upper limb function after stroke. J NeuroEngineering Rehabil 2020;17:83.

35. Conroy SS, Wittenberg GF, Krebs HI, et al. Robot-assisted arm training in chronic stroke: addition of transition-to-task practice. Neurorehabilitation Neural Repair 2019;33(9):751–61.

36. Platz T, Eickhof C, van Kaick S, et al. Impairment-oriented training or Bobath therapy for severe arm paresis after stroke: a single-blind, multicentre randomized controlled trial. Clin Rehabil 2005;19(7):714–24.

37. Krebs HI, Mernoff S, Fasoli SE, et al. A comparison of functional and impairment-based robotic training in severe to moderate chronic stroke: a pilot study. NeuroRehabilitation 2008;23(1):81–7.

38. Comino-Suárez N, Moreno JC, Gómez-Soriano J, et al. Transcranial direct current stimulation combined with robotic therapy for upper and lower limb function after stroke: a systematic review and meta-analysis of randomized control trials. J Neuroengineering Rehabil 2021;18(1):148.

39. Hsu HY, Chiu HY, Kuan TS, et al. Robotic-assisted therapy with bilateral practice improves task and motor performance in the upper extremities of chronic stroke patients: a randomised controlled trial. Aust Occup Ther J 2019;66(5):637–47.

40. Kuo LC, Yang KC, Lin YC, et al. Internet of things (iot) enables robot-assisted therapy as a home program for training upper limb functions in chronic stroke: a randomized control crossover study. Arch Phys Med Rehabil 2023;104(3):363–71.

41. Morone G, Capone F, Iosa M, et al. May dual transcranial direct current stimulation enhance the efficacy of robot-assisted therapy for promoting upper limb recovery in chronic stroke? Neurorehabilitation Neural Repair 2022;36(12):800–9.

42. Kinoshita S, Abo M, Okamoto T, et al. Utility of the revised version of the ability for basic movement scale in predicting ambulation during rehabilitation in post-stroke patients. J Stroke Cerebrovasc Dis 2017;26(8):1663–9.

43. van Nunen MPM, Gerrits KHL, Konijnenbelt M, et al. Recovery of walking ability using a robotic device in subacute stroke patients: a randomized controlled study. Disabil Rehabil Assist Technol 2015;10(2):141–8.

44. Tamburella F, Moreno JC, Herrera Valenzuela DS, et al. Influences of the biofeedback content on robotic post-stroke gait rehabilitation: electromyographic vs joint torque biofeedback. J Neuroengineering Rehabil 2019;16(1):95.

45. Hesse S, Werner C, von Frankenberg S, et al. Treadmill training with partial body weight support after stroke. Phys Med Rehabil Clin N Am 2003;14(1 Supplement):S111–23.

46. Louie DR, Mortenson WB, Durocher M, et al. Exoskeleton for post-stroke recovery of ambulation (ExStRA): study protocol for a mixed-methods study investigating the efficacy and acceptance of an exoskeleton-based physical therapy program during stroke inpatient rehabilitation. BMC Neurol 2020;20(1):35.

47. Louie DR, Mortenson WB, Durocher M, et al. Efficacy of an exoskeleton-based physical therapy program for non-ambulatory patients during subacute stroke rehabilitation: a randomized controlled trial. J Neuroengineering Rehabil 2021; 18(1):149.

48. Awad LN, Esquenazi A, Francisco GE, et al. The ReWalk ReStore™ soft robotic exosuit: a multi-site clinical trial of the safety, reliability, and feasibility of exosuit-augmented post-stroke gait rehabilitation. J Neuroengineering Rehabil 2020; 17(1):80.

49. Tefertiller C, Hays K, Jones J, et al. Initial outcomes from a multicenter study utilizing the indego powered exoskeleton in spinal cord injury. Top Spinal Cord Inj Rehabil 2018;24(1):78–85.

50. Nilsson A, Vreede KS, Häglund V, et al. Gait training early after stroke with a new exoskeleton–the hybrid assistive limb: a study of safety and feasibility. J Neuroengineering Rehabil 2014;11:92.

51. Hobbs B, Artemiadis P. A review of robot-assisted lower-limb stroke therapy: unexplored paths and future directions in gait rehabilitation. Front Neurorobotics 2020;14:19.

52. Zhu YH, Ruan M, Yun RS, et al. Is leg-driven treadmill-based exoskeleton robot training beneficial to poststroke patients: a systematic review and meta-analysis. Am J Phys Med Rehabil 2023;102(4):331–9.

53. Bruni MF, Melegari C, De Cola MC, et al. What does best evidence tell us about robotic gait rehabilitation in stroke patients: a systematic review and meta-analysis. J Clin Neurosci 2018;48:11–7.

54. Zhang X, Yue Z, Wang J. Robotics in lower-limb rehabilitation after stroke. Behav Neurol 2017;2017:3731802.

55. Shakti D, Mathew L, Kumar N, et al. Effectiveness of robo-assisted lower limb rehabilitation for spastic patients: a systematic review. Biosens Bioelectron 2018;117:403–15.

56. Rodríguez-Fernández A, Lobo-Prat J, Font-Llagunes JM. Systematic review on wearable lower-limb exoskeletons for gait training in neuromuscular impairments. J Neuroengineering Rehabil 2021;18(1):22.

57. Buesing C, Fisch G, O'Donnell M, et al. Effects of a wearable exoskeleton stride management assist system (SMA®) on spatiotemporal gait characteristics in individuals after stroke: a randomized controlled trial. J NeuroEngineering Rehabil 2015;12(1):69.

58. Jayaraman A, O'Brien MK, Madhavan S, et al. Stride management assist exoskeleton vs functional gait training in stroke: A randomized trial. Neurology 2019;92(3):e263–73.

59. Yeung LF, Ockenfeld C, Pang MK, et al. Randomized controlled trial of robot-assisted gait training with dorsiflexion assistance on chronic stroke patients wearing ankle-foot-orthosis. J NeuroEngineering Rehabil 2018;15(1):51.

60. Carpino G, Pezzola A, Urbano M, et al. Assessing effectiveness and costs in robot-mediated lower limbs rehabilitation: a meta-analysis and state of the art. J Healthc Eng 2018;2018:7492024.

61. Lo K, Stephenson M, Lockwood C. The economic cost of robotic rehabilitation for adult stroke patients: a systematic review. JBI Database Syst Rev Implement Rep 2019;17(4):520–47.

62. Bhardwaj S, Khan AA, Muzammil M. Lower limb rehabilitation robotics: The current understanding and technology. Work Read Mass 2021;69(3):775–93.

63. Campagnini S, Liuzzi P, Mannini A, et al. Effects of control strategies on gait in robot-assisted post-stroke lower limb rehabilitation: a systematic review. J NeuroEngineering Rehabil 2022;19:52.

64. Naro A, Billeri L, Manuli A, et al. Breaking the ice to improve motor outcomes in patients with chronic stroke: a retrospective clinical study on neuromodulation plus robotics. Neurol Sci Off J Ital Neurol Soc Ital Soc Clin Neurophysiol 2021; 42(7):2785–93.

65. Gigante MA. Virtual reality: definitions, history and applications. In: Virtual reality systems. Academic Press; 1993. p. 3–14.

66. Bergmann J, Krewer C, Bauer P, et al. Virtual reality to augment robot-assisted gait training in non-ambulatory patients with a subacute stroke: a pilot randomized controlled trial. Eur J Phys Rehabil Med 2018;54(3):397–407.

67. Cruz-Neira C, Sandin DJ, DeFanti TA, et al. The CAVE: audio visual experience automatic virtual environment. Commun ACM 1992;35(6):64–72.

68. Yoshida T, Otaka Y, Osu R, et al. Motivation for rehabilitation in patients with subacute stroke: a qualitative study. Front Rehabil Sci 2021;2.

69. Laver KE, Lange B, George S, et al. Virtual reality for stroke rehabilitation. Cochrane Database Syst Rev 2017;11.

70. Leong SC, Tang YM, Toh FM, et al. Examining the effectiveness of virtual, augmented, and mixed reality (VAMR) therapy for upper limb recovery and activities of daily living in stroke patients: a systematic review and meta-analysis. J Neuroengineering Rehabil 2022;19(1):93.

71. Lyu T, Yan K, Lyu J, et al. Comparative efficacy of gait training for balance outcomes in patients with stroke: A systematic review and network meta-analysis. Front Neurol 2023;14.

72. Virtual reality training enhances gait poststroke: a systematic review and meta-analysis. Ann N Y Acad Sci 2020;1478(1):18–42.

73. De Keersmaecker E, Lefeber N, Geys M, et al. Virtual reality during gait training: does it improve gait function in persons with central nervous system movement disorders? A systematic review and meta-analysis. NeuroRehabilitation 2019; 44(1):43–66.

74. Luque-Moreno C, Ferragut-Garcías A, Rodríguez-Blanco C, et al. A decade of progress using virtual reality for poststroke lower extremity rehabilitation: systematic review of the intervention methods. BioMed Res Int 2015;2015:342529.

75. Zhang B, Li D, Liu Y, et al. Virtual reality for limb motor function, balance, gait, cognition and daily function of stroke patients: a systematic review and meta-analysis. J Adv Nurs 2021;77(8):3255–73.

76. Wiley E, Khattab S, Tang A. Examining the effect of virtual reality therapy on cognition post-stroke: a systematic review and meta-analysis. Disabil Rehabil Assist Technol 2022;17(1):50–60.

77. Saposnik G, Cohen LG, Mamdani M, et al. Efficacy and safety of non-immersive virtual reality exercising in stroke rehabilitation (EVREST): a randomised, multicentre, single-blind, controlled trial. Lancet Neurol 2016;15(10):1019–27.

78. Thomson K, Pollock A, Bugge C, et al. Commercial gaming devices for stroke upper limb rehabilitation: a survey of current practice. Disabil Rehabil Assist Technol 2016;11(6):454–61.
79. Clark WE, Sivan M, O'Connor RJ. Evaluating the use of robotic and virtual reality rehabilitation technologies to improve function in stroke survivors: A narrative review. J Rehabil Assist Technol Eng 2019;6. https://doi.org/10.1177/2055668319863557. 2055668319863557.
80. Mubin O, Alnajjar F, Jishtu N, et al. Exoskeletons with virtual reality, augmented reality, and gamification for stroke patients' rehabilitation: systematic review. JMIR Rehabil Assist Technol 2019;6(2):e12010.
81. Zanatta F, Farhane-Medina NZ, Adorni R, et al. Combining robot-assisted therapy with virtual reality or using it alone? A systematic review on health-related quality of life in neurological patients. Health Qual Life Outcomes 2023;21(1):18.
82. McIntyre A, Viana R, Cao P, et al. A national survey of evidence-based stroke rehabilitation intervention use in clinical practice among Canadian occupational therapists. NeuroRehabilitation 2023;52(3):463–75.
83. Glover W. Work-related strain injuries in physiotherapists: prevalence and prevention of musculoskeletal disorders. Physiotherapy 2002;88(6):364–72.
84. Masiero S, Armani M, Ferlini G, et al. Randomized trial of a robotic assistive device for the upper extremity during early inpatient stroke rehabilitation. Neurorehabilitation Neural Repair 2014;28(4):377–86.
85. Timmermans AA, Lemmens RJ, Monfrance M, et al. Effects of task-oriented robot training on arm function, activity, and quality of life in chronic stroke patients: a randomized controlled trial. J NeuroEngineering Rehabil 2014;11:45.
86. Olczak A, Truszczyńska-Baszak A, Stępień A. The use of armeo®spring device to assess the effect of trunk stabilization exercises on the functional capabilities of the upper limb—an observational study of patients after stroke. Sensors 2022;22(12):4336.
87. Wu C, Yang C, Chen Mde, et al. Unilateral versus bilateral robot-assisted rehabilitation on arm-trunk control and functions post stroke: a randomized controlled trial. J NeuroEngineering Rehabil 2013;10(1):35.
88. Housman SJ, Scott KM, Reinkensmeyer DJ. A randomized controlled trial of gravity-supported, computer-enhanced arm exercise for individuals with severe hemiparesis. Neurorehabilitation Neural Repair 2009;23(5):505–14.
89. Mayr A, Kofler M, Saltuari L. [ARMOR: an electromechanical robot for upper limb training following stroke. A prospective randomised controlled pilot study]. Handchir Mikrochir Plast Chir Organ Deutschsprachigen Arbeitsgemeinschaft Handchir Organ Deutschsprachigen Arbeitsgemeinschaft Mikrochir Peripher Nerven Gefasse Organ V 2008;40(1):66–73.
90. Polygerinos P, Wang Z, Galloway KC, et al. Soft robotic glove for combined assistance and at-home rehabilitation. Robot Auton Syst 2015;73:135–43.
91. Gassert R, Dietz V. Rehabilitation robots for the treatment of sensorimotor deficits: a neurophysiological perspective. J NeuroEngineering Rehabil 2018;15(1):46.
92. Hesse S, Tomelleri C, Bardeleben A, et al. Robot-assisted practice of gait and stair climbing in nonambulatory stroke patients. J Rehabil Res Dev 2012;49(4):613–22.
93. Ochi M, Wada F, Saeki S, et al. Gait training in subacute non-ambulatory stroke patients using a full weight-bearing gait-assistance robot: A prospective, randomized, open, blinded-endpoint trial. J Neurol Sci 2015;353(1–2):130–6.

94. End-effector-based Gaittrainer | LEXO®. Tyromotion. Available at: https://tyromotion.com/en/products/lexo/. Accessed May 1, 2023.
95. Ronchi R, Perez-Marcos D, Giroux A, et al. Use of immersive virtual reality to detect unilateral spatial neglect in chronic stroke. Ann Phys Rehabil Med 2018;61:e90–1.
96. Mekbib DB, Zhao Z, Wang J, et al. Proactive motor functional recovery following immersive virtual reality-based limb mirroring therapy in patients with subacute stroke. Neurother J Am Soc Exp Neurother 2020;17(4):1919–30.
97. Bahadori S, Williams JM, Wainwright TW. Lower limb kinematic, kinetic and spatial-temporal gait data for healthy adults using a self-paced treadmill. Data Brief 2021;34:106613.
98. Isaacson BM, Swanson TM, Pasquina PF. The use of a computer-assisted rehabilitation environment (CAREN) for enhancing wounded warrior rehabilitation regimens. J Spinal Cord Med 2013;36(4):296–9.
99. Timmermans C, Roerdink M, Meskers CGM, et al. Walking-adaptability therapy after stroke: results of a randomized controlled trial. Trials 2021;22(1):923.
100. Park DS, Lee DG, Lee K, et al. Effects of virtual reality training using xbox kinect on motor function in stroke survivors: a preliminary study. J Stroke Cerebrovasc Dis 2017;26(10):2313–9.
101. Yavuzer G, Senel A, Atay MB, et al. "Playstation eyetoy games'" improve upper extremity-related motor functioning in subacute stroke: a randomized controlled clinical trial. Eur J Phys Rehabil Med 2008;44(3):237–44.
102. Lee MM, Shin DC, Song CH. Canoe game-based virtual reality training to improve trunk postural stability, balance, and upper limb motor function in subacute stroke patients: a randomized controlled pilot study. J Phys Ther Sci 2016;28(7):2019–24.
103. Wang ZR, Wang P, Xing L, et al. Leap Motion-based virtual reality training for improving motor functional recovery of upper limbs and neural reorganization in subacute stroke patients. Neural Regen Res 2017;12(11):1823–31.

Spasticity Treatment Beyond Botulinum Toxins

Sheng Li, MD, PhD[a,b],*, Paul Winston, MD[c,d], Manuel F. Mas, MD[e]

KEYWORDS

- Spasticity • Stroke • Phenol neurolysis • Cryoneurolysis
- Extracorporeal shock wave therapy (ESWT)

KEY POINTS

- Botulinum toxin (BoNT) therapy is the mainstream treatment option for post-stroke spasticity. Phenol neurolysis, cryoneurolysis, and extracorporeal shock wave therapy (ESWT) can be alternative and/or complementary to BoNT therapy.
- Phenol neurolysis to nerves and/or motor branches provide greater spasticity reduction with longer effective duration, as compared to BoNT therapy. The possibility of long-term side effects, especially neuropathic pain following mixed nerve injections, needs to be taken into account.
- Cryoneurolysis is an innovative intervention. Feasibility and safety have been demonstrated through case series and an analysis of 113 patients. Cryoneurolysis can be used to target both spasticity and pain as primary goals. There is no maximal dose as no drugs are administered. Further clinical trials on its efficacy are needed.
- ESWT is a safe and promising physical modality for spasticity management, likely related changes in the rheological properties of spastic muscles. It could be used as an effective adjunctive therapy with other interventions.

INTRODUCTION

Post-stroke spasticity is a common complication that gradually develops in the course of motor recovery, and often persists if there is incomplete motor recovery.[1] Reports of incidence and prevalence vary widely due to different definitions and clinical measurements of spasticity in varying populations of stroke survivors. It occurs in anywhere from 19%[2] to 98%[3] of stroke survivors. Spasticity is clinically significant as it causes problems directly, such as pain, distorted joint position, posture, and hygiene

[a] Department of Physical Medicine and Rehabilitation, McGovern Medical School, University of Texas Health Science Center – Houston, Houston, TX, USA; [b] TIRR Memorial Herman; [c] Division of Physical Medicine and Rehabilitation, University of British Columbia, Victoria, British Columbia, Canada; [d] Canadian Advances in Neuro-Orthopedics for Spasticity Consortium, Victoria, British Columbia, Canada; [e] Department of Physical Medicine and Rehabilitation, School of Medicine, University of Puerto Rico, San Juan, Puerto Rico
* Corresponding author.
E-mail address: sheng.li@uth.tmc.edu

Phys Med Rehabil Clin N Am 35 (2024) 399–418
https://doi.org/10.1016/j.pmr.2023.06.009
1047-9651/24/© 2023 Elsevier Inc. All rights reserved.

difficulties, as well as predisposes to other complications, such as musculotendinous retractions, joint contractures, and permanent deformities. Spasticity interacts with and amplifies the effects of other impairments, such as weakness, exaggerated stretch reflexes, clonus, impaired coordination, and motor control and planning, contributing to limitations in activity and participation.[4] These abnormalities and impairments interact with each other and evolve over time, resulting in a dynamic picture of varying clinical presentations after stroke.[5,6] These motor impairments limit vocational and social participation in more than half of stroke survivors at age 65 years and over.[7,8]

The main goals of spasticity treatment are to reduce spasticity and its associated involuntary muscle activity, and to prevent secondary complications that lead to pain, deformity, and barriers to performing activities of daily living.[9] There are a number of treatment options for management of spasticity, including physical modalities, oral medications, chemodenervation with botulinum toxins (BoNT), phenol or alcohol injections, intrathecal baclofen therapy, and surgical interventions.[10] BoNT therapy is widely used and is the first-line treatment for focal spasticity management after stroke.[11] BoNT exerts its effect through inhibition of acetylcholine release at the neuromuscular junction via a complex process, that is, resulting in muscle paralysis and thus spasticity reduction.[12–14] The profile of clinical effects of BoNT is well recognized. The BoNT effect starts to manifest within several days following an injection, and reaches its peak in 2 to 3 weeks. The clinical effects last about 3 months, and spasticity returns. The reversible BoNT effect is likely due to turnover of the neuromuscular junctions, replacing those paralyzed by the toxin.[15] Therefore, patients require repeated BoNT injections every 3 to 4 months to maintain therapeutic effects.[16,17] The efficacy and safety of BoNT therapy in spasticity reduction is well established over last 30 years. In a meta-analysis study that included 40 clinical trials, including 2718 stroke patients,[18] the authors reported robust evidence of BoNT on reducing resistance to passive movement and on self-care, as measured with the (Modified) Ashworth Score, and improving self-care ability for the affected side after intervention and at follow-up. Similarly, evidence of the absence of effect on the "arm-hand capacity" at follow-up was also robust. BoNT significantly reduced "involuntary movements," "spasticity-related pain," "care burden," and improved "passive range of motion," whereas no evidence was found for improved "arm and hand use" after the intervention.

Despite its favorable safety and efficacy profile, BoNT therapy alone is often inadequate to fully control symptoms. Typical insurance coverage and US. Food and Drug Administration approval for spasticity limits the use of onabotulinumtoxin A to 400 to 600 units no more than every 3 months. In those with moderate to severe spasticity, BoNT therapy may not be effective even with a high dose of BoNT. There are a number of emerging treatment options for spasticity management. In this paper, we focus on innovative and revived treatment options that can be alternative or complementary to BoNT therapy, including phenol neurolysis, cryoneurolysis, and extracorporeal shock wave therapy (ESWT).

Phenol Neurolysis

Phenol has been used in spasticity since the late 1950 by intrathecal administration.[19] Peripheral neurolysis with phenol to reduce spasticity was first reported in 1964.[20] Phenol neurolysis has since been used for spasticity management.[21–24] Phenol neurolysis was largely replaced by BoNT therapy since its approval for spasticity management about 30 years ago in the United States despite phenol neurolysis having significantly lower cost and longer treatment duration.[25] Limiting factors include difficulty in obtaining medical grade phenol solution, potential adverse effects, and the procedure skills required for injection. Advances in combined ultrasound and electrical stimulation guidance have greatly improved procedure techniques and have expanded clinical use of phenol neurolysis in recent years.[26–29]

Mechanisms of Action

Phenol, a benzene derivative, is also known as carbolic acid. Phenol is typically prepared as a sterile aqueous solution. An aqueous solution containing less than 2% phenol will produce only short-term anesthetic effects, whereas 3% phenol or more typically induces Wallerian degeneration. For neurolysis, concentration of phenol usually ranges for 5% to 7% to produce neurolysis.[30] Phenol denatures proteins in axons and membranes nonselectively in both afferent and efferent nerve fibers, leading to denervation and degeneration of spindles.[31] When injected into muscle, it can cause myonecrosis. Both nonselective nerve destruction and local muscle damage can occur near the site of injection.[30] Additionally, phenol can cause occlusion and fibrosis in the microcirculation around the nerve.[32] However, animal studies have shown that both nerves and muscles regenerate and have near complete recovery after phenol is injected either into peripheral nerves[33] or intramuscularly.[34]

Clinical Application

Phenol neurolysis usually produces immediate anesthesic effects and a later neurolytic effect on spasticity reduction. The immediate effect is about 50% of its peak which occurs 1 week after injection.[35] Its longer-term improvement occurs with Wallerian degeneration. The duration depends on the dose, accuracy of injection, and repeated injections, ranging from 3 to 9 months. The effects can even last years until axonal regrowth occurs.[32,36]

Guidance techniques

The accuracy of phenol injection into the nerve is the most important factor determining the relief of spasticity.[23] It requires precise localization and injection of these agents to the nerve fibers at the trunk, branch, or motor points of the target nerves. Precise localization is usually achieved with guidance combining ultrasound imaging and electrical stimulation. With advanced guidance techniques, motor branches of median, ulnar, and radial nerves can be precisely blocked for management of focal spasticity in distal muscles of upper extremities with desirable outcomes.[27] As such, phenol neurolysis can be used to block main nerves (pectoral and musculocutaneous nerves) to reduce spasticity in large muscles to correct shoulder and elbow joint abnormalities (**Fig. 1**A). It can also be used to precisely block motor branches of tibial nerve to flexor digitorum longus and flexor hallucis longus muscles for toe curling (**Fig. 1**B). All peripheral nerves and their motor branches can be blocked with phenol for management of limb spasticity[26,27]

Dosing

Previous studies have reported 8.5 g as the lethal dose in humans, whereas the Agency for Toxic Substances and Disease Registry states that the fatal dose for ingestion of phenol ranges from 1.0 to 32 g.[37] The maximum daily dose of phenol is 1 g per session, and caution must be taken in patients with liver disease since the liver metabolizes phenol.[19] A general rule for clinicians is to use no more than 20 mL of 5% aqueous phenol solution, which is equivalent to 1 g of phenol.[30] In a recent retrospective study of 185 patients, a mean of 3.48 mL of 6% phenol was injected per nerve and 10.95 mL of phenol was used per procedure.[26]

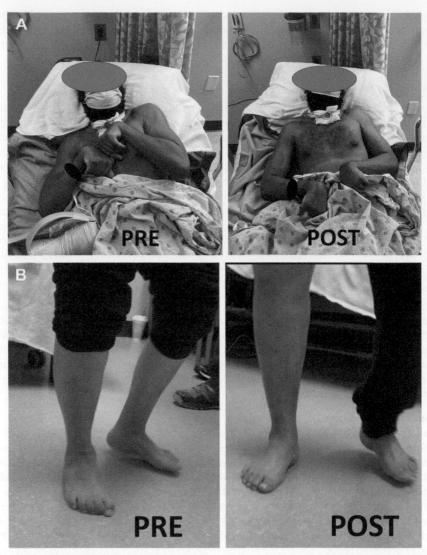

Fig. 1. Immediate effects of phenol neurolysis. (*A*) Correction of shoulder and elbow joint postures after nerve blocks with a total of 12 mL 6% phenol to bilateral pectoral nerves and bilateral musculocutaneous nerves in a patient with disorders of consciousness after anoxic brain injury. (*B*) Correction of toe positions after nerve blocks with 1.5 mL 6% phenol to tibial nerve motor branches to flexor hallucis longus and flexor digitorum longus muscles in a chronic stroke patient with spastic right hemiplegia.

Efficacy

As compared to BoNT therapy, there is paucity of evidence of efficacy and safety based on randomized controlled studies on phenol neurolysis for spasticity management. Multiple studies have demonstrated that phenol has the potential to last longer with greater clinical efficacy compared with BoNT.[26,27,36,38–40] In a study by Halpern and Meelhuysen,[36] 5% phenol was injected into 95 patients and the effects lasted for 3 to 17 months. Furthermore, they found 60% of muscles demonstrated persistence of relaxation for 6 months or more.[36]

The magnitude and duration of response after phenol neurolysis is related to the concentration. One study demonstrated successful treatment in spasticity of hip adductors and/or ankle flexors in 89% of patients who received 4.5% phenol compared to 18% benefit in those who received 3% phenol.[38] In addition, the efficacy of phenol neurolysis also depends on the site of blocks, that is, motor point blocks versus nerve blocks. BoNT therapy demonstrated superior treatment in spasticity reduction and gait improvement in ambulatory children with cerebral palsy and spastic diplegia and less severe side effects, as compared to phenol motor point blocks.[41,42] In contrast, phenol neurolysis with blocks of nerve or nerve branches has similar[23] or better[39,40] clinical outcomes than BoNT therapy. Manca and colleagues[40] compared the efficacy of phenol nerve block to motor branch of tibial nerve and 300 units of onabotulinum toxin injection in triceps surae muscles in the inhibition of ankle clonus in stroke patients. Both groups had significant clonus reduction over time, but the effect of phenol was greater than that of BoNT. In a recent chart review study, Li and colleagues[39] reported that the amount of BoNT in the subsequent treatment (ie, second cycle of injection) was significantly higher in stroke patients who received BoNT treatment first as compared to those who received phenol treatment first.

Patients with severe spasticity many need an amount of BoNT beyond the maximal recommended dose if used alone. Combined use of phenol and BoNT is effective in managing spasticity in these patients. The most common pattern is that phenol and BoNT are used for different muscles. Phenol neurolysis is used for large muscle groups, such as shoulder adductors, elbow flexors and hip adductors, and hamstrings, whereas BoNT is reserved for distal muscles.[26,43,44]

Repeat injections

Unlike BoNT-A injections, nerve blocks can be repeated as early as several days. Phenol injections can be safely repeated over time as needed clinically. However, there is limited data on repeated nerve blocks with phenol for chronic spasticity management. Repeated phenol neurolysis can achieve similar effects and duration of spasticity reduction.[45] Possibly due to muscle fibrosis, motor branch localization with electrical stimulation (e-stim) in patients who have received multiple injections is more difficult.[46] Large volumes of phenol (5 mL) can produce a longer-lasting block but are more likely to cause muscle fibrosis, thus making repeat injections more difficulty. Combined ultrasound and electrical stimulation guidance allows a smaller volume due to improved accuracy in up to 8 repeated injections with similar clinical effects and duration.[47]

Side Effects

The side effects of phenol range from mild to severe. A few patients may experience transient bitter taste, sometimes metallic, during or immediately after the procedure for 2 or 3 minutes.[48] Mild side effects include injection pain, bleeding, and bruising that are similar to other interventional procedures.[19] Local post-injection pain is usually resolved in 24 to 48 hours.[32] Because peripheral nerves contain both motor and sensory fibers, the injection of phenol into a mixed nerve can result in the undesirable loss of sensation, chemical neuritis, and severe burning pain in the distribution of the nerve.[23] The rate of dysesthesia and neuropathic pain is highly variable between 2% and 32%.[32] Nerves with larger sensory territory such as the tibial nerve may have a higher rate of dysesthesia compared to the musculocutaneous or obturator nerves, where there is a lower incidence and severity of dysesthesia.[47] Systemic complications of phenol administration usually occur from accidental intravascular injection, which may result in potentially fatal cardiac dysrhythmias, hypotension, cardiovascular collapse, seizures, and respiratory depression. In addition, phenol can cause serious vascular and nerve lesions such as thrombosis, ischemia, and tissue sloughing.[32] An overdose can cause tremors, central nervous system (CNS) depression, and cardiovascular collapse.[49] Given that phenol undergoes hepatic metabolism, it is generally avoided in patients with advanced liver disease.[19]

Overall, severe side effects are uncommon when using proper technique and dosing. In a recent retrospective chart review of 293 procedures with combined ultrasound and electrical stimulation guidance, phenol neurolysis has a relatively favorable safety profile, including pain (4.0%), swelling and inflammation (2.7%), dysesthesia (0.7%), and hypotension (0.7%).[26]

CRYONEUROLYSIS

The practice of pain medicine has demonstrated that it is possible to perform neurolysis without chemical agents including using radiofrequency ablation or cryoneurolysis. In the 1960s, Lloyd used liquid nitrogen to cool a probe and later coined the term cryoanalgesia. He described an absence of neuritis or neuralgia with treatment.[50] Cryoneurolysis has decades of established efficacy in the analgesic literature. There are historically few mentions of percutaneous neurolysis for spasticity. This includes one published case report of using percutaneous radiofrequency ablation on a motor nerve for spasticity[51] and one for cryoneurolysis.[52] An additional published abstract documented improvements in elbow spasticity using cryoneurolysis to the musculocutaneous nerve.[53] With recent advances in ultrasound guidance for diagnostic nerve blocks (DNBs), Winston and colleagues have demonstrated feasibility and effectiveness of cryoneurolysis in spasticity management in recent years.[54–57]

Mechanism of Action

The procedure begins with identifying a nerve target with ultrasound guidance. A cryoprobe is inserted percutaneously through a recommended angiocatheter after a weal of lidocaine is placed subcutaneously. The cryoprobe is placed against the nerve target and electrical stimulation at low frequency, less than 1 mA, is used to stimulate the target and not the surrounding muscle similar to phenol neurolysis. Cryoneurolysis occurs due to the process of throttling a gas through an orifice from high to low pressure area, which results in rapid expansion of the gas, leading to a drop in temperature, known as the Joule-Thomson effect.[50] The temperature is determined by the boiling point of the gas, carbon dioxide or nitrous oxide, used as the cryogen, typically between $-60°C$ and $-88°C$ for pain or spasticity.[50] At this temperature, the surrounding fluid forms an ice ball with a diameter between 3.5 and 18 mm in seconds along the distal cryoprobe (**Fig. 2**). No fluid passes from the probe into the body. The ice ball causes a local zone of axon and myelin disruption leading to a secondary axonotmesis and Wallerian degeneration of the targeted nerve, extending bidirectionally outward from the lesion. A distinct property of cryoneurolysis is that the basal lamina, epineurium, and perineurium of the targeted nerve are not damaged and serve as a conduit for neural regeneration. Depending on the size of the nerve, the axon will regrow after 3 to 6 months.[58] Unlike other neurolytic techniques, there is little risk of damage to surrounding structures, which usually results in perineural and muscular fibrosis.[58] With cryoneurolysis there is no dispersion of fluid away from the ice ball toward unwanted targets, the ice ball will freeze in place. A cycle can last from seconds to minutes. We have most experience with 106 second cycles, 1 to 3 cycles per nerve depending on

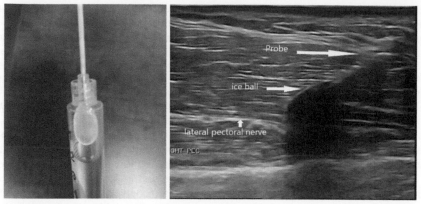

Fig. 2. Demonstration of ice ball. Left: Ice ball formed in water; Right: Ice ball formed in the pectoralis major muscle targeting the lateral pectoral nerve.

its circumference.[59] Experimental rat studies have shown the need for a 60 second cycle to produce analgesia and hypoesthesia.[60] Blood vessels are typically not affected by the cryoneurolysis at the temperatures used. They serve as a heat sink and are not thrombosed as is described with phenol.[61] It is hypothesized that the maintenance of the perineurium prevents the release of the chemical agent, neurotropin, which is implicated in the formation of painful neuromas and explains why Lloyd noted the absence of the neuritis or neuralgia formation.[62] Cryoneurolysis is a treatment in itself for neuromas and neuropathic pain.[63,64]

Clinical Application

Cryoneurolysis for spasticity is modeled on anesthetic DNBs using 1% to 2% lidocaine.[65,66] The protocol of cryoneurolysis was originally created by Dr. Daniel Vincent, an anesthesiologist of the University of British Columbia. The protocol has been recently published.[57]

A cornerstone of the protocol is to first perform a DNB. Through temporary paralysis, the DNB can isolate the contribution of each muscle to a spastic pattern.[56] Most importantly, it will distinguish if a muscle has a musculotendinous contracture versus a fully or partial reducible deformity, that only relaxes with a nerve block. For example, assessing the contribution of the brachialis, biceps, or brachioradialis in elbow flexion.[67] The DNB can be used to predict the outcomes for spasticity triage from simple to complex patterns, including those with the adducted shoulder, flexed elbow, thumb-in-palm, stiff-knee, adducted thighs, and equinovarus foot.[68] Once the DNB is performed and the outcomes are evaluated, the optimal targets can be selected for cryoneurolysis.

Cryoneurolysis has numerous targets for spastic patients, including spasticity, spastic dystonia, and pain. Both cryoneurolysis and the DNB are recommended to use electrical stimulation and ultrasound guidance.[55,56] As cryoneurolysis was designed to target sensory nerves, it offers numerous targets in spasticity, a whole mixed motor sensory nerve trunk, primary motor nerve branches, intramuscular motor branches, and primary sensory. A recent analysis of spasticity noted that 35.75% of 277 nerves targeted included mixed motor sensory nerves, which differs from other neurolytic techniques.[59]

A clinical assessment may reveal that some patients with spasticity are hemiesthetic, whereas others have neuropathic pain or pain associated with contractures such as a claw hand. The patient thus first undergoes a DNB to see if there will be a sensory disturbance or excessive weakness with the anesthetic. This knowledge allows to preplan the targets for cryoneurolysis (**Table 1**). Specific anatomic targets for cryoneurolysis can be found in a recent Atlas on this topic.[57]

Efficacy

Cryoneurolysis for spasticity is novel with numerous ongoing studies (NCT04670783, NCT05147441, NCT04907201, NCT05674604). There are numerous case studies and published videos demonstrating the technique and patient outcomes.[55,69–71] An accompanying video demonstrates several clinical outcomes in patients for cryoneurolysis on both the upper and lower extremity. Emerging literature demonstrates the reproducibility and durability of this technique. The published case series show potential for long-lasting results, including improvements on the Modified Ashworth Scale and the Modified Tardieu Scale.[54,69,70] The first prospective cases series found statistically significant improvement in shoulder range of motion, with reductions in pain in follow-up to 1 year.[72] As a novel intervention, much more data are required to determine the efficacy of this treatment.

Side Effects

Cryoneurolysis has an established history in the pain literature. Side effects include have been noted to be localized skin effects, unwanted numbness, paresthesias, and numbness. Most are considered mild and limited to a few weeks to months.[73,74] Cryoneurolysis causes immediate damage to the nerve. Patients may experience burning and cramping and a painful dysesthesia as the procedure takes place. In clinical experience, cryoneurolysis is more painful than other spasticity treatments but ends quickly as the nerve is fully neurolyzed. The presence of dysesthesia indicates that further cycles should be pursued to ensure a complete neurolysis. The first analysis of side effects on 277 nerves in 113 patients found 96.75% of nerves had no side effects after the treatment.[59] Among 113 patients, there were 3 skin events that healed. Nine patients reported nerve pain or dysesthesia (in 3.25% of the 277 nerves; 2 motor nerves and 7 mixed motor sensory targets) with 4 patients requiring a medical treatment for this. All patients reported resolution on follow-up. Three patients' symptoms remained at 3 months, resolving at 6 months. No patients withdrew from the study due to side effects.

Extracorporeal Shock Wave Therapy

ESWT is a noninvasive modality that applies high-pressure waves to different targeted parts of the body. It is defined as a sequence of single acoustic pulses characterized by a high peak of pressure, fast pressure rise, short duration, and rapid propagation in 3-dimensional space.[75] It has emerged as a treatment option for musculoskeletal injuries, such as plantar fasciitis and calcific tendinitis of the shoulder. It does not require any analgesia, sedation, or anesthesia. ESWT includes 2 types of shockwave therapies: focused and radial. These 2 types differ in their physical properties, depth of penetration, and mode of generation.[76] Focused ESWT (fESWT) is generated by electromagnetic, electrohydraulic, and piezoelectric sources. It rapidly increases pressure at the targeted treatment site and is more invasive. Radial ESWT (rESWT) is a low-to medium-energy type of shock wave produced by pneumatic devices inside a generator. It produces a wider effective region due to eccentric wave dispersion from the application site.[77] It has a lower depth of penetration than that of fESWT (up to 3 vs 12 cm) which makes it less invasive and better tolerated.[78] There is emerging evidence showing that ESWT may be an effective method to reduce spasticity. Earliest

Table 1
Recommended target nerves and nerve branches for cryoneurolysis

	Nerve / nerve branches	Target muscles
Shoulder Girdle	Suprascapular nerve Lateral pectoral motor branch Medial pectoral motor branch Thoracodorsal motor branch Subscapular intramuscular nerve branches	70% of sensory fibers shoulder. Pectoralis major Pectoralis minor Latissimus dorsi Subscapularis
Elbow	Musculocutaneous motor branch or intramuscular motor branch Radial nerve branch or intramuscular motor branch	Biceps brachii and or brachialis Brachioradialis
Wrist and fingers	Median nerve trunk above the elbow for a clawed or nonfunctioning hand if no sensory disturbance. Or selective intramuscular motor branches to each extrinsic muscle Ulnar nerve trunk above the elbow for a clawed or nonfunctioning hand if no sensory disturbance, Or selective intramuscular motor branches to each extrinsic muscle Intrinsic muscles may be too small for cryoprobe to target intramuscularly	Pronator teres, flexor carpi radialis, flexor digitorum superficialis, flexor digitorum profundus (radial half), flexor pollicis longus, and pronator quadratus, and intrinsic muscles Flexor carpi ulnaris, flexor digitorum profundus (ulnar half), intrinsic muscles
Hip	Femoral nerve intramuscular branches Obturator nerve: Anterior division Posterior divisions	Rectus femoris, sartorius Adductor longus, gracilis, adductor brevis Adductor magnus, adductor brevis *may have hip and genicular sensory changes
Knee	Femoral nerve intramuscular motor branches Sciatic nerve trunk Sciatic nerve intramuscular motor branches	Rectus femoris, sartorius All hamstrings, and all muscles innervated by tibial and peroneal nerves in severe spasticity Biceps femoris, semitendinosus and semimembranosus, adductor magnus
Foot and ankle	Tibial nerve trunk Intramuscular motor branches Peroneal nerve motor branches	All muscles if no sensory changes Medial and lateral gastrocnemius, soleus, tibialis posterior, flexor hallucis longus, flexor digitorum longus Tibialis anterior muscles, extensor hallucis longus

published data on ESWT and spasticity dates back to 1997, a pilot study on the effects of shock wave therapy on muscular dysfunction in children with spastic movement disorders.[79] Later, in 2005, Manganotti and Amelio[80] reported the beneficial effects of ESWT on upper limb hypertonia in 20 stroke patients lasting up to 12 weeks following one active session to ESWT treatment. Since then, research on ESWT and spasticity has grown significantly.

Mechanism of Action

The mechanism of action of ESWT on spasticity reduction is still in dispute, though multiple mechanisms have been proposed. Relevant mechanisms of action have been attributed to alterations in muscle elasticity and extensibility, as well as ability to induce nitric oxide to act on neuromuscular junctions.[81] ESWT may alter the elasticity and extensibility of spastic muscles and tendons by inducing nitric oxide synthesis, which can enhance neovascularization and reduce muscle stiffness.[82] Nitric oxide may also modulate neurotransmission and synaptic plasticity in the central nervous system, affecting spasticity at the cortical and spinal levels.[83] ESWT can affect rheological properties and fibrosis of chronic hypertonic muscles. This may reduce the passive resistance and stiffness of spastic muscles, as evidenced by infrared thermal imaging and electrical impedance myography.[84,85] Other mechanisms proposed include the reduction of motor neuron excitability, specifically reducing alpha motor neuron hyperexcitability.[86]

Clinical Application

Parameters of extracorporeal shock wave therapy for spasticity management

As with any other intervention, ESWT has multiple modifiable factors during treatment. Each of these may affect the outcome, such as spasticity reduction. Some of these include location of ESWT application, intensity, frequency, dosage, among others. Data on optimal ESWT location are limited. Although the myotendinous junction might be the logical location to reduce motor neuron excitability more effectively with ESWT,[87] there were no differences between applying treatment to the muscle belly or the myotendinous junction, with both groups achieving reduction in spasticity.[88] Likewise, applying ESWT in either the agonist or antagonist muscles in patients suffering from elbow flexor spasticity showed reduction in modified Ashworth scale (MAS) scores in both groups, but no difference in active function.[89] Generally, the number of pulses is applied in a range of 1000 to 2000. The frequency is usually set at 4 to 5 Hz and the pressure at 1.5 bars. The total energy flux density varies among studies, with lower energy (-0.03 mJ/mm^2) for upper extremity muscles and higher energy (-0.1 mJ/mm^2) for lower limb muscles. Interestingly, studies analyzing patients with cerebral palsy use a higher frequency than those involving stroke survivors.[87] The effect of different dosing parameters, such as the number of pulses of ESWT, has also been investigated. When cerebral palsy patients were divided into 4 groups with different total amount of ESWT pulses (500, 1000, 1500, 2000), they all improved throughout a 4-week follow-up period, as measured by the Australian Spasticity Assessment Scale.[90]

Therapeutic effects of extracorporeal shock wave therapy in spasticity reduction

Interest in the effectiveness of ESWT for spasticity after stroke has increased in recent years. There are numerous studies for both upper and lower-body stroke-related spasticity. Stroke-related ankle plantarflexor spasticity significantly decreased after 2 sessions per week for 2 weeks of radial ESWT and physical therapy.[91] This was compared to a sham ESWT and a control group. There was also significant improvement in walking times in the 6 m timed walk test for those treated with radial ESWT.[91] In a separate study, both focal and radial ESWT showed significant improvement in ankle plantarflexor spasticity after stroke in both MAS and Tardieu scale measurements. There was no difference between groups in any outcomes, except for ankle passive range of motion in favor of radial ESWT.[92] When applying rESWT to stroke patients with ankle plantar flexor spasticity, spasticity as measured by the MAS had immediate improvement following treatment but had no lasting effect at 2-week follow-up.[91] Treatment was compared to a sham and control group, when combined with conventional rehabilitation. Others have found similar results in spasticity reduction of lower-limb muscles.[93,94] Yet, data on functional improvement are inconclusive.[87]

After analysis of 16 randomized controlled trials, ESWT was concluded to be effective in reducing upper limb spasticity and improving upper limb function, when combined with conventional physiotherapy.[95] As previously discussed, early studies by Manganotti used ESWT to treat stroke patients suffering from upper limb dystonia. Finger flexor spasms improved at 1, 4 and 12, weeks following one active session of treatment whereas wrist flexors improved at 1 and 4 weeks, but not at 12 weeks.[80] Kim and colleagues[96] treated stroke patients suffering from subscapularis spasm with ESWT for 2 weeks. Subscapular muscle spasm, shoulder pain, and joint range of motion all improved significantly at 4 weeks following treatment. Radial ESWT to either agonist or antagonist elbow flexor muscles was effective in reducing spasticity after 4 weeks following the completion of treatment.[89] Like studies focusing on lower limb spasticity, even though upper limb spasticity improves after treatment with ESWT, studies have generally failed to demonstrate improvement in functionality.[97]

ESWT has been proven to have an immediate effect in spasticity. However, as with other interventions, the effective timeframe is limited. Oh and colleagues[98] conducted a recent meta-analysis to understand the duration of treatment effect of ESWT on spasticity as measured by MAS, combining different pathologies such as stroke, multiple sclerosis, and cerebral palsy. Analyzing 9 trials that met inclusion criteria, there was statistically significant reduction in MAS grade immediately after treatment. Spasticity reduction was also significant at week 1, 4, and 12, suggesting that duration of treatment could last up to 12 weeks. In addition, the number of shocks or site of application had no significant effect on reducing spasticity. In a separate study, ESWT was proposed as a long-lasting effective treatment for post-stroke spasticity, as defined by follow-up of 4 weeks and later.[99]

As with other interventions, optimal timing is an important factor to consider when studying ESWT for post-stroke spasticity management. A recent meta-analysis concluded that it could reduce spasticity for up to 3 months and that patients who had a stroke for less than 45 months could benefit from treatment with ESWT for spasticity throughout all follow-up periods analyzed (up to 3 months).[77] The number of total sessions and frequency of ESWT varied among the studies analyzed. When compared to other common interventions such as BoNT injections, ESWT has an immediate effect on spasticity. Notably, a recent systematic review concluded that ESWT was comparable to BoNT injections for post-stroke spasticity, with radial ESWT potentially being superior to all interventions using a ranking probability.[81] Zhang and colleagues[78] proposed that the efficacy of rESWT appears to be higher than that of fESWT for spasticity treatment.

ESWT has been combined with other spasticity interventions, such as BoNT injections, for a proposed synergistic effect. BoNT uptake has been found to be muscle activity dependent, with more receptors available for BoNT uptake in activated muscles.[100] Thus, clinicians are suggested to encourage activation of the injected

Table 2
Summary and comparisons among botulinum toxin, phenol neurolysis, cryoneurolysis, and extracorporeal shock wave therapy

	Botulinum Toxin (BoNT)	Phenol Neurolysis	Cryoneurolysis	Extracorporeal Shock Wave Therapy (ESWT)
Mechanism of action	Blockade of acetylcholine release into neuromuscular junction	Nonselective protein denaturation of nerves and muscles at the injection site	Axonotmesis and Wallerien degeneration from cold temperature without affecting surrounding tissues	Multiple: Improving muscle rheologic properties, nitric oxide synthesis, reduction of motor neuron excitability
Injection technique	Target muscles, using anatomic landmarks, intramuscular EMG, electrical stimulation, or sonographic guidance	Target nerves, preferably motor branches, using electrical stimulation and sonographic guidance	Target nerves, preferably motor branches, using electrical stimulation and sonographic guidance	Apply at the belly of the muscle or myotendinous junction.
Onset	3–7 d	Immediate, about 60% of peak effect	Immediate	Immediate
Peak effect	~2–3 wk	~1~2 wk	Not yet established	Not yet established
Duration	~3 mo	Variable, > 3 mo in general	Variable, > 3 mo in general	Variable, 4–12 wk
Dose titration to desired effect	Yes	Yes	Usually 1–3 cycles per nerve or nerve branch	Not described
Ease of administration	Relatively easy	Requires advanced training and expertise	Requires advanced training and experience	Relatively easy
Evidence of efficacy	Robust, RCTs published	Several RCTs	No RCT, ongoing trials	RCTs published
Pain during injection	Some	More	More	Some
Pain days after injection	Rare	More	Rare, 96.75% of 277 nerves had none in a recent study	Rare
Adverse events	Less common	Higher incidence of dysesthetic pain and swelling (<4%)	Negligible for motor nerves; whole mixed motor sensory nerves have increased incidence.	Rare
Use during pregnancy	Not recommended. Category C drug per FDA	Not recommended. Birth defects observed in animals, but not reported in humans	Not contraindicated	Contraindicated
Cost	Expensive	Very affordable	Significantly less than BoNT	High out of pocket

muscles. ESWT could play a role in muscle activation and improving BoNT uptake in injected muscles. In 2021, Marinaro and colleagues[101] studied the synergic use of BoNT and rESWT in spasticity of patients suffering from multiple sclerosis. rESWT was applied 4 months following BoNT injection to the triceps surae muscles, 1 session per week for a total of 4 weeks. Patients showed a statistically significant decrease in MAS after the last session of rESWT when compared to evaluation prior to starting this adjunct treatment. These values were not maintained when measured 1 and 3 months following ESWT. The goal of this study was to analyze the addition of rESWT when the efficacy of BoNT was decreasing, with positive results. Yet, based on the hypothesis of increased BoNT uptake in activated muscles, an earlier ESWT intervention immediately following injection could prove beneficial.

In 2021, Ip and colleagues[102] analyzed the practice patterns of Canadian physicians using adjunct therapies with BoNT injections for spasticity management. Only one physician was prescribing delayed ESWT following BoNT injection. Most physicians reported several barriers to use ESWT including physician and clinic resources, lack of evidence, or patient preference. Future studies are necessary to continue to analyze the synergistic effect of different spasticity treatments, including ESWT.

SIDE EFFECTS

Shock waves are considered a safe modality, but bleeding disorders and pregnancy are considered a contraindication for treatment. Most studies do not report major adverse effects with the most common ones being pain, muscular weakness, petechiae, and small bullae. These were all well-tolerated and resolved within days.[87] ESWT has also been shown as a safe alternative in other pathologies, such as cerebral palsy, with a similar safety profile as in stroke patients.[103–107] Thus, ESWT is a promising and safe intervention for spasticity reduction, but more research is needed to determine the optimal parameters and locations of application.

SUMMARY

BoNT therapy remains the mainstream treatment for post-stroke spasticity. Phenol neurolysis has become more practical due to advances in combined use of ultrasound imaging and electrical stimulation. Cryoneurolysis is an innovative intervention for spasticity management. Case series studies have demonstrated its feasibility and safety. ESWT is an emerging physical modality with promising evidence in spasticity reduction. Brief history, mechanism of activation, efficacy, and safety of each treatment are discussed in detail in each section. **Table 2** provides a succinct summary of comparisons among these treatments with BoNT therapy.

CLINICS CARE POINTS

- BoNT therapy is the mainstream treatment option for post-stroke spasticity. It may not be adequate due to dose limitations, however.

- Phenol neurolysis, cryoneurolysis, and ESWT can be alternative and/or complementary to BoNT therapy.

- Phenol neurolysis to nerves and/or motor branches provides greater spasticity reduction with longer effective duration, as compared to BoNT therapy. The possibility of long-term side effects, especially neuropathic pain following mixed nerve injections need to be taken into account.

- Cryoneurolysis is an innovative intervention. Feasibility and safety have been demonstrated through case series and an analysis of 113 patients. Cryoneurolysis can be used to target both spasticity and pain as primary goals. There is no maximal dose as no drugs are administered. Further clinical trials on its efficacy are needed.

- ESWT is a safe and promising physical modality for spasticity management, likely related changes in the rheological properties of spastic muscles. It could be used as an effective adjunctive therapy with other interventions.

DISCLOSURE

S. Li receives a research grant from SAOL Therapeutics, and is a consultant for Pacira Biosciences. P. Winston receives honoraria and educational grants from Abbvie, Ipsen, Merz and Pacira. M. Mas have nothing to disclose.

REFERENCES

1. Li S, Francisco GE, Rymer WZ. A New Definition of Poststroke Spasticity and the Interference of Spasticity With Motor Recovery From Acute to Chronic Stages. Neurorehabil Neural Repair 2021;35(7):601–10.
2. Sommerfeld DK, Eek EU, Svensson AK, et al. Spasticity after stroke: its occurrence and association with motor impairments and activity limitations. Stroke 2004;35(1):134–9.
3. Wissel J, Schelosky LD, Scott J, et al. Early development of spasticity following stroke: a prospective, observational trial. J Neurol 2010;257(7):1067–72.
4. Mayer NH, Esquenazi A. Muscle overactivity and movement dysfunction in the upper motoneuron syndrome. Phys Med Rehabil Clin N Am 2003;14(4):855–83, vii-viii.
5. Gracies JM. Pathophysiology of spastic paresis. II: Emergence of muscle overactivity. Muscle Nerve 2005;31(5):552–71.
6. Gracies JM. Pathophysiology of spastic paresis. I: Paresis and soft tissue changes. Muscle Nerve 2005;31(5):535–51.
7. Benjamin EJ, Blaha MJ, Chiuve SE, et al. Heart Disease and Stroke Statistics-2017 Update: A Report From the American Heart Association. Circulation 2017;135(10):e146–603.
8. Murphy MP, Carmine H. Long-term health implications of individuals with TBI: a rehabilitation perspective. NeuroRehabilitation 2012;31(1):85–94.
9. Turner-Stokes L, Ashford S, Esquenazi A, et al. A comprehensive person-centered approach to adult spastic paresis: a consensus-based framework. Eur J Phys Rehabil Med 2018;54(4):605–17.
10. Francisco GE, Li S. Spasticity. In: Cifu DX, editor. Braddom physical medicine and rehabilitation. 6th edition; 2020.
11. Simon O, Yelnik AP. Managing spasticity with drugs. Eur J Phys Rehabil Med 2010;46(3):401–10.
12. Wheeler A, Smith HS. Botulinum toxins: Mechanisms of action, antinociception and clinical applications. Toxicology 2013;306:124–46.
13. Pirazzini M, Rossetto O, Eleopra R, et al. Botulinum neurotoxins: Biology, pharmacology, and toxicology. Pharmacol Rev 2017;69(2):200–35.
14. Jankovic J. Botulinum toxin: State of the art. Movement Disorders 2017;32(8):1131–8.
15. de Paiva A, Meunier FA, Molgó J, et al. Functional repair of motor endplates after botulinum neurotoxin type A poisoning: biphasic switch of synaptic activity

between nerve sprouts and their parent terminals. Proc Natl Acad Sci USA 1999;96(6):3200–5.

16. Simpson DM, Hallett M, Ashman EJ, et al. Practice guideline update summary: Botulinum neurotoxin for the treatment of blepharospasm, cervical dystonia, adult spasticity, and headache Report of the Guideline Development Subcommittee of the American Academy of Neurology. Neurology 2016;86(19):1818–26.

17. Moeini-Naghani I, Hashemi-Zonouz T, Jabbari B. Botulinum Toxin Treatment of Spasticity in Adults and Children. Semin Neurol 2016;36(1):64–72.

18. Andringa A, van de Port I, van Wegen E, et al. Effectiveness of botulinum toxin treatment for upper limb spasticity after stroke over different ICF domains: a systematic review and meta-analysis. Arch Phys Med Rehabil 2019;100(9): 1703–25.

19. D'Souza RS, Warner NS. Phenol Nerve Block. 2023; https://www.ncbi.nlm.nih. gov/books/NBK525978/. Accessed April 16, 2023.

20. Khalili AA, Harmel MH, Forster S, et al. Management of Spasticity by Selective Peripheral Nerve Block with Dilute Phenol Solutions in Clinical Rehabilitation. Arch Phys Med Rehabil 1964;45:513–9.

21. Petrillo CR, Knoploch S. Phenol block of the tibial nerve for spasticity: a long-term follow-up study. Int Disabil Stud 1988;10(3):97–100.

22. Petrillo CR, Chu DS, Davis SW. Phenol block of the tibial nerve in the hemiplegic patient. Orthopedics 1980;3(9):871–4.

23. Kirazli Y, On AY, Kismali B, et al. Comparison of phenol block and botulinus toxin type a in the treatment of spastic foot after stroke: A randomized, double-blind trial. Am J Phys Med Rehab 1998;77(6):510–5.

24. Gündüz S, Kalyon TA, Dursun H, et al. Peripheral nerve block with phenol to treat spasticity in spinal cord injured patients. Paraplegia 1992;30(11):808–11.

25. Kim H, Tenaglia A, Munin MC. Nerve-target procedures. In: Winston P, Vincent D, editors. Altas of ultrasound-guided nerve-targetd procedures for spasticity. Surrey (United Kingdom): Quintessence Publishing Co, Ltd; 2023. p. 53–9.

26. Karri J, Mas MF, Francisco GE, et al. Practice patterns for spasticity management with phenol neurolysis. J Rehabil Med 2017;49(6):482–8.

27. Karri J, Zhang B, Li S. Phenol neurolysis for management of focal spasticity in the distal upper extremity. PM R 2019;12(3):246–50.

28. Demir Y, Şan AU, Kesikburun S, et al. The short-term effect of ultrasound and peripheral nerve stimulator-guided femoral nerve block with phenol on the outcomes of patients with traumatic spinal cord injury. Spinal Cord 2018;56(9): 907–12.

29. Korupolu R, Malik A, Pemberton E, et al. Phenol neurolysis in people with spinal cord injury: a descriptive study. Spinal cord series and cases 2022;8(1):90.

30. Zafonte RD, Munin MC. Phenol and alcohol blocks for the treatment of spasticity. Phys Med Rehabil Clin N Am 2001;12(4):817–32.

31. Bodine-Fowler SC, Allsing S, Botte MJ. Time course of muscle atrophy and recovery following a phenol-induced nerve block. Muscle Nerve 1996;19(4): 497–504.

32. Kocabas H, Salli A, Demir AH, et al. Comparison of phenol and alcohol neurolysis of tibial nerve motor branches to the gastrocnemius muscle for treatment of spastic foot after stroke: A randomized controlled pilot study. Eur J Phys Rehabil Med 2010;46(1):5–10.

33. Burkel WE, McPhee M. Effect of phenol injection into peripheral nerve of rat: electron microscope studies. Arch Phys Med Rehabil 1970;51(7):391–7.

34. Halpern D. Histologic studies in animals after intramuscular neurolysis with phenol. Arch Phys Med Rehabil 1977;58(10):438–43.
35. Zhang B, Darji N, Francisco GE, et al. The Time Course of Onset and Peak Effects of Phenol Neurolysis. Am J Phys Med Rehabil 2021;100(3):266–70.
36. Halpern D, Meelhuysen FE. Duration of relaxation after intramuscular neurolysis with phenol. JAMA 1967;200(13):1152–4.
37. Wood KM. The use of phenol as a neurolytic agent: a review. Pain 1978;5(3): 205–29.
38. Bakheit A, Badwan D, McLellan D. The effectiveness of chemical neurolysis in the treatment of lower limb muscle spasticity. Clin Rehabil 1996;10(1):40–3.
39. Li S, Woo J, Mas MF. Early Use of Phenol Neurolysis Likely Reduces the Total Amount of Botulinum Toxin in Management of Post-Stroke Spasticity. Frontiers in rehabilitation sciences 2021;2:729178.
40. Manca M, Merlo A, Ferraresi G, et al. Botulinum toxin type a versus phenol. A clinical and neurophysiological study in the treatment of ankle clonus. Eur J Phys Rehabil Med 2010;46(1):11–8.
41. Wong AM, Chen CL, Chen CP, et al. Clinical effects of botulinum toxin A and phenol block on gait in children with cerebral palsy. Am J Phys Med Rehabil 2004;83(4):284–91.
42. Gonnade N, Lokhande V, Ajij M, et al. Phenol versus botulinum toxin a injection in ambulatory cerebral palsy spastic diplegia: A comparative study. J Pediatr Neurosci 2017;12(4):338–43.
43. Gooch JL, Patton CP. Combining botulinum toxin and phenol to manage spasticity in children. Arch Phys Med Rehabil 2004;85(7):1121–4.
44. Anwar F, Ramanathan S. Combined botulinum toxin injections and phenol nerve/ motor point blocks to manage multifocal spasticity in adults. Br J Med Pract 2017;10(1):a1002.
45. Helweg-Larsen J, Jacobsen E. Treatment of spasticity in cerebral palsy by means of phenol nerve block of peripheral nerves. Dan Med Bull 1969; 16(1):20–5.
46. Halpern D, Meelhuysen FE. Phenol motor point block in the management of muscular hypertonia. Arch Phys Med Rehabil 1966;47(10):659–64.
47. Matsumoto ME, Berry J, Yung H, et al. Comparing Electrical Stimulation With and Without Ultrasound Guidance for Phenol Neurolysis to the Musculocutaneous Nerve. Pm r 2018;10(4):357–64.
48. Trainer N, Bowser BL, Dahm L. Obturator nerve block for painful hip in adult cerebral palsy. Arch Phys Med Rehabil 1986;67(11):829–30.
49. Kumar R, Venugopal K, Tharion G, et al. A study to evaluate the effectiveness of phenol blocks to peripheral nerves in reducing spasticity in patients with paraplegia and brain injury. IJPMR 2008;19(1):13–7.
50. Ilfeld BM, Gabriel RA, Trescot AM. Ultrasound-guided percutaneous cryoneurolysis for treatment of acute pain: could cryoanalgesia replace continuous peripheral nerve blocks? Br J Anaesth 2017;119(4):703–6.
51. Kanpolat Y, Cağlar C, Akiş E, et al. Percutaneous selective RF neurotomy in spasticity. Acta neurochirurgica Supplementum 1987;39:96–8.
52. Kim PS, Ferrante FM. Cryoanalgesia: a novel treatment for hip adductor spasticity and obturator neuralgia. Anesthesiology 1998;89(2):534–6.
53. Paulin MH, Patel AT. Cryodenervation for the Treatment of Upper Limb Spasticity : A Prospective Open Proof-of-Concept Study. Am J Phys Med 2015;94(3):12.
54. MacRae F, Boissonnault E, Hashemi M, et al. Bilateral Suprascapular Nerve Cryoneurolysis for Pain Associated With Glenohumeral Osteoarthritis: A Case

Report. Archives of rehabilitation research and clinical translation 2023;5(1): 100256.

55. Winston P, Mills PB, Reebye R, et al. Cryoneurotomy as a Percutaneous Mini-invasive Therapy for the Treatment of the Spastic Limb: Case Presentation, Review of the Literature, and Proposed Approach for Use. Archives of rehabilitation research and clinical translation 2019;1(3–4):100030.

56. Winston P, Reebye R, Picelli A, et al. Recommendations for Ultrasound Guidance for Diagnostic Nerve Blocks for Spasticity. What are the Benefits? Arch Phys Med Rehabil 2023;S0003-9993(23):00086–92.

57. Winston P, Vincent D. Atlas of ultrasound-guided nerve-targeted procedures for spasticity. Berlin: Quintessence publishing; 2023.

58. Hsu M, Stevenson FF. Wallerian degeneration and recovery of motor nerves after multiple focused cold therapies. Muscle Nerve 2015;51(2):268–75.

59. Winston P, MacRae F, Raiapakshe S, et al. Analysis of side effects of cryoneurolysis for the treatment of spasticity. Am J Phys Med Rehabil 2023. https://doi. org/10.1097/PHM.0000000000002267.

60. Myers RR, Heckman HM, Powell HC. Axonal viability and the persistence of thermal hyperalgesia after partial freeze lesions of nerve. J Neurol Sci 1996;139(1): 28–38.

61. Gage AA, Baust JM, Baust JG. Experimental cryosurgery investigations in vivo. Cryobiology 2009;59(3):229–43.

62. Trescot AM. Peripheral nerve entrapments. Cham (Switzerland): Springer International Publishing; 2016.

63. Cheng J-G. Cryoanalgesia for refractory neuralgia. Journal of PerioperativeScience 2015;2:2.

64. Friedman T, Richman D, Adler R. Sonographically guided cryoneurolysis: preliminary experience and clinical outcomes. J Ultrasound Med 2012;31(12): 2025–34.

65. Tardieu G, Hariga J. [treatment of muscular rigidity of cerebral origin by infiltration of dilute alcohol. (results of 500 injections)]. Arch Fr Pediatr 1964;21:25–41.

66. Deltombe T, De Wispelaere JF, Gustin T, et al. Selective blocks of the motor nerve branches to the soleus and tibialis posterior muscles in the management of the spastic equinovarus foot. Arch Phys Med Rehabil 2004;85(1):54–8.

67. Genet F, Schnitzler A, Droz-Bartholet F, et al. Successive motor nerve blocks to identify the muscles causing a spasticity pattern: example of the arm flexion pattern. J Anat 2017;230(1):106–16.

68. Elovic EP, Esquenazi A, Alter KE, et al. Chemodenervation and Nerve Blocks in the Diagnosis and Management of Spasticity and Muscle Overactivity. PM and R 2009;1(9):842–51.

69. Scobie J, Winston P. Case Report: Perspective of a Caregiver on Functional Outcomes Following Bilateral Lateral Pectoral Nerve Cryoneurotomy to Treat Spasticity in a Pediatric Patient With Cerebral Palsy. Frontiers in rehabilitation sciences 2021;2:719054.

70. Rubenstein J, Harvey AW, Vincent D, et al. Cryoneurotomy to Reduce Spasticity and Improve Range of Motion in Spastic Flexed Elbow: A Visual Vignette. Am J Phys Med Rehabil 2021;100(5):e65.

71. MacRae F, Brar A, Boissonnault E, et al. Cryoneurolysis of Anterior and Posterior Divisions of the Obturator Nerve. Am J Phys Med Rehabil 2023;102(1):e1–2.

72. Winston P, Hashemi M, Boissonnault E, et al. Measuring the efficacy of percutaneous cryoneurolysis in the management of patients. Am J Phys Med Rehabil 2023. in press.

73. Perry TA, Segal NA. An open-label, single-arm trial of cryoneurolysis for improvements in pain, activities of daily living and quality of life in patients with symptomatic ankle osteoarthritis. Osteoarthritis and cartilage open 2022;4(3): 100272.

74. Radnovich R, Scott D, Patel AT, et al. Cryoneurolysis to treat the pain and symptoms of knee osteoarthritis: a multicenter, randomized, double-blind, sham-controlled trial. Osteoarthritis Cartilage 2017;25(8):1247–56.

75. Dymarek R, Ptaszkowski K, Słupska L, et al. Effects of extracorporeal shock wave on upper and lower limb spasticity in post-stroke patients: A narrative review. Top Stroke Rehabil 2016;23(4):293–303.

76. Walewicz K, Taradaj J, Rajfur K, et al. The Effectiveness Of Radial Extracorporeal Shock Wave Therapy In Patients With Chronic Low Back Pain: A Prospective, Randomized, Single-Blinded Pilot Study. Clin Interv Aging 2019;14: 1859–69.

77. Ou-Yang LJ, Chen PH, Lee CH, et al. Effect and Optimal Timing of Extracorporeal Shock-Wave Intervention to Patients With Spasticity After Stroke: A Systematic Review and Meta-analysis. Am J Phys Med Rehabil 2023;102(1):43–51.

78. Zhang HL, Jin RJ, Guan L, et al. Extracorporeal Shock Wave Therapy on Spasticity After Upper Motor Neuron Injury: A Systematic Review and Meta-analysis. Am J Phys Med Rehabil 2022;101(7):615–23.

79. Lohse-Busch H, Kraemer M, Reime U. [A pilot investigation into the effects of extracorporeal shock waves on muscular dysfunction in children with spastic movement disorders]. Schmerz 1997;11(2):108–12.

80. Manganotti P, Amelio E. Long-Term Effect of Shock Wave Therapy on Upper Limb Hypertonia in Patients Affected by Stroke. Stroke 2005;36(9):1967–71.

81. Hsu PC, Chang KV, Chiu YH, et al. Comparative Effectiveness of Botulinum Toxin Injections and Extracorporeal Shockwave Therapy for Post-Stroke Spasticity: A Systematic Review and Network Meta-Analysis. EClinicalMedicine 2022;43: 101222.

82. Xiang J, Wang W, Jiang W, et al. Effects of extracorporeal shock wave therapy on spasticity in post-stroke patients: A systematic review and meta-analysis of randomized controlled trials. J Rehabil Med 2018;50(10):852–9.

83. Blottner D, Lück G. Just in time and place: NOS/NO system assembly in neuromuscular junction formation. Microsc Res Tech 2001;55(3):171–80.

84. Dymarek R, Taradaj J, Rosińczuk J. The Effect of Radial Extracorporeal Shock Wave Stimulation on Upper Limb Spasticity in Chronic Stroke Patients: A Single-Blind, Randomized, Placebo-Controlled Study. Ultrasound Med Biol 2016;42(8):1862–75.

85. Leng Y, Lo WLA, Hu C, et al. The Effects of Extracorporeal Shock Wave Therapy on Spastic Muscle of the Wrist Joint in Stroke Survivors: Evidence From Neuromechanical Analysis. Front Neurosci 2020;14:580762.

86. Bae H, Lee JM, Lee KH. The Effects of Extracorporeal Shock Wave Therapy on Spasticity in Chronic Stroke Patients. Ann Rehabil Med 2010;34(6):663–9.

87. Yang E, Lew HL, Özçakar L, et al. Recent Advances in the Treatment of Spasticity: Extracorporeal Shock Wave Therapy. J Clin Med 2021;10(20).

88. Yoon SH, Shin MK, Choi EJ, et al. Effective site for the application of extracorporeal shock-wave therapy on spasticity in chronic stroke: Muscle belly or myotendinous junction. Annals of Rehabilitation Medicine 2017;41(4):547–55.

89. Li G, Yuan W, Liu G, et al. Effects of radial extracorporeal shockwave therapy on spasticity of upper-limb agonist/antagonist muscles in patients affected by stroke: a randomized, single-blind clinical trial. Age Ageing 2020;49(2):246–52.

90. Wardhani RK, Wahyuni LK, Laksmitasari B, et al. Effect of total number of pulses of radial extracorporeal shock wave therapy (rESWT) on hamstring muscle spasticity in children with spastic type cerebral palsy: A randomized clinical trial. J Pediatr Rehabil Med 2022;15(1):159–64.

91. Aslan Ş Yoldaş, Kutlay S, Düsünceli Atman E, et al. Does extracorporeal shock wave therapy decrease spasticity of ankle plantar flexor muscles in patients with stroke: A randomized controlled trial. Clin Rehabil 2021;35(10):1442–53.

92. Wu YT, Chang CN, Chen YM, et al. Comparison of the effect of focused and radial extracorporeal shock waves on spastic equinus in patients with stroke: a randomized controlled trial. Eur J Phys Rehabil Med 2018;54(4):518–25.

93. Lee CH, Lee SH, Yoo JI, et al. Ultrasonographic Evaluation for the Effect of Extracorporeal Shock Wave Therapy on Gastrocnemius Muscle Spasticity in Patients With Chronic Stroke. PM and R 2019;11(4):363–71.

94. Taheri P, Vahdatpour B, Mellat M, et al. Effect of extracorporeal shock wave therapy on lower limb spasticity in stroke patients. Arch Iran Med 2017;20(6):338–43.

95. Cabanas-Valdés R, Serra-Llobet P, Rodriguez-Rubio PR, et al. The effectiveness of extracorporeal shock wave therapy for improving upper limb spasticity and functionality in stroke patients: a systematic review and meta-analysis. Clin Rehabil 2020;34(9):1141–56.

96. Kim YW, Shin JC, Yoon JG, et al. Usefulness of radial extracorporeal shock wave therapy for the spasticity of the subscapularis in patients with stroke: a pilot study. Chin Med J (Engl) 2013;126(24):4638–43.

97. Duan H, Lian Y, Jing Y, et al. Research progress in extracorporeal shock wave therapy for upper limb spasticity after stroke. Front Neurol 2023;14:1121026.

98. Oh JH, Park HD, Han SH, et al. Duration of treatment effect of extracorporeal shock wave on spasticity and subgroup-analysis according to number of shocks and application site: A meta-analysis. Annals of Rehabilitation Medicine 2019;43(2):163–77.

99. Jia G, Ma J, Wang S, et al. Long-term Effects of Extracorporeal Shock Wave Therapy on Poststroke Spasticity: A Meta-analysis of Randomized Controlled Trials. J Stroke Cerebrovasc Dis 2020;29(3):104591.

100. Hallett M. Explanation of timing of botulinum neurotoxin effects, onset and duration, and clinical ways of influencing them. Toxicon : official journal of the International Society on Toxinology 2015;107(Pt A):64–7.

101. Marinaro C, Costantino C, D'Esposito O, et al. Synergic use of botulinum toxin injection and radial extracorporeal shockwave therapy in Multiple Sclerosis spasticity. Acta Biomed Atenei Parmensis 2021;92(1):e2021076.

102. Ip AH, Phadke CP, Boulias C, et al. Practice Patterns of Physicians Using Adjunct Therapies with Botulinum Toxin Injection for Spasticity: A Canadian Multicenter Cross-Sectional Survey. Pm r 2021;13(4):372–8.

103. Chang MC, Choo YJ, Kwak SG, et al. Effectiveness of Extracorporeal Shockwave Therapy on Controlling Spasticity in Cerebral Palsy Patients: A Meta-Analysis of Timing of Outcome Measurement. Children 2023;10(2).

104. Corrado B, Di Luise C, Servodio Iammarrone C. Management of Muscle Spasticity in Children with Cerebral Palsy by Means of Extracorporeal Shockwave Therapy: A Systematic Review of the Literature. Dev Neurorehabil 2021;24(1):1–7.

105. Kim HJ, Park JW, Nam K. Effect of extracorporeal shockwave therapy on muscle spasticity in patients with cerebral palsy: meta-analysis and systematic review. Eur J Phys Rehabil Med 2019;55(6):761–71.

106. Kudva A, Abraham ME, Gold J, et al. Intrathecal baclofen, selective dorsal rhizotomy, and extracorporeal shockwave therapy for the treatment of spasticity in cerebral palsy: a systematic review. Neurosurg Rev 2021;44(6):3209–28.
107. Vidal X, Martí-Fàbregas J, Canet O, et al. Efficacy of radial extracorporeal shock wave therapy compared with botulinum toxin type A injection in treatment of lower extremity spasticity in subjects with cerebral palsy: A randomized, controlled, cross-over study. J Rehabil Med 2020;52(6):jrm00076.

A Review of Poststroke Aphasia Recovery and Treatment Options

Victoria E. Tilton-Bolowsky, PhD[a], Argye E. Hillis, MD, MA[a],*

KEYWORDS

- Stroke • Aphasia • Recovery • Treatment

KEY POINTS

- Recovery from aphasia is variable and depends on baseline severity and amount of speech and language intervention.
- Baseline severity of aphasia depends on size and site of stroke and less so on demographic variables.
- Behavioral speech and language treatment is the mainstay of intervention for poststroke aphasia and might be augmented by noninvasive brain stimulation, medications, and/or computer practice, but further trials are needed to support the efficacy of specific approaches.

INTRODUCTION

Aphasia is a language-based communication disorder that occurs when the brain regions responsible for language processes incur damage. This damage can occur from stroke, traumatic brain injury, gunshot wound, infectious process, or neurodegenerative disease. Of these, stroke is the leading cause of aphasia in the United States.[1] In reports across lower middle-income to high-income countries, aphasia is reported to occur in as low as 7% and as high as 77% of stroke survivors, with an estimate of aphasia occurring in ~18% of stroke survivors in the United States.[2,3] This incidence rate equates to ~180,000 new cases of poststroke aphasia (PSA) in the United States per year.[4] Estimates from lower income/developing countries are underreported, and thus, the global impact of aphasia remains unknown.[2]

People with aphasia experience changes to their expressive language abilities, including spoken and written language, receptive language abilities, including spoken and written word comprehension, or a combination of these. Humans are a heavily language-driven species, and therefore, aphasia—whether temporary or long-

[a] Department of Neurology, Johns Hopkins School of Medicine, 600 North Wolfe Street, Phipps 446F, Baltimore, MD 21287, USA
* Corresponding author.
E-mail address: argye@jhmi.edu

Phys Med Rehabil Clin N Am 35 (2024) 419–431
https://doi.org/10.1016/j.pmr.2023.06.010
1047-9651/24/© 2023 Elsevier Inc. All rights reserved.

term—can have profound effects on one's life. Many who acquire aphasia experience depression and require supports to address their psychosocial well-being at higher rates and for different reasons than those who do not acquire aphasia following stroke.[5-8] Reports of feeling fear and shock, changes to one's self-identity, and negative changes within social relationships[6] emphasize the important role of aphasia rehabilitation.

APHASIA RECOVERY

Presently, aphasia recovery can best be characterized as variable, heterogeneous, and multidimensional.[9] Many experience rapid improvements within the first 2 weeks following stroke.[10] Improvements in language function in the acute to early subacute phases of recovery are attributed to reperfusion of the tissue surrounding the core infarct(s) and resolution of diaschisis effects, that is, dysfunction in distant, spared brain regions connected to damaged regions.[11] Language recovery in this phase is highly variable; ~30% to 40% of those who experience aphasia following stroke will live with their aphasia as a chronic disability for the rest of their lives.[9] Importantly, however, people with chronic aphasia can continue to experience improvements in their language function for many years. Improvements in the chronic phase are attributed to residual language network reorganization, contralesional cortex recruitment, domain-general network compensation, and the development of compensatory mechanisms for lost function.[11-14] Roughly half of people with PSA continue to experience improvements in their language function well into the chronic phase of recovery, while the remaining half either reach relative stability or experience decline over time.[15,16] Overall, recovery is extremely variable, making prognostication challenging. Therefore, many studies attempt to identify which factors are associated with, or predictive of, long-term recovery. The aim of such work is to improve clinicians' and practitioners' ability to predict outcomes and facilitate recovery, with the ultimate goal of improving the quality of life of people with aphasia.

Baseline Predictors

Chronologic age is sometimes linked to outcomes. Some studies find that older age is associated with more severe aphasia and negatively correlated with outcomes,[16-19] whereas others report no relationship between age and outcomes.[19,20] Findings that older age is associated with worse severity and outcomes have been attributed to gradual reductions in neural plasticity and brain/cognitive reserve that occur with normal aging.[21,22] Relatedly, studies have begun to explore estimations of brain age—an approximation of brain tissue integrity that takes into account gray matter, white matter connections, and functional connectivity[21,23]—as a meaningful predictor in addition to chronologic age. There is emerging evidence that those with delayed brain aging (brain age < chronologic age) demonstrate greater improvements than those with advanced brain aging (brain age > chronologic age).[21,23] The distinction between chronologic age and brain age seems to be an important one, as there is evidence that estimated brain age explains significant proportions of additional variance in certain language outcomes after controlling for chronologic age and lesion volume.[23] Overall, emerging evidence supports that brain age methodology may have facilitative prognostic value and requires further evaluation.

In the United States, people from minoritized groups experience worse health-related outcomes than White, non-Hispanic people.[24] These health disparities can be attributed to inequalities across social, political, and economic spheres, which in turn impact one's environment, resources, support, and access to care.[25] Patterns of racial and ethnic disparities that exist in general health-related outcomes are also observed in stroke and aphasia outcomes.[26–29] For example, Black/African American stroke survivors are found to experience more severe aphasia and worse aphasia-related outcomes compared with their White, non-Hispanic peers, even when matched on other demographic and language variables, and despite greater speech–language pathology (SLP) service utilization.[3,26] Racial disparities in aphasia outcomes are well-documented, but have yet to gain wide-spread attention or ubiquitous use as important variables in observational and interventional studies,[30,31] which may be obfuscating critical findings related to the variability seen in outcomes. Overall, the extent to which aphasia outcomes vary based on race and ethnicity and the factors underlying those disparate outcomes warrant prioritization and further investigation. The National Institutes on Deafness and Other Communication Disorders—a major funding mechanism for aphasia research—has made reducing health disparities part of their 2023 to 2027 Strategy Plan and has multiple research opportunities that support this priority. Therefore, research aiming to examine and mitigate racial and ethnic disparities in aphasia will hopefully accelerate in the coming years.

The presence of coexistent cerebrovascular conditions (eg, hypertension, diabetes) is shown to be associated with worse aphasia symptoms and declines in language function over time.[16,32] As mentioned, improvements in language function are partially attributed to reorganization within the residual language network and recruitment of contralesional cortex, mechanisms which rely on healthy brain tissue in ipsilesional and contralesional cortices. Therefore, the presence of microvascular and macrovascular changes that reduce the amount of healthy tissue and thus one's cognitive reserve[22] can negatively impact recovery. For instance, the extent of leukoaraiosis at baseline, that is, diffuse changes to white matter, has been found to be an independent predictor of stroke outcomes and has even been linked to worsening scores on aphasia assessments over time.[33]

There is mixed evidence that other baseline factors such as handedness, education, and gender are associated with outcomes.[19,20,32,34] More consistent evidence is needed to establish whether these factors are reliable/meaningful predictors of outcomes.

Stroke-Related Predictors

Stroke-related factors—namely lesion volume and location—have emerged as primary predictors of aphasia recovery. Larger lesion volume is shown to be negatively correlated with measures of overall aphasia severity, scores on individual speech and language domains (eg, auditory comprehension), and treatment response, such that greater lesion volume is associated with lower standardized scores, less response to certain types of treatment, and worse overall recovery.[15,18–20,35–39] Relatedly, recent work finds further evidence that greater damage to the posterior superior temporal gyrus, superior longitudinal fasciculus, insula, supramarginal gyrus, angular gyrus, postcentral gyrus, superior parietal lobe, and inferior parietal lobe is associated with aphasia severity and performance on naming tasks.[20,36,40] People with more extensive tissue damage throughout the middle cerebral artery distribution and temporoparietal regions have been found to have longer persisting moderate–severe aphasia symptoms than those with less or no damage to these areas.[9,20] Taken together, larger lesions within key language regions result in worse initial aphasia severity—which in itself is another strong predictor of later performance. Initial aphasia severity is found to be associated with future naming performance, response to treatment, and overall language recovery.[17,34,41]

Treatment Predictors

The REhabilitation and recovery of peopLE with Aphasia after StrokE (RELEASE) Collaboration conducted a meta-analysis evaluating associations between speech–language therapy (SLT) regimens and several aphasia outcomes. Their meta-analysis compiled data from 25 randomized control trials, with greater than 900 individual participants' data. After controlling for age, sex, aphasia severity, and time poststroke, the greatest improvements in overall language (as quantified by the Western Aphasia Battery-Revised Aphasia Quotient[42]) and functional communication (as quantified by the Aachen Aphasia Test's Spontaneous Speech Communication subscore) were associated with a dosage of ~20 to 50 total hours of SLT, at an intensity of about 2 hours per week, and a frequency of five+ days per week, with clinically similar gains at intensities of 2 to 3 and 3 to 4 h/wk.[43] In addition, mixed expressive-receptive approaches, prescribed home practice, functionally-tailored, and difficulty-level tailored approaches were associated with greater overall language recovery.[43] Their findings are consistent with prior work finding that more therapy is associated with greater recovery in those with chronic aphasia.[16,44] The RELEASE Collaborators make note that the dose, frequency, and intensity regimens they found to be associated with the greatest improvements are higher than current clinical practice provision.[43] There is a notable research practice-dosage gap, with published intervention studies delivering higher therapy doses than estimates of clinical service provision.[45,46] These findings highlight the need for better alignment between clinical service delivery constraints and research-based treatment regimens, and identification of viable, alternative treatment delivery methods to increase treatment delivery at the clinical level.

Time-post onset is another factor of interest. The most rapid language recovery occurs within the first year of stroke and decelerates over time.[20] Thus, it has become a common refrain that earlier initiation of therapy is best. However, studies investigating the effectiveness of earlier and more intensive SLT engagement on acute and subacute outcomes generally do not find significant benefit or large positive effects. In studies comparing outcomes between groups that received no SLT versus impairment-based SLT, and standard SLT versus intensive SLT, significant group differences at 1, 3, and 6 months post-onset demonstrating the benefit of early intensive SLT remain mixed.[47–49] This is not to say that early intervention aiming to capitalize on the period of spontaneous recovery immediately following stroke are not worthwhile or do not warrant further investigation. Rather, optimal timing for initiating SLT and/or an optimal SLT intensity in the acute to subacute phases have not been identified.

THERAPEUTIC OPTIONS

Behavioral SLT is the most common and widely-consumed form of treatment for aphasia. SLT is delivered face-to-face and one-on-one with an SLP, via telepractice, and in group settings (which can also be virtual). Evidence supports SLT as effective from the acute to chronic phases of recovery.[34,44,50,51] There are many ways in which SLT approaches are dichotomized—restitutive versus substitutive, restorative versus compensatory, semantic versus phonological, impairment-based versus functionally-oriented, theory-driven (impairment-based and functional SLT) versus social approaches (participation and counseling-based), and so on. All of these approaches share the common goals of improving people's language function and increasing their communication participation in daily life, but they differ in the specific skills they aim to improve, the ways in which those skills are targeted, and the mechanisms through which they are thought to promote change. In reviews and discussions of SLT approaches, Treatment of Underlying Forms, Constraint-Induced Language Therapy,

Semantic Feature Analysis (SFA), Melodic Intonation Therapy (MIT), and Verb Network Strengthening Treatment (VNeST) are often identified as the more "established" of the SLT approaches. Interestingly, examinations of current clinical practice patterns show only partial overlap with these oft-cited approaches.

A 2021 survey of US-based SLPs across acute, subacute, outpatient, and university clinic settings asked SLPs to identify their most frequently used treatment approaches to target eight specific language skills. Over half of the respondents reported using SFA to target *word finding*; Response Elaboration Training (RET), MIT, and Script training to target *expansion of verbal productions*; Commands, Yes/No questions, and word-to-item matching/object discrimination to target *auditory comprehension*; Narrative productions and VNeST to target *syntax and fluency*; Reading comprehension with increasing complexity to target *reading comprehension*; Writing with demands of increasing complexity to target *written expression*; Training in external communication aids to target *multimodal communication*; and patient and caregiver-supportive communication education/training to target *participation, caregiver, and quality of life skills*.[52] These findings highlight another gap between research and clinical practice: interventions used by clinicians may not be the predominant interventions being evaluated in interventional studies, and vice versa—with the exceptions of SFA, MIT, RET, and VNeST, which have been extensively investigated. Again, better alignment with clinical service practices would be beneficial to research efforts.

Importantly, the wants, needs, and desires of people with aphasia should remain at the forefront of practitioners' minds when creating treatment plans and selecting treatment activities. Frameworks and models such as SMARTER Goal Setting,[53] the FOURC model,[54] and Goal Attainment Scaling[55] can be used to facilitate collaboration between practitioners and their patients—along with their care partners—during rehabilitation planning. Engaging in collaborative goal setting can ensure that time spent in therapy is spent working toward the goals that matter most to patients and will have a meaningful positive impact on patients' communication participation in everyday life.

Several approaches intended to augment the effects of behavioral SLT have emerged in recent decades. Noninvasive brain stimulation (NIBS) methodologies, including transcranial direct current stimulation (tDCS), repetitive transcranial magnetic stimulation (rTMS), and more recently, transcranial alternating current stimulation (tACS), are thought to modulate neuronal activity, enhance synaptic plasticity, and support reorganization within the residual language network.[41] There is evidence of positive effects (eg, reduced aphasia severity, improved naming accuracy) of tDCS and rTMS when delivered synchronously (for tDCS and rTMS), or immediately before SLT (rTMS).[56] However, positive effects on functional communication are mixed.[57–60] Studies examining the comparative effectiveness of tDCS versus rTMS are just beginning to emerge[61,62] and thus warrant ongoing investigation. The few studies examining the effectiveness of tACS, which is thought to improve anterior–posterior functional connectivity, have found improved speech output for patients with non-fluent aphasia[63] and significantly greater improvements in overall language severity and auditory verbal comprehension when compared with sham conditions.[64] However, these are the only two studies reporting on tACS in chronic PSA, so further investigation is necessary. Future investigations will continue to explore the effectiveness of NIBS with manipulations to NIBS type, stimulation site, targeted brain region(s), type of concurrent SLT, NIBS dosage (eg, frequency, amount of sessions), and temporal implementation (subacute vs chronic) on language performance.

Pharmacologic approaches are thought to facilitate adaptive neuroplasticity and network reorganization, although the specific mechanisms through which these changes are hypothesized to be achieved are presently underspecified.[65] Similar to

NIBS, most of the drug therapies investigated in PSA (eg, reversible acetylcholines-terase inhibitors, N-methyl-D-aspartate (NMDA) receptor antagonists, dopamine precursors, dopamine agonists) are administered in combination with SLT, with the goal of bolstering its effects. Broadly, some studies have found that drug therapies can improve patient's language functioning across various domains (eg, naming, comprehension, spontaneous speech), but results are mixed.[65–67] Larger samples and double-blind, placebo-controlled trials are required to address questions regarding efficacy and safety.

Interventional approaches focused on improving mental health and facilitating acceptance and adjustment to living with aphasia have reported benefits on emotional well-being and companionship (eg, SUPERB[68]). Such work has also identified the importance of early communication regarding aphasia as a condition, aphasia treatment, and prognosis, as well as humanizing treatment (eg, using humor, being treated as "normal") on one's adjustment to living with aphasia.[69] Related interventional studies focused on psychosocial adjustment and successful communication participation are ongoing (eg, NCT04984239).

Tablet-based therapy applications, computerized SLT, and free online therapy tools have been on the rise, with accelerated integration into clinical care as an effect of the COVID-19 pandemic. Technology-assisted therapy options reduce certain logistical barriers to accessing therapeutic activity (eg, transportation), do not impose time caps on therapy minutes, have relative ease of use, comparatively lower costs, and have been shown to have clinical effectiveness.[69] However, they require some baseline technological literacy and ownership of/access to a smart device or computer and have not been extensively evaluated in comparative effectiveness studies. Overall, technology-assisted options are safe and can increase the amount of therapeutic activity people with aphasia can access and engage in. Other approaches, such as music-based interventions (eg, vocal music listening[70,71]), acupuncture,[72] and virtual reality[73] have been studied as complimentary treatments to SLT. However, the efficacy of such therapies is presently unclear and requires further evaluation.

RECOMMENDATIONS FOR RESEARCH

Three areas of growth for aphasia research are: (1) systematic characterization of treatments; (2) reporting of race and ethnicity, and (3) recruitment, retention, and representation of people from systematically marginalized groups,[74] and those with cultural backgrounds different from European-American culture[75] and linguistic backgrounds different from standardized American English.[76]

As reflected above, there are many aphasia treatment approaches used across research and clinical care. The delivery of said treatments varies from study to study and from SLP to SLP due to the complexities of behavioral treatment as well as individual variability that necessitate tailoring of treatments in clinical care. Such variations and manipulations to aspects of a treatment (eg, feedback provision) are shown to impact learning success and retention.[77] This means that even minor variations in a treatment's delivery can influence outcomes. To compare outcomes across treatment delivery methods and evaluate which aspects of a treatment can or should be manipulated to ensure successful learning, all aspects of a treatment must be adequately characterized. The Rehabilitation Treatment Specification System (RTSS)[78] has been proposed as a way to characterize treatments across the rehabilitation disciplines. Through the RTSS, one can characterize a treatment's target(s) (ie, measurable aspects of functioning expected to change as a result of treatment), active ingredients (ie, aspects of a treatment thought to result in change in the target), and mechanisms of action (ie, the hypothesized mechanisms through which the active ingredients act to make changes in the target).[78] Collective use of the RTSS by researchers to describe interventions would allow for better comparison across studies and better evaluation of individual ingredient's effectiveness and importance within treatments.

A foundational principle of clinical research is that study samples should be representative of the larger populations that they intend to represent and reflect the relevant characteristics of the larger population in similar proportions.[79] Considering that language/communication is deeply influenced by a person's culture and environment[80] and is affected by aphasia, adequate representation of people from heterogeneous cultural–linguistic backgrounds in aphasia study samples is essential. Race and ethnicity become important to consider in relation to cultural–linguistic background because although racial and ethnic representation will not necessarily equate with cultural/cultural–linguistic representation, often members of a given culture share the same race.[81] Therefore, it is important for aphasia study samples to be reflective of the racial and ethnic diversity that exists in the United States. Investigations of whether aphasia study samples are reflective of the racial and ethnic diversity within the United States have been challenging, however, because these two variables are vastly underreported.

In 2009, Ellis reviewed studies of neurogenic communication disorders published between 1997 and 2007 in two of the American Speech-Language and Hearing Association's journals. Ellis found that only ~14% of the identified studies reported participants' race and ethnicity.[30] Ellis highlights that stroke-related differences between people from different races and ethnicities (eg, initial level of residual impairment) and their potential influence on communication following stroke makes reporting race and ethnicity—among other key demographic variables—essential to the external validity of studies of neurogenic communication disorders.[30] Of note, reporting insurance status, comorbidities, and socioeconomic status may also be relevant, especially in observational studies. Ellis generously ends the article by pointing readers to several existing guidelines related to demographic variable reporting. About a decade later, Nguy and colleagues examined whether race and ethnicity reporting had improved since Ellis's article. They conducted a scoping review of US-based aphasia treatment studies published between 2009 and 2019 and found a marginal improvement in reporting race—up to 28% of the identified studies—whereas other demographic variables such as age and sex (which as discussed above are comparatively weaker predictors of outcomes) continue to be reported in greater than 90% of published studies.[31]

From the studies that reported participants' race, Nguy and colleagues further examined whether the samples were racially representative of the population of stroke survivors in the United States.[31] They compared the proportions of Black and White participants in the studies' samples to those from a large sample of US stroke survivors and found that they were significantly different, with fewer Black participants represented in aphasia treatment studies compared with their percentage within the population. Of note, they did not examine proportions of American Indian or Alaska Native, Asian, or Native Hawaiian or Other Pacific Islander (the other three categories included in the US Office of Management and Budget's five minimum categories for data on race), or ethnicity proportions. Therefore, the extent to which aphasia treatment study samples lack members of these groups remains unknown. However, it would be reasonable to assume they are also underrepresented, as the underrepresentation of systematically marginalized group members plagues many fields of study, such as multiple sclerosis,[82] diabetes,[83] and adverse pregnancy outcomes.[84]

For researchers invested in (1) responsible collection and reporting of race and ethnicity and (2) improving recruitment, retention, and representation of people from systematically marginalized groups in their studies, a plethora of resources exist.[29,85,86] Addressing these two areas of growth will improve our ability to measure long-term aphasia recovery, more adequately test treatments' effectiveness, and address persistent health disparities. To be clear, the need to address these issues is rooted in the indisputable necessity to improve the quality, external validity, and generalizability of our vital work, rather than for aesthetic or compulsory purposes.[75] Until then, the generalizability of findings remains unclear. Therefore, it remains important for clinicians to continue exercising critical discernment when selecting materials for their clients in cases where cultural–linguistic factors are at play.

DISCUSSION AND SUMMARY

The impact aphasia has on one's communication abilities can be detrimental to psychosocial well-being and quality of life. Recent work highlights the importance of early discussions with patients regarding aphasia as a condition, treatment options, and prognosis, in addition to humanizing care practices.[6] Practitioners should consider stroke size, stroke location, initial aphasia severity, race and ethnicity, preexisting cerebrovascular conditions/cognitive–linguistic deficits, and time post-onset to guide discussions regarding prognosis—while also acknowledging the variable nature of recovery. Behavioral SLT remains the most common treatment for aphasia. Including patients and care partners in treatment planning is important to the rehabilitation process. NIBS and drug therapies as adjuvants to behavioral SLT may bolster the positive effects of behavioral SLT, but more evidence is needed.

CLINICS CARE POINTS

- Stroke size and location, initial aphasia severity, race and ethnicity, presence of preexisting cerebrovascular conditions/cognitive–linguistic deficits, and time post-onset are all important factors to consider when discussing a patient's prognosis.

- Early discussions about aphasia as a disorder, treatment options, and prognosis, humanizing practices, and including patients in treatment selection/goal planning are all important parts of the aphasia rehabilitation process.

- People with aphasia can continue to experience improvements in their language function for many years following onset and should be encouraged to engage in speech–language therapy throughout the phases of recovery. Group therapy and support groups, sometimes free-of-cost, should also be encouraged.

DISCLOSURE

Research reported in this publication was supported by the National Institute on Deafness and Other Communication Disorders, United States of the National Institutes of Health under award numbers R01 DC05375 and P50 014664. The content is solely the responsibility of the authors and does not necessarily represent the official views of the National Institutes of Health.

REFERENCES

1. National Institute of Deafness and Other Communication Disorders (NIDCD). What is aphasia? Types, causes and treatment. Available at: https://www.nidcd.nih.gov/health/aphasia. Published December 2015. Accessed April 13, 2023.

2. Frederick A, Jacobs M, Adams-Mitchell CJ, et al. The global rate of post-stroke aphasia. Perspect ASHA Special Interest Groups 2022;7(5):1567–72.
3. Jacobs M, Ellis C. Racial disparities in post-stroke aphasia: A need to look beyond the base analysis. J Natl Med Assoc 2022;114(3):258–64.
4. National Aphasia Association. Aphasia FAQs. Available at: https://www.aphasia.org/aphasia-faqs/. Accessed March 18, 2023.
5. Lin HL, Sung FC, Muo CH, et al. Depression risk in post-stroke aphasia patients: A nationwide population-based cohort study. Neuroepidemiology 2023. https://doi.org/10.1159/000530070.
6. Moss B, Northcott S, Behn N, et al. 'Emotion is of the essence.... Number one priority': A nested qualitative study exploring psychosocial adjustment to stroke and aphasia. Int J Lang Commun Disord 2021;56(3):594–608.
7. Pompon RH, Fassbinder W, Mcneil MR, et al. Associations among depression, demographic variables, and language impairments in chronic post-stroke aphasia. J Commun Disord 2022;100:106266.
8. Wilson C, Jones A, Schick-Makaroff K, et al. Understanding the impact of group therapy on health-related quality of life of people with Aphasia: a scoping review. Speech Lang Hear 2021;1–14.
9. Stefaniak JD, Geranmayeh F, Lambon Ralph MA. The multidimensional nature of aphasia recovery post-stroke. Brain 2022;145(4):1354–67.
10. Wilson SM, Eriksson DK, Brandt TH, et al. Patterns of recovery from aphasia in the first 2 weeks after stroke. J Speech Lang Hear Res 2019;62(3):723–32.
11. Wawrzyniak M, Schneider HR, Klingbeil J, et al. Resolution of diaschisis contributes to early recovery from post-stroke aphasia. Neuroimage 2022;251:119001.
12. Hillis AE, Heidler J. Mechanisms of early aphasia recovery. Aphasiology 2002; 16(9):885–95.
13. Saur D, Lange R, Baumgaertner A, et al. Dynamics of language reorganization after stroke. Brain 2006;129(6):1371–84.
14. Wilson SM, Schneck SM. Neuroplasticity in post-stroke aphasia: A systematic review and meta-analysis of functional imaging studies of reorganization of language processing. Neurobiol Lang 2020;2(1):22–82.
15. Hope TM, Leff AP, Prejawa S, et al. Right hemisphere structural adaptation and changing language skills years after left hemisphere stroke. Brain 2017;140(6): 1718–28.
16. Johnson L, Basilakos A, Yourganov G, et al. Progression of aphasia severity in the chronic stages of stroke. Am J Speech Lang Pathol 2019;28(2):639–49.
17. Kristinsson S, Basilakos A, Den Ouden DB, et al. Predicting Outcomes of Language Rehabilitation: Prognostic Factors for Immediate and Long-Term Outcomes After Aphasia Therapy. J Speech Lang Hear Res 2023;66(3):1068–84.
18. Laska AC, Hellblom A, Murray V, et al. Aphasia in acute stroke and relation to outcome. J Intern Med 2001;249(5):413–22.
19. Watila MM, Balarabe SA. Factors predicting post-stroke aphasia recovery. J Neurol Sci 2015;352(1–2):12–8.
20. Wilson SM, Entrup JL, Schneck SM, et al. Recovery from aphasia in the first year after stroke. Brain 2023;146(3):1021–39.
21. Kristinsson S, Busby N, Rorden C, et al. Brain age predicts long-term recovery in post-stroke aphasia. Brain Communications 2022;4(5):fcac252.
22. Varkanitsa M, Kiran S. Understanding, facilitating and predicting aphasia recovery after rehabilitation. Int J Speech Lang Pathol 2022;24(3):248–59.
23. Busby N, Wilmskoetter J, Gleichgerrcht E, et al. Advanced brain age and chronic poststroke aphasia severity. Neurology 2022;100(11):e1166–76.

24. Agency for Healthcare Research and Quality (AHRQ). 2016 National healthcare quality and disparities report. Available at: https://www.ahrq.gov/research/findings/nhqrdr/nhqdr16/index.html. Published October 2017. Accessed April 13, 2023.

25. Ellis C, Jacobs M. The complexity of health disparities: More than just black–white differences. Perspectives of the ASHA Special Interest Groups 2021;6(1):112–21.

26. Ellis C. African Americans and aphasia: A 25-year review. Journal of the National Black Association for Speech-Language and Hearing 2018;13(1):31–42.

27. Hoshino T, Uchiyama S, Wong LK, et al. Differences in characteristics and outcomes between Asian and non-Asian patients in the TIAregistry. Stroke 2017; 48(7):1779–87.

28. Penn C, Armstrong E, Brewer K, et al. Decolonizing speech-language pathology practice in acquired neurogenic disorders. Perspectives of the ASHA Special Interest Groups 2017;2(2):91–9.

29. Scimeca M, Abdollahi F, Peñaloza C, et al. Clinical perspectives and strategies for confronting disparities in social determinants of health for Hispanic bilinguals with aphasia. J Commun Disord 2022;98:106231.

30. Ellis C. Does Race/Ethnicity Really Matter in Adult Neurogenics? Am J Speech Lang Pathol 2009;18:310–4.

31. Nguy B, Quique YM, Cavanaugh R, et al. Representation in aphasia research: An examination of US treatment studies published between 2009 and 2019. Am J Speech Lang Pathol 2022;31(3):1424–30.

32. Mokhtar HM, Sawahel HM. Diffusion tensor imaging (DTI) and fractional anisotropy (FA) for arcuate fasciculus in predicting post-stroke aphasia outcome. The Egyptian Journal of Hospital Medicine 2021;85(1):3284–90.

33. Basilakos A, Stark BC, Johnson L, et al. Leukoaraiosis is associated with a decline in language abilities in chronic aphasia. Neurorehabilitation Neural Repair 2019;33(9):718–29.

34. RELEASE Collaborators, Brady MC, Ali M, VandenBerg K, et al. Precision rehabilitation for aphasia by patient age, sex, aphasia severity, and time since stroke? A prespecified, systematic review-based, individual participant data, network, subgroup meta-analysis. Int J Stroke 2022;17(10):1067–77.

35. Benghanem S, Rosso C, Arbizu C, et al. Aphasia outcome: the interactions between initial severity, lesion size and location. J Neurol 2019;266:1303–9.

36. Døli H, Andersen Helland W, Helland T, et al. Associations between lesion size, lesion location and aphasia in acute stroke. Aphasiology 2021;35(6):745–63.

37. Gadson DS, Wesley DB, van der Stelt CM, et al. Aphasia severity is modulated by race and lesion size in chronic survivors: A retrospective study. J Commun Disord 2022;100:106270.

38. Kristinsson S, Basilakos A, Elm J, et al. Individualized response to semantic versus phonological aphasia therapies in stroke. Brain Communications 2021; 3(3):fcab174.

39. Lee S, Na Y, Tae WS, et al. Clinical and neuroimaging factors associated with aphasia severity in stroke patients: diffusion tensor imaging study. Sci Rep 2020;10(1):12874.

40. Hillis AE, Beh YY, Sebastian R, et al. Predicting recovery in acute poststroke aphasia. Ann Neurol 2018;83(3):612–22.

41. Fridriksson J, Hillis AE. Current approaches to the treatment of post-stroke aphasia. Journal of Stroke 2021;23(2):183–201.

42. Kertesz A. The Western aphasia Battery – Revised. New York: Grune & Stratton; 2007.

43. RELEASE Collaborators. Dosage, intensity, and frequency of language therapy for aphasia: A systematic review–based, individual participant data network meta-analysis. Stroke 2022;53(3):956–67.

44. Breitenstein C, Grewe T, Flöel A, et al. Intensive speech and language therapy in patients with chronic aphasia after stroke: A randomised, open-label, blinded-endpoint, controlled trial in a health-care setting. Lancet 2017;389(10078):1528–38.

45. Guo YE, Togher L, Power E. Speech pathology services for people with aphasia: what is the current practice in Singapore? Disabil Rehabil 2014;36(8):691–704.

46. Cavanaugh R, Kravetz C, Jarold L, et al. Is there a research–practice dosage gap in aphasia rehabilitation? Am J Speech Lang Pathol 2021;30(5):2115–29.

47. Godecke E, Armstrong E, Rai T, et al. A randomized control trial of intensive aphasia therapy after acute stroke: The Very Early Rehabilitation for SpEech (VERSE) study. Int J Stroke 2021;16(5):556–72.

48. Husak RS, Wallace SE, Marshall RC, et al. A systematic review of aphasia therapy provided in the early period of post-stroke recovery. Aphasiology 2022;1–34.

49. Nouwens F, Dippel DW, de Jong-Hagelstein M, et al. RATS-3 investigators. Rotterdam Aphasia Therapy Study (RATS)-3: "The efficacy of intensive cognitive-linguistic therapy in the acute stage of aphasia"; design of a randomized controlled trial. Trials 2013;14:1–8.

50. Attard MC, Loupis Y, Togher L, et al. The efficacy of an interdisciplinary community aphasia group for living well with aphasia. Aphasiology 2018;32(2):105–38.

51. Brady MC, Kelly H, Godwin J, et al. Speech and language therapy for aphasia following stroke. Cochrane Database Syst Rev 2016;6:CD000425.

52. Tierney-Hendricks C, Schliep ME, Vallila-Rohter S. Using an implementation framework to survey outcome measurement and treatment practices in aphasia. Am J Speech Lang Pathol 2022;31(3):1133–62.

53. Hersh D, Worrall L, Howe T, et al. SMARTER goal setting in aphasia rehabilitation. Aphasiology 2012;26(2):220–33.

54. Haley KL, Cunningham KT, Barry J, et al. Collaborative goals for communicative life participation in aphasia: The FOURC model. Am J Speech Lang Pathol 2019;28(1):1–13.

55. Turner-Stokes L. Goal attainment scaling (GAS) in rehabilitation: a practical guide. Clin Rehabil 2009;23(4):362–70.

56. Berube S, Hillis AE. Advances and innovations in aphasia treatment trials. Stroke 2019;50(10):2977–84.

57. Biou E, Cassoudesalle H, Cogné M, et al. Transcranial direct current stimulation in post-stroke aphasia rehabilitation: A systematic review. Ann Phys Rehabil Med 2019;62(2):104–21.

58. Elsner B, Kugler J, Pohl M, et al. Transcranial direct current stimulation (tDCS) for improving aphasia in adults with aphasia after stroke. Cochrane Database Syst Rev 2019;5.

59. Zhang J, Zhong D, Xiao X, et al. Effects of repetitive transcranial magnetic stimulation (rTMS) on aphasia in stroke patients: A systematic review and meta-analysis. Clin Rehabil 2021;35(8):1103–16.

60. Gholami M, Pourbaghi N, Taghvatalab S. Evaluation of rTMS in patients with post-stroke aphasia: a systematic review and focused meta-analysis. Neurol Sci 2022;43(8):4685–94.

61. Ding X, Zhang S, Huang W, et al. Comparative efficacy of non-invasive brain stimulation for post-stroke aphasia: a network meta-analysis and meta-regression of moderators. Neurosci Biobehav Rev 2022;104804.

62. Zumbansen A, Black SE, Chen JL, et al. NORTHSTAR-study group. Non-invasive brain stimulation as add-on therapy for subacute post-stroke aphasia: a randomized trial (NORTHSTAR). Eur Stroke J 2020;5(4):402–13.
63. Keator L.M., Transcranial Alternating Current Stimulation as an Adjuvant for Nonfluent Aphasia Therapy: A Proof-Of-Concept Study. (Doctoral dissertation). 2022, Available at: https://scholarcommons.sc.edu/etd/7002.
64. Xie X, Hu P, Tian Y, et al. Transcranial alternating current stimulation enhances speech comprehension in chronic post-stroke aphasia patients: A single-blind sham-controlled study. Brain Stimul 2022;15(6):1538–40.
65. Picano C, Quadrini A, Pisano F, et al. Adjunctive approaches to aphasia rehabilitation: a review on efficacy and safety. Brain Sci 2021;11(1):41.
66. Berthier ML. Ten key reasons for continuing research on pharmacotherapy for post-stroke aphasia. Aphasiology 2021;35(6):824–58.
67. Stockbridge MD. Better language through chemistry: augmenting speech-language therapy with pharmacotherapy in the treatment of aphasia. In: Aminoff MJ, Boller F, Swaab DF, editors. Handbook of clinical neurology, vol. 185. Amsterdam: Elsevier; 2022. p. 261–72.
68. Hilari K, Behn N, James K, et al. Supporting wellbeing through peer-befriending (SUPERB) for people with aphasia: a feasibility randomised controlled trial. Clin Rehabil 2021;35(8):1151–63.
69. Palmer R, Dimairo M, Cooper C, et al. Self-managed, computerised speech and language therapy for patients with chronic aphasia post-stroke compared with usual care or attention control (Big CACTUS): a multicentre, single-blinded, randomised controlled trial. Lancet Neurol 2019;18(9):821–33.
70. Sihvonen AJ, Leo V, Ripollés P, et al. Vocal music enhances memory and language recovery after stroke: pooled results from two RCTs. Ann Clin Transl Neurol 2020;7(11):2272–87.
71. Sihvonen AJ, Pitkäniemi A, Leo V, et al. Resting-state language network neuroplasticity in post-stroke music listening: A randomized controlled trial. Eur J Neurosci 2021;54(11):7886–98.
72. Huang J, Qin X, Shen M, et al. An overview of systematic reviews and meta-analyses on acupuncture for post-stroke aphasia. Eur J Integr Med 2020;37:101133.
73. Devane N, Behn N, Marshall J, et al. The use of virtual reality in the rehabilitation of aphasia: a systematic review. Disabil Rehabil 2022;1–20.
74. Jeffries-EL M. How do we mitigate the impact of systemic bias on faculty from underrepresented groups? AAAS. Available at: https://www.aaas-iuse.org/mitigate-the-impact-of-systemic-bias/. Published December 14, 2022. Accessed March 18, 2023.
75. Fletcher-Janzen E, Strickland TL, Reynolds CR, editors. Handbook of cross-cultural neuropsychology. New York: Kluwer Academic/Plenum Publishers; 2000.
76. Hudley AHC, Mallinson C. Understanding English language variation in US schools. New York, New York: Teachers College Press; 2015.
77. Nunn K, Vallila-Rohter S, Middleton EL. Errorless, errorful, and retrieval practice for naming treatment in aphasia: a scoping review of learning mechanisms and treatment ingredients. J Speech Lang Hear Res 2023;66(2):668–87.
78. Hart T, Dijkers MP, Whyte J, et al. A theory-driven system for the specification of rehabilitation treatments. Arch Phys Med Rehabil 2019;100(1):172–80.
79. Portney LG, Watkins MP. Foundations of clinical research: applications to practice, vol. 892. Hoboken, NJ: Pearson/Prentice Hall; 2009.

80. Penn C, Armstrong E. Intercultural aphasia: new models of understanding for Indigenous populations. Aphasiology 2017;31(5):563–94.
81. Taylor OL, Payne KT. Culturally valid testing: A proactive approach. Top Lang Disord 1983;3(3):8–20.
82. Onuorah HM, Charron O, Meltzer E, et al. Enrollment of non-White participants and reporting of race and ethnicity in phase III trials of multiple sclerosis DMTs: A systematic review. Neurology 2022;98(9):e880–92.
83. Akturk HK, Agarwal S, Hoffecker L, et al. Inequity in racial-ethnic representation in randomized controlled trials of diabetes technologies in type 1 diabetes: Critical need for new standards. Diabetes Care 2021;44(6):e121–3.
84. Gomez SE, Sarraju A, Rodriguez F. Racial and ethnic group underrepresentation in studies of adverse pregnancy outcomes and cardiovascular risk. J Am Heart Assoc 2022;11(5):e024776.
85. Flanagin A, Frey T, Christiansen SL, AMA Manual of Style Committee. Updated guidance on the reporting of race and ethnicity in medical and science journals. JAMA 2021;326(7):621–7.
86. Magwood GS, Ellis C, Buie JN, et al. High tech and high touch: Recruitment strategies for enrolling African American stroke survivors in Community Based Intervention under Nurse Guidance after stroke (CINGS) trial. Contemp Clin Trials Commun 2021;24:100844.

Dysphagia and Enteral Feeding After Stroke in the Rehabilitation Setting

Robynne G. Braun, MD, PhD[a,b,c,*], Jodi Arata, MS, CCC-SLP[d],
Marlis Gonzalez-Fernandez, MD, PhD[e,f]

KEYWORDS

- Stroke • Dysphagia • Enteral feeding • Prognosis • Physiatry • Neurorehabilitation

KEY POINTS

- There is growing clinical and research interest in the study of post-stroke dysphagia recovery based on trends identified in the literature.
- The complex decision-making around enteral access options is another area where physiatrists can make a major contribution.
- Swallow screening tests are primarily focused on determining whether the patient can safely tolerate oral nutrition, hydration, or medications, which may reflect factors other than dysphagia (eg, decreased level of arousal).

INTRODUCTION, BACKGROUND, AND DEFINITIONS

Disease Burden of Dysphagia After Stroke

Dysphagia is a common post-stroke complication that affects more than 50% of stroke survivors[1] and is associated with higher mortality rates, aspiration pneumonia, malnutrition, and worse patient outcomes.[2] A recent systematic review estimated health care–related costs for oropharyngeal dysphagia of up to $16,900 in the acute phase, and additional costs with aspiration pneumonia of $27,600.[3] Dysphagia also has profound effects on patients' quality of life, in many cases causing mealtime distress and avoidance of social eating.[4] Although the majority of dysphagic patients

[a] Department of Neurology, University of Maryland School of Medicine, Baltimore, MD, USA; [b] University of Maryland Rehabilitation and Orthopedic Institute, Baltimore, MD, USA; [c] Brain Rehab and Recovery Lab, University of Maryland School of Medicine, Bressler Research Building, Suite 12-019, 655 West Baltimore Street, Baltimore, MD 21201, USA; [d] Rehabilitation Research Lab, University of Maryland Rehabilitation and Orthopedic Institute, 2200 Kernan Drive, Baltimore, MD 21207, USA; [e] Department of PM&R, Johns Hopkins University School of Medicine, 600 North Wolf Street, Phipps 184, Baltimore, MD 21287, USA; [f] Outpatient PM&R Clinics, Johns Hopkins Hospital, 600 North Wolfe Street Phipps 174, Baltimore, MD 21287, USA
* Corresponding author. Brain Rehab and Recovery LabUniversity of Maryland School of MedicineBressler Research Building, Suite 12-019655 West Baltimore Street, Baltimore, MD 21201
E-mail address: Robynne.Braun@umm.edu

Phys Med Rehabil Clin N Am 35 (2024) 433–443
https://doi.org/10.1016/j.pmr.2023.07.001
1047-9651/24/© 2023 Elsevier Inc. All rights reserved.

will recover swallowing function within the first week after stroke with up to 86% swallowing normally by 14 days,[5] 11% to13% will have persistent dysphagia at 6 months and beyond.[6,7]

As physicians who aim to add "life to years," physiatrists play a vital role in post-stroke dysphagia management not only by providing guidance on the risks, benefits, and efficacy of various treatment options but also as advocates for patient independence and quality of life. While swallow study results are often discussed broadly by acute stroke clinicians as "pass/fail" findings, physiatrists need a more nuanced working knowledge of dysphagia diagnosis and treatment that encompasses swallow pathophysiology, targeted treatment strategies, and prognosis for recovery. To that end, this review summarizes current clinical practice guidelines on dysphagia, nutrition and oral care, risks and benefits of differing enteral access routes, prognostic factors, and approaches to rehabilitation.

Swallow screening tests versus diagnostic assessments

It is important to distinguish between *swallow screening tests* and *diagnostic assessments* for dysphagia. This can be a source of confusion since some screening tests include elements that overlap with diagnostic dysphagia assessments. However, swallow screening tests are primarily focused on determining whether the patient can safely tolerate oral nutrition, hydration, or medications, which may reflect factors other than dysphagia (eg, decreased level of arousal). They are not considered appropriate as standardized tests for the diagnosis of dysphagia *per se*. There are multiple screening tests available in clinical practice as summarized in **Fig. 1** including the Burke Dysphagia Screening Test,[8] Simple Standardized Bedside Swallowing Assessment,[9] Timed Test of Hinds and Wiles,[10] Toronto Bedside Swallowing Screening Test,[11] Yale Swallow Protocol,[12] Gugging Swallow Screen,[13] Modified Mann Assessment of Swallowing,[14] and Barnes Jewish Hospital Swallow Screen/Acute Stroke Dysphagia Screen.[15] There is no established consensus on a single best instrument, but important considerations when selecting a screening tool include its validity, reliability, sensitivity and specificity, ease of administration, ease of documentation, and training requirements. Several comprehensive reviews comparing the clinimetric properties of these instruments have been published.[16–18]

By contrast, *diagnostic assessments* of dysphagia focus on techniques to characterize swallowing pathomechanics and identify aspiration. The gold standard test is the Modified Barium Swallowing study ("MBS"), also known as the videofluorographic swallowing study, ("VFSS"). The MBS is typically performed by a speech-language

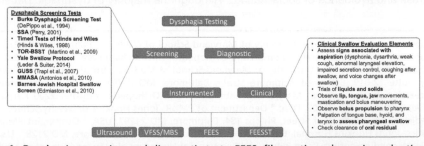

Fig. 1. Dysphagia screening and diagnostic tests. FEES, fiberoptic endoscopic evaluation of swallowing; FEESST, fiberoptic endoscopic evaluation of swallowing with sensory testing; GUSS, Gugging Swallowing Screen; MBS, Modified Barium Swallowing Study; MMASA, Modified Mann Assessment of Swallowing; SSA, simple standardized bedside swallowing assessment; TOR-BSST, Toronto Bedside Swallowing Screening Test; VFSS, video fluoroscopic swallow study.

pathologist together with a physiatrist or radiologist, and allows direct, real-time visualization of bolus flow, swallowing physiology, and airway invasion. The ability to directly observe the oropharyngeal phase of swallowing allows clinicians to characterize the mechanism and severity of impairment. The VFSS also allows the clinician to observe relationships between swallowing, food consistency, positioning, and ventilation. Other instrumental tools for the diagnosis of dysphagia have been developed (see **Fig. 1**) that assess the strength, pressure and range of structural movements, airway protection, sensation, bolus clearance and efficiency, and bolus flow patterns. These include ultrasound, fiberoptic endoscopic evaluation of swallowing (FEES) and fiberoptic endoscopic evaluation of swallowing with sensory testing (FEESST). Less commonly, pharyngeal manometry can be used if VFSS or endoscopy has not yielded a diagnosis and there is concern for problems with the esophageal sphincter or impaired peristalsis.

Non-instrumented clinical swallowing examinations are also performed by speech-language pathologists, and typically include motor and sensory assessments of the oral, pharyngeal, and laryngeal stages of swallow. Liquids and solid foods are trialed with close surveillance of the patient's lip, tongue, and jaw movements, mastication and maneuvering of liquid and solid boluses, ability to propel boluses into the pharynx, and clearance of oral residual. The timing and strength of the swallow is often assessed through palpation of the tongue base, hyoid, and larynx, though the reliability and validity of this approach has been questioned.[18] Patients are monitored for signs of overt aspiration before, during, and after swallowing. Although silent aspiration cannot be reliably detected during a bedside examination and remains a risk, several clinical signs associated with aspiration can be monitored including dysphonia, dysarthria, weak cough, abnormal laryngeal elevation, impaired secretion control, coughing after swallow, and voice changes after swallow.[19–21]

Current guidelines
Swallow screening and enteral feeding decisions. Current American Heart Association (AHA) guidelines[2] state that a swallow screen should be completed before the patient begins eating, drinking, or receiving oral medications, and if not cleared for oral intake, an enteral diet should be started within 7 days post-stroke. For the purposes of our discussion, enteral feeding refers to the delivery of nutrition and hydration directly into the gastrointestinal tract (stomach, duodenum, or jejunum) by a tube inserted either via an anatomic aperture (nose or mouth) or one created surgically (percutaneous insertion). Many types of enteral feeding tubes can be used depending on the expected period of feeding, clinical condition, and anatomy. Nasogastric tubes (NGT) are perhaps the most frequently used, while others include nasoduodenal or nasojejunal tubes (passing beyond the pyloric sphincter), and gastrostomies or jejunostomies (placed by endoscopic, radiologic, or surgical means). The AHA guidelines designate initial use of nasogastric tube during the first 2 to 3 weeks of enteral feeding.[2] When enteral feeding is expected for more than 28 days, percutaneous endoscopic gastrostomy (PEG) tubes should be placed after 14 to 28 days during a stable clinical phase.[22]

Decision-making on enteral access routes. Clinicians, patients, and caregivers often struggle when weighing the risks/benefits and quality-of-life considerations involved in decisions about enteral access routes. Oral intake is a major issue affecting quality of life, with >50% of seriously ill hospitalized patients viewing reliance on a feeding tube to live as a state equal to or worse than death.[23] Unfortunately, there is a relative dearth of high-quality evidence on dysphagia recovery to guide practice and patient/

family discussions. The complexity of these discussions—not to mention time spent planning for potentially invasive procedures—can significantly prolong length of stay.

Further challenge for informed decision-making includes the inherent heterogeneity of recovery trajectories in stroke. Due to variability in the timing and methods of assessment, and definitions of recovery used across studies, estimated rates of dysphagia occurrence span a remarkably wide range from 37% to 78%.[1] The relative lack of well-designed longitudinal studies on dysphagia has also limited our understanding of the prognosis for recovery, though more recent research has recognized and begun to bridge this gap.

Comparative risks and benefits of nasogastric tubes and percutaneous endoscopic gastrostomy

Overall, the choice of enteral feeding method for dysphagia after stroke should be based on the individual patient's medical condition, preferences, prognosis, and goals of care. Some factors that may influence the decision are the expected duration of tube feeding, the availability and expertise of locally available endoscopic/radiologic/surgical services, the risk of tube-related complications, and the patient's comfort and quality of life. A multidisciplinary team approach involving physicians, nurses, speech-language pathologists, dietitians, and caregivers is recommended to ensure optimal care planning. To help guide team discussions with patients and families, information comparing risk factors, relative contraindications, and positives and negatives for NGT versus PEG is provided in **Table 1**.

NGT is a well-established feeding method, but prolonged use can lead to complications such as nasal erosions, sinusitis, and gastro-esophageal reflux, among others. PEG is generally used when enteral nutrition is needed for a longer time period, and there is a high demand for PEG in patients with swallowing disorders, but there has been a lack of consistent evidence about the effectiveness and safety of PEG as compared to NGT.[24] An initial Cochrane meta-analysis[25] suggested that PEG feeding may improve mortality and nutrition (ie, weight, albumin levels) compared with NGT feeding, but overall the review was inconclusive, stating that too few studies with too few patients had been performed. A later randomized controlled trial (RCT) of 22 stroke patients showed that serum albumin levels were significantly higher for patients with PEG compared to NGT.[26] However, the validity of albumin as a metric of nutritional status has been criticized due to low specificity,[27,28] and there were no corresponding differences in anthropometric parameters (weight, arm circumference) between-groups or within-groups over time.

To date, the largest RCT on enteral feeding post-stroke is the Feed Or Ordinary Diet (FOOD) trial.[29] Allocating patients to NGT or PEG within days of admission, the trial found no difference in survival rates between groups at 6 months, but a 7.8% increase in the absolute risk of death or poor outcome was observed with PEG (borderline significance, $P = 0.05$). A subsequent Cochrane meta-analysis on NGT vs. PEG[24] that included 11 randomized controlled trials showed no significant difference in mortality rates or adverse events, including pneumonia related to aspiration. However, PEG was associated with a lower probability of intervention failure, defined as feeding interruption, blockage, or leakage of the feeding tube. The posited rationale for this finding is that the larger caliber of PEG and more secure insertion site leads to less interruption due to tube dislodgement and/or blockage. Individual factors must be taken into consideration since either enteral access route may create differing degrees of physical and emotional discomfort for a given patient. Some patients may be more prone to the risk of accidental nasogastric tube displacement with increased risk of aspiration due to behavioral factors (eg,

Table 1
Positives, negatives, risks, and relative contraindications for percutaneous endoscopic gastrostomy versus nasogastric tubes

	Percutaneous Endoscopic Gastrostomy (PEG)	Nasogastric Tubes (NGT)
Positives	• Less easily dislodged • Better cosmesis than NGT • Most rehabilitation sites accept	• Bedside procedure • Readily reversible • Less costly to place than PEG • May be less distressing decision for patient/family (temporary tube)
Negatives	• Difficult to remove (if traction type) • More costly to place than NGT • May be distressing decision for patient/family (longerterm tube) • May prolong LOS [family discussions, serial Modified Barium Swallowing study (MBS), procedure scheduling, titrating feeds]	• Social concerns for cosmesis • More easily dislodged (may require bridle) • Greater risk of blockage than PEG • May limit discharge options/prolong length of stay (LOS) (if rehab site cannot accept NGT)
Risks	• Potential for pain, discomfort • Operative risks • Stoma site infection • Gastric ulceration/bleeding • Peristomal bleeding • Peritonitis • Buried bumper syndrome • Colonic injury • Gastrocolocutaneous fistula	• Potential for pain, discomfort • Sinusitis • Laryngeal ulcerations • Pneumothorax • Tracheoesophagic fistula • Nasal damage • Gastroesophageal reflux disease (GERD) • Bronchial placement
Relative Contraindications	• High cardiovascular operative risk • Ascites (difficult placement window) • Cirrhosis (abnormal hemostasis) • Bleeding disorders • Anticoagulation/antiplatelet use	• Esophageal stricture (risk of esophageal perforation) • Basilar skull or facial fracture (risk of intracranial misplacement) • Esophageal varices (may trigger variceal bleeding)

agitation, degree of preserved hand motor function) and anatomy (eg, deviated nasal septum leading to malpositioning). It is also worth noting patient and caregiver perceptions that PEG is more convenient and comfortable than NGT [30] and may therefore offer benefits for quality of life.

The importance of oral care

Patients with neurodisability who are enterally fed often have difficulty attending to their own oral care due to physical, perceptual, and cognitive difficulties. The flora of the oral cavity after stroke can be altered by candida infections, build-up of oropharyngeal residues and dental plaque, and antibiotic treatment.[31] The probable relationship between stroke-associated pneumonia and patients' oral health has received increasing attention. Unfortunately, oral care is often delegated to junior nursing staff who may be inadequately trained to safely or optimally provide it.[32,33] A more effective strategy for the provision of oral care could involve the broader multidisciplinary stroke team, including dietetic, dental, and occupational therapy professionals.[34] The reader is referred to latest Cochrane review on interventions for improving oral hygiene following stroke[35] for further details. Scheduling the application of chlorhexidine and/or artificial saliva by oral swab (rather than ordering them for oral care on an as-needed basis) is helpful in establishing a consistent oral hygiene schedule.

Approaches to dysphagia rehabilitation treatments

Dysphagia rehabilitation encompasses both compensatory strategies and restorative treatments.[36] Compensatory strategies focus on reducing the symptoms of dysphagia without necessarily altering the underlying pathophysiology. These include postural adjustments; altering the consistency, viscosity, or volume of the bolus; and increased volitional control. Restorative treatments, by contrast, are focused on improving the swallowing physiology, swallow safety, and tolerance of the least restrictive diet.[37] These include tongue hold exercises, Shaker exercise (head-raise), lingual exercises, resistance training, expiratory muscle strength training, Lee Silverman Voice Therapy, and neuromuscular electrical stimulation (NMES). Some rehabilitative approaches are both compensatory and restorative since they can be used initially to reduce the acute symptoms of dysphagia, but over time will also improve the swallowing physiology. These include effortful swallow, Mendelsohn maneuver, sensory enhancement, Supraglottic Safety Swallow, and Super Supraglottic Safety Swallow (breath hold). Descriptions of these exercises and the associated stages of swallowing they address are depicted in **Fig. 2**.

The types of treatment available for dysphagia have evolved greatly over the years. Traditional therapies have focused more on mechanical interventions and compensatory strategies such as the use of thickened fluids, modified texture diet, and postural maneuvers to improve swallowing biomechanics and minimize aspiration risk. More

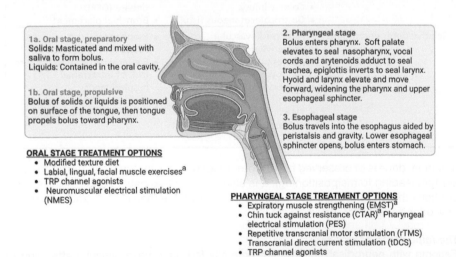

1a. Oral stage, preparatory
Solids: Masticated and mixed with saliva to form bolus.
Liquids: Contained in the oral cavity.

1b. Oral stage, propulsive
Bolus of solids or liquids is positioned on surface of the tongue, then tongue propels bolus toward pharynx.

2. Pharyngeal stage
Bolus enters pharynx. Soft palate elevates to seal nasopharynx, vocal cords and arytenoids adduct to seal trachea, epiglottis inverts to seal larynx. Hyoid and larynx elevate and move forward, widening the pharynx and upper esophageal sphincter.

3. Esophageal stage
Bolus travels into the esophagus aided by peristalsis and gravity. Lower esophageal sphincter opens, bolus enters stomach.

ORAL STAGE TREATMENT OPTIONS
• Modified texture diet
• Labial, lingual, facial muscle exercises[a]
• TRP channel agonists
• Neuromuscular electrical stimulation (NMES)

PHARYNGEAL STAGE TREATMENT OPTIONS
• Expiratory muscle strengthening (EMST)[a]
• Chin tuck against resistance (CTAR)[a] Pharyngeal electrical stimulation (PES)
• Repetitive transcranial motor stimulation (rTMS)
• Transcranial direct current stimulation (tDCS)
• TRP channel agonists

LARYNGEAL STAGE TREATMENT OPTIONS
• Esophageal stents or dilatation for strictures

Fig. 2. Treatment options by swallow stage affected. Blue font: Voluntary Control. Red font: Involuntary Control. [a]Exercises ± biofeedback. (Portions of the figure are created using Biorender.)

recent innovations have included advances in the use of peripheral and central stimulation methods. Central stimulation methods studied to date include neuromodulation via transcranial direct current stimulation (tDCS) and repetitive transcranial magnetic stimulation (rTMS).[38] While both rTMS and tDCS have shown promise as treatments,[39] rTMS was recently reported to have greater efficacy.[40] There is still considerable work to be done on standardizing treatment protocols, outcome metrics, and study designs in this area of research.

Peripheral stimulation methods have also been investigated. For example, transcutaneous electrical stimulation (TES) is endorsed as a beneficial therapy by the National Institute for Health and Care Excellence[41] and there is a relatively high quality of evidence to support efficacy with several RCTs completed to date. For example, a recent RCT by Arreola and colleagues[42] showed that both sensory [sensory electrical stimulation (SES)] and motor (NMES) applications of TES improved the safety of swallow and reduced the need for thickened fluids compared to treatment with compensatory strategies alone. These effects were furthermore retained at the 12-month follow-up. One challenge in interpreting the literature on TES has been the lack of a uniform measurement to assess swallow function, though in many cases the functional oral intake scale (FOIS) or similar measures have been documented.

Dysphagia prognosis and rehabilitation planning
An important aspect of medical decision-making for stroke rehabilitation is selecting candidates who are likely to respond to intensive dysphagia therapy in the acute rehabilitation setting versus those with a poor swallow prognosis that warrants skilled nursing admission. Previous studies have identified multiple indicators associated with prolonged swallowing problems. These include age,[43,44] signs of aspiration,[44–46] presence of bilateral infarcts,[44,46,47] frontal lobe involvement,[48,49] and severity on the National Institutes of Health Stroke Scale (NIHSS) score.[43,46–48,50] However, there are inherent challenges for interpreting the literature on predicting dysphagia recovery after stroke. Notably, definitions of recovery in the research have varied widely, with some studies considering PEG removal to be the marker of recovery (despite confounds based on delays for tract maturation) or have defined recovery in terms of clearance for an oral diet (despite continued supplemental nutrition/hydration). Similarly, inconsistent methods are used for defining the presence of dysphagia and dysphagia recovery. Metrics intended for differing applications may be conflated, including screening measures performed by nurses, bedside/clinical swallow evaluations by speech-language pathologists, instrumental assessments, or some combination thereof.

An ambitious study by Galovic and colleagues in 2019 evaluated many of the prognostic factors described earlier to generate an algorithmic tool for clinical decision-making (the Predictive Swallowing Score, "PRESS"). This study greatly raised awareness of the need for prognostic tools in post-stroke dysphagia. However, the generalizability of this approach depends upon whether clinical sites are able to reliably obtain measures of the same prognostic indicators, including the FOIS,[16] which may not be possible depending on local practice patterns. PRESS also defined aspiration risk based on the Any 2 Scale,[19] which is not currently accepted by the Joint Commission as a validated dysphagia screening measure. More recently, a systematic review on dysphagia prognosis was published that defined recovery more comprehensively based on multiple metrics (standardized scales, upgrade to oral diet, and discontinuation of enteral feeding). Overall, in reviewing the prior research, we identified a consensus from 2 or more studies for predictors of persistent dysphagia and negative recovery including penetration or aspiration on instrumental assessment, age, bilateral lesions, initial FOIS score, and stroke severity measured by the NIHSS.

Based on the evidence outlined earlier, we recently implemented a clinical pathway at our comprehensive stroke center developed collaboratively by Physical Medicine and Rehabilitation (PM&R), Stroke Neurology, Speech Language Pathology, and Executive leadership with the intention to improve the quality of stroke care, bring practice patterns into better alignment with existing AHA guidelines, and improve the efficiency of stroke patient transitions to rehabilitation. We hypothesized that a PM&R consultation including an assessment of age, stroke severity, unilateral versus bilateral stroke, the presence of pharyngeal versus oral dysphagia, stroke location (frontal lobe vs. brainstem involvement), and command following for oral/facial/lingual movements would allow identification of patients who were likely to recover swallowing function during their subsequent inpatient rehabilitation stay. Our physiatrists' assessments also incorporated additional key elements that rely on PM&R expertise including determination of the anticipated rehabilitation length of stay and potential barriers to discharge from the rehabilitation hospital. The initial results were presented at the American Academy of Physical Medicine and Rehabilitation (AAPM&R) 2022, and a related article is forthcoming.

DISCUSSION

There is growing clinical and research interest in the study of post-stroke dysphagia recovery based on trends identified in the literature. However, consensus building and comparison of outcomes to date have been hampered by methodological differences in the follow-up time points, recovery metrics, and choice of dysphagia assessment methods. There has also been a relative lack of data on hemorrhagic versus ischemic stroke, and large vessel occlusion versus other stroke subtypes. Future research will benefit from uniform usage of standardized scales, broader representation of stroke types, and well-documented data collection time points across the acute and post-acute care continuum. As physicians whose expertise spans the continuum of care, physiatrists can contribute much-needed longitudinal data on dysphagia recovery. The American Academy of Physical Medicine and Rehabilitation's strategic initiative on the future of care across the rehabilitation care continuum (PM&R Bold)[51] furthermore emphasizes physiatrists' expertise in managing the utilization of resources across the continuum of care. The complex decision-making around enteral access options is another area where physiatrists can make a major contribution.

CLINICS CARE POINTS

- Swallow screens and dysphagia diagnositc assessments differ in their ability to identify pathophysiology, inform therapy choices, and determine recovery prognosis.
- Predictors of persistent dysphagia identified to date include: (i) penetration or aspiration on instrumental assessment, (ii) age, (iii) bilateral lesions, (iv) initial FOIS score, and (v) stroke severity on the NIHSS.
- American Heart Association Guidelines recommend nasogastric tube for the first 2-3 weeks post-stroke, while PEG is considered for dysphagia that persists longer.
- Oral hygiene with chlorhexidine and/or artificial saliva should be scheduled to reduce the risk of aspiration pneumonia and improve patient comfort while NPO.

DISCLOSURE

The authors declare no relevant conflicts of interest.

REFERENCES

1. Martino R, Foley N, Bhogal S, et al. Dysphagia after stroke: incidence, diagnosis, and pulmonary complications. Stroke 2005;36(12):2756–63.
2. Powers WJ, Rabinstein AA, Ackerson T, et al. Guidelines for the early management of patients with acute ischemic stroke: 2019 update to the 2018 guidelines for the early management of acute ischemic stroke: a guideline for healthcare professionals from the American heart association/American stroke association. Stroke 2019;50(12):e344–418.
3. Marin S, Serra-Prat M, Ortega O, et al. Healthcare-related cost of oropharyngeal dysphagia and its complications pneumonia and malnutrition after stroke: a systematic review. BMJ Open 2020;10(8):e031629.
4. Ekberg O, Hamdy S, Woisard V, et al. Social and psychological burden of dysphagia: its impact on diagnosis and treatment. Dysphagia 2002;17(2):139–46.
5. Gordon C, Hewer RL, Wade DT. Dysphagia in acute stroke. Br Med J 1987;295(6595):411–4.
6. Smithard DG, O'Neill PA, England RE, et al. The natural history of dysphagia following a stroke. Dysphagia 1997;12(4):188–93.
7. Mann G, Hankey GJ, Cameron D. Swallowing function after stroke: prognosis and prognostic factors at 6 months. Stroke 1999;30(4):744–8.
8. DePippo KL, Holas MA, Reding MJ. The Burke dysphagia screening test: validation of its use in patients with stroke. Arch Phys Med Rehabil 1994;75(12):1284–6.
9. Perry L. Screening swallowing function of patients with acute stroke. Part two: detailed evaluation of the tool used by nurses. J Clin Nurs 2001;10(4):474–81.
10. Hinds NP, Wiles CM. Assessment of swallowing and referral to speech and language therapists in acute stroke. QJM 1998;91(12):829–35.
11. Martino R, Silver F, Teasell R, et al. The toronto bedside swallowing screening test (TOR-BSST): development and validation of a dysphagia screening tool for patients with stroke. Stroke 2009;40(2):555–61.
12. Leder SB, Suiter DM. The yale swallow protocol: an evidence-based approach to decision making. Switzerland: Springer International Publishing; 2014.
13. Trapl M, Enderle P, Nowotny M, et al. Dysphagia bedside screening for acute-stroke patients: the Gugging Swallowing Screen. Stroke 2007;38(11):2948–52.
14. Antonios N, Carnaby-Mann G, Crary M, et al. Analysis of a physician tool for evaluating dysphagia on an inpatient stroke unit: the modified Mann Assessment of Swallowing Ability. J Stroke Cerebrovasc Dis 2010;19(1):49–57.
15. Edmiaston J, Connor LT, Loehr L, et al. Validation of a dysphagia screening tool in acute stroke patients. Am J Crit Care 2010;19(4):357–64.
16. Crary MA, Mann GDC, Groher ME. Initial psychometric assessment of a functional oral intake scale for dysphagia in stroke patients. Arch Phys Med Rehabil 2005;86(8):1516–20.
17. Everton LF, Benfield JK, Hedstrom A, et al. Psychometric assessment and validation of the dysphagia severity rating scale in stroke patients. Sci Rep 2020;10(1):7268.
18. McCullough GH, Wertz RT, Rosenbek JC, et al. Inter- and intrajudge reliability of a clinical examination of swallowing in adults. Dysphagia 2000;15(2):58–67.

19. Daniels S, McAdam C, Brailey K, et al. Clinical assessment of swallowing and prediction of dysphagia severity. Am J Speech Lang Pathol 1997;6:17.
20. Linden P, Kuhlemeier KV, Patterson C. The probability of correctly predicting subglottic penetration from clinical observations. Dysphagia 1993;8(3):170–9.
21. Ramsey DJC, Smithard DG, Kalra L. Early assessments of dysphagia and aspiration risk in acute stroke patients. Stroke 2003;34(5):1252–7.
22. Wirth R, Smoliner C, Jäger M, et al. Guideline clinical nutrition in patients with stroke. Exp Transl Stroke Med 2013;5(1):14.
23. Rubin EB, Buehler AE, Halpern SD. States worse than death among hospitalized patients with serious illnesses. JAMA Intern Med 2016;176(10):1557–9.
24. Gomes CAR, Andriolo RB, Bennett C, et al. Percutaneous endoscopic gastrostomy versus nasogastric tube feeding for adults with swallowing disturbances. Cochrane Database Syst Rev 2015;2015(5):CD008096.
25. Bath PM, Bath-Hextall FJ, Smithard D. Interventions for dysphagia in acute stroke. Cochrane Database Syst Rev 1999;4. https://doi.org/10.1002/14651858. CD000323.
26. Hamidon BB, Abdullah SA, Zawawi MF, et al. A prospective comparison of percutaneous endoscopic gastrostomy and nasogastric tube feeding in patients with acute dysphagic stroke. Med J Malaysia 2006;61(1):59–66.
27. Levitt DG, Levitt MD. Human serum albumin homeostasis: a new look at the roles of synthesis, catabolism, renal and gastrointestinal excretion, and the clinical value of serum albumin measurements. Int J Gen Med 2016;9:229–55.
28. Takeda H, Ishihama K, Fukui T, et al. Significance of rapid turnover proteins in protein-losing gastroenteropathy. Hepato-Gastroenterology 2003;50(54): 1963–5.
29. Dennis MS, Lewis SC, Warlow C, FOOD Trial Collaboration. Effect of timing and method of enteral tube feeding for dysphagic stroke patients (FOOD): a multicentre randomised controlled trial. Lancet 2005;365(9461):764–72.
30. Anis MK, Abid S, Jafri W, et al. Acceptability and outcomes of the percutaneous endoscopic gastrostomy (PEG) tube placement- patients' and care givers' perspectives. BMC Gastroenterol 2006;6(1):37.
31. Gosney M, Martin MV, Wright AE. The role of selective decontamination of the digestive tract in acute stroke. Age Ageing 2006;35(1):42–7.
32. Horne M, McCracken G, Walls A, et al. Organisation, practice and experiences of mouth hygiene in stroke unit care: a mixed-methods study. J Clin Nurs 2015; 24(5–6):728–38.
33. Talbot A, Brady M, Furlanetto DLC, et al. Oral care and stroke units. Gerodontology 2005;22(2):77–83.
34. Bellomo F, de Preux F, Chung JP, et al. The advantages of occupational therapy in oral hygiene measures for institutionalised elderly adults. Gerodontology 2005; 22(1):24–31.
35. Campbell P, Bain B, Furlanetto DL, et al. Interventions for improving oral health in people after stroke. Cochrane Database Syst Rev 2020;2020(12). https://doi.org/ 10.1002/14651858.CD003864.pub3. Cochrane Stroke Group.
36. Huckabee M, Pelletier CA. Management of Adult Neurogenic Dysphagia. In: ; 1998. Available at: https://www.semanticscholar.org/paper/Management-of-Adult-Neurogenic-Dysphagia-Huckabee-Pelletier/9125b657044483f1386e5961d df8ed47a4b11cca. Accessed April 27, 2023.
37. Carnaby G, Lenius K, Crary M. Update on assessment and management of dysphagia post stroke. Northeast Florida Med 2007;58:31–4.

38. Cabib C, Ortega O, Kumru H, et al. Neurorehabilitation strategies for poststroke oropharyngeal dysphagia: from compensation to the recovery of swallowing function. Ann N Y Acad Sci 2016;1380(1):121–38.
39. Cheng I, Hamdy S. Current perspectives on the benefits, risks, and limitations of noninvasive brain stimulation (NIBS) for post-stroke dysphagia. Expert Rev Neurother 2021;21(10):1135–46.
40. Chiang CF, Lin MT, Hsiao MY, et al. Comparative efficacy of noninvasive neurostimulation therapies for acute and subacute poststroke dysphagia: a systematic review and network meta-analysis. Arch Phys Med Rehabil 2019;100(4):739–50.e4.
41. Tools and resources | Transcutaneous neuromuscular electrical stimulation for oropharyngeal dysphagia in adults | Guidance | NICE. Published December 19, 2018. Available at: https://www.nice.org.uk/guidance/ipg634/resources. Accessed April 26, 2023.
42. Arreola V, Ortega O, Álvarez-Berdugo D, et al. Effect of transcutaneous electrical stimulation in chronic poststroke patients with oropharyngeal dysphagia: 1-year results of a randomized controlled trial. Neurorehabil Neural Repair 2021;35(9):778–89.
43. Dubin PH, Boehme AK, Siegler JE, et al. New model for predicting surgical feeding tube placement in patients with an acute stroke event. Stroke 2013;44(11):3232–4.
44. Ickenstein GW, Kelly PJ, Furie KL, et al. Predictors of feeding gastrostomy tube removal in stroke patients with dysphagia. J Stroke Cerebrovasc Dis 2003;12(4):169–74.
45. Ickenstein GW, Höhlig C, Prosiegel M, et al. Prediction of outcome in neurogenic oropharyngeal dysphagia within 72 hours of acute stroke. J Stroke Cerebrovasc Dis 2012;21(7):569–76.
46. Kumar S, Doughty C, Doros G, et al. Recovery of swallowing after dysphagic stroke: an analysis of prognostic factors. J Stroke Cerebrovasc Dis 2014;23(1):56–62.
47. Kumar S, Langmore S, Goddeau RP, et al. Predictors of percutaneous endoscopic gastrostomy tube placement in patients with severe dysphagia from an acute-subacute hemispheric infarction. J Stroke Cerebrovasc Dis 2012;21(2):114–20.
48. Galovic M, Leisi N, Müller M, et al. Lesion location predicts transient and extended risk of aspiration after supratentorial ischemic stroke. Stroke 2013;44(10):2760–7.
49. Galovic M, Leisi N, Pastore-Wapp M, et al. Diverging lesion and connectivity patterns influence early and late swallowing recovery after hemispheric stroke. Hum Brain Mapp 2017;38(4):2165–76.
50. San Luis COV, Staff I, Ollenschleger MD, et al. Percutaneous endoscopic gastrostomy tube placement in left versus right middle cerebral artery stroke: effects of laterality. NeuroRehabilitation 2013;33(2):201–8.
51. Moon CH, Groman R, Jasak RS, et al. PM&R BOLD: the American academy of physical medicine and rehabilitation's strategic initiative to envision – and effectuate – the future of care across the rehabilitation care continuum. PM&R 2022;14(12):1497–508.

Innovations in Stroke Recovery and Rehabilitation
Poststroke Pain

Juliet Zakel, MD*, John Chae, MD, Richard D. Wilson, MD

KEYWORDS

- Poststroke pain • Stroke sequelae • Pain • Shoulder pain
- Complex regional pain syndrome • Quality of life

KEY POINTS

- Poststroke pain impairs function and decreases quality of life.
- Common pain syndromes after stroke include headache, musculoskeletal pain, spasticity-related pain, complex regional pain syndrome, and central poststroke pain.
- Future research focusing on treatment strategies for poststroke pain syndromes is needed.

INTRODUCTION

Pain after stroke is a common condition associated with worsened health outcomes.[1–4] The prevalence of poststroke pain has been reported as high as 66%, although estimates vary depending on study methods.[5] A prospective, cross-sectional, multicenter study documented the prevalence of poststroke pain in the acute stage (within 14 days of stroke) at 14%; at 42% in the subacute setting (15–90 days after stroke); and at 31% in the chronic period (>90 days after stroke).[6] Stroke survivors who experience pain have greater rates of depression, suicide, disability, fatigue, cognitive impairment, and functional decline compared with those without pain after stroke.[1,3,5,7] Pain can be a significant barrier to a stroke survivors' rehabilitation, and uncontrolled pain can prevent stroke survivors from reaching their maximal functional potential. As with pain in nonstroke populations, having pain after stroke is associated with decreased quality of life.[7]

The severity of stroke and premorbid depression are the most significant risk factors associated with poststroke pain.[1,2,8] In addition to risk factors that increase the risk of pain in the general population, risk factors for developing pain after stroke include

MetroHealth Rehabilitation Institute, MetroHealth System, Case Western Reserve University, 4229 Pearl Road, Cleveland, OH 44109, USA
* Corresponding author.
E-mail address: jzakel@metrohealth.org

Phys Med Rehabil Clin N Am 35 (2024) 445–462
https://doi.org/10.1016/j.pmr.2023.06.027
pmr.theclinics.com

female sex, alcohol use, tobacco use, sensory impairment, spasticity, ischemic stroke, brainstem or thalamic stroke localization, and chronic comorbid conditions such as diabetes mellitus, peripheral vascular disease, and hyperlipidemia.[1,5]

Despite the common occurrence of poststroke pain, it is often not recognized, is underdiagnosed, and is inadequately treated.[5,6] Impairments in cognition and communication may contribute to the challenge clinicians have when diagnosing and treating poststroke pain conditions. Research shows that people with cognitive impairment are prescribed fewer medications for pain.[9–12] Similarly, stroke survivors with aphasia receive less pain medication than those without impairments in communication, not because they experience less pain but are less able to notify caregivers that pain is present.[13] The Abbey pain scale is a psychometrically valid tool used to assess pain in those who have communication impairments.[14] The Abbey pain scale generates a pain score by observing a patients' vocalization (whimpering, crying), facial expression (grimace, tense, frightened), body language (restless, rocking, guarding, withdrawn), behavior (confusion, refusing to eat), physiology (vital sign changes, perspiration, flush, pallor), and physical changes (skin break down, arthritis, contractures, injury).[15,16] The Abbey pain scale can help providers recognize pain in those who cannot verbally express their discomfort.[14,17,18]

Pain after stroke can be complex and multifactorial in nature. Common types of pain that are related to the stroke include headache, musculoskeletal, spasticity-related pain, complex regional pain syndrome (CRPS), and central poststroke pain (CPSP). Paolucci and colleagues, studied the prevalence of pain occurring after stroke and found headache pain to be the most prevalent in the acute stage; whereas, shoulder, other musculoskeletal, and CPSP were more prevalent during the subacute phase, and spasticity related pain occurred most often in the chronic stage after stroke.[6] The purpose of this review is to discuss common types of poststroke pain and evaluate the current evidence for identifying, managing, and treating these conditions.

POSTSTROKE PAIN SYNDROMES

Pain is a common condition in the general population, and it is well established that pain is associated with increased disability and morbidity along with decreased function and quality of life. Not only can a stroke cause abrupt devastating consequences to a person's function and independence but can also cause additional challenges due to pain syndromes that are related to the stroke itself, which can further affect recovery and worsen functional outcomes. Special considerations are essential when treating pain in stroke survivors and prominent poststroke pain syndromes are discussed in the following sections of this evidence-based review.

Headache After Stroke

Headache after stroke is more likely to occur in the acute setting (within 14 days); however, persistent headache, defined as a headache greater than 3 months after stroke, has a reported prevalence of 1% to 23% depending on study methods.[19,20] The pathophysiology of poststroke headache is not well established. Among headache types, tension and migraine are the most common after stroke.[20] Ischemic infarcts in the posterior circulation are associated with increased incidence of headache compared with ischemic infarcts in the anterior circulation.[19,20]

Treatment considerations of acute headache after stroke
Poststroke headache management has a paucity of research and no defined clinical guidelines, which can make relieving headache after stroke a challenge. Although there are no clinical guidelines for treating headache after stroke, minimizing known

headache triggers can be a starting point. For example, lack of sleep is associated with acute and chronic headache after stroke.[20] Evaluating sleep patterns, improving sleep hygiene, and treating sleep disorders may help improve poststroke headache. Melatonin at night, which some studies have associated with improved sleep, can be effective in decreasing migraine frequency.[21] Additionally, a thorough review of a person's medication history can help identify potential drugs that have a side effect of headache. For example, dipyridamole, an antiplatelet medication commonly prescribed for secondary stroke prevention, can cause headache as a side effect in approximately one-third of people.[22–24] If the headache coincides with initiation of dipyridamole, then providers may consider the risks and benefits of switching to another antiplatelet agent. Limited studies suggest that aspirin and clopidogrel, antiplatelet agents commonly prescribed for secondary prevention of stroke, may decrease migraine, and thus a better choice than dipyridamole for someone with headaches after stroke.[25,26]

In the general population, first-line treatment options for acute headache are NonSteroidal Anti-Inflammatory Drugs (NSAIDs) or acetaminophen.[27–29] Nonaspirin NSAID use after acute stroke is not advised—due to side effects of hypertension, edema, heart failure, gastritis, and the increased risk of myocardial infarction and stroke.[27,28,30,31] With very few exceptions, acetaminophen is a more appropriate first-line treatment option for acute headache after stroke. Attention should be paid to the duration of acetaminophen use since frequent consumption (more than 15 days per month) can cause headache due to overuse.[32]

Second-line management of acute headache with migrainous features in the general population include abortive therapies, ergotamine and triptans, which are contraindicated after stroke due to risk of vasoconstriction of intracranial arteries that could increase the risk of recurrent stroke.[23] Recently, the Food and Drug Administration (FDA) approved ubrogepant and rimegepant (calcitonin gene-related peptide receptor antagonists) and lasmiditan (a serotonin agonist) as acute headache therapies, and these medications do not cause constriction of intracranial arteries. Consequently, ubrogepant, rimegepant, and lasmiditan may be more appropriate options for aborting headache with migrainous features in stroke survivors after first-line options are exhausted.[28,29] **Fig. 1** illustrates acute headache treatment strategies after stroke.

Prophylactic treatment considerations of headache after stroke

Current guidelines recommend initiating prophylactic headache medication for those who have 2 or more headache days a month despite optimized acute therapy or when symptoms are disabling despite acute management.[28] Initial preventative headache medications for the general population include propranolol, metoprolol, nadolol,

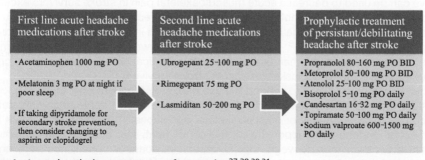

First line acute headache medications after stroke	Second line acute headache medications after stroke	Prophylactic treatment of persistant/debilitating headache after stroke
• Acetaminophen 1000 mg PO	• Ubrogepant 25–100 mg PO	• Propranolol 80–160 mg PO BID
		• Metoprolol 50–100 mg PO BID
• Melatonin 3 mg PO at night if poor sleep	• Rimegepant 75 mg PO	• Atenolol 25–100 mg PO BID
		• Bisoprolol 5–10 mg PO daily
	• Lasmiditan 50–200 mg PO	• Candesartan 16–32 mg PO daily
• If taking dipyridamole for secondary stroke prevention, then consider changing to aspirin or clopidogrel		• Topiramate 50–100 mg PO daily
		• Sodium valproate 600–1500 mg PO daily

Fig. 1. Acute headache treatments after stroke.[27,28,30,31]

atenolol, bisoprolol, candesartan, amitriptyline, nortriptyline, topiramate, and sodium valproate.[27,28] Special consideration should be taken when prescribing prophylactic headache medications for stroke survivors to minimize interactions with current medications, minimize side effects, and maximize treatment of comorbid conditions. In stroke survivors who have headache and hypertension, the following antihypertensive medications—propranolol, metoprolol, nadolol, atenolol, bisoprolol, and candesartan—can be advantageous to manage both conditions. Antiepileptic drugs, topiramate and sodium valproate, may be useful to treat both seizure and headache; however, the associated cognitive side of topiramate and hepatotoxicity of sodium valproate may limit use.[33,34] Caution is advised when using tricyclic antidepressants, amitriptyline and nortriptyline, after stroke due to potential side effects of drowsiness, confusion, constipation, orthostasis, cardiac arrhythmia, and urinary retention.[35] The care of stroke survivors would benefit from further studies that allow creation of clinical guidelines for treatment of poststroke headache.

Musculoskeletal Pain After Stroke

Musculoskeletal pain is one of the most common causes of disability in the United States. Stroke survivors aged older than 55 years have a higher prevalence of joint pain, stiffness, and swelling compared with aged-matched adults without stroke.[36] Joint pain during stroke recovery is associated with an increased hospital length of stay and worse functional outcomes.[2,37] Stroke survivors with joint pain have more difficulty performing activities of daily living (ADLs), such as, transferring, standing, walking, holding objects, donning socks/shoes, brushing teeth, and combing hair than stroke survivors without joint pain.[2,37] The effect of the pain on functional outcomes varies by the side of stroke deficit and location of musculoskeletal pain. For example, upper extremity hemiparesis combined with contralateral upper extremity joint pain results in poorer functional outcomes than if joint pain was located on the paretic limb. Conversely, lower extremity hemiparesis combined with ipsilateral lower extremity joint pain causes decreased functional impairment than if the joint pain was located contralaterally to the paretic leg.[36] Adequately controlling musculoskeletal pain during stroke recovery is imperative to maximize recovery and functional outcomes.

Careful consideration of treatment options and potential side effects is warranted when managing acute and chronic musculoskeletal pain in stroke survivors compared with the general population. In the nonstroke population, treatment guidelines for acute musculoskeletal pain advise topical NSAIDs with or without menthol gel as first-line therapy.[38] Additionally, the literature supports the use of oral NSAIDs, acetaminophen, acupressure, and transcutaneous electrical nerve stimulation to decrease acute musculoskeletal pain in the otherwise healthy individuals.[38] These guidelines above can be used to decrease acute musculoskeletal pain in stroke survivors except for oral NSAIDs, which are not advised due to side effects of hypertension, edema, heart failure, gastritis, and the black box warning for an increased risk of myocardial infarction and stroke.[27,28,30,31] Topical NSAIDs have lower systemic absorption and fewer adverse side effects than oral NSAIDs; thus, topical NSAIDs can be beneficial in decreasing acute musculoskeletal pain in stroke survivors.[39]

There is strong evidence to support the use of exercise, weight loss, tai chi, topical NSAIDs, oral NSAIDs, and intra-articular steroid injections to improve chronic pain secondary to osteoarthritis or musculoskeletal conditions.[40–42] Additionally, there is conditional evidence to support the utilization of heat, ice, acupuncture, paraffin, cognitive behavior therapy, yoga, topical capsaicin, acetaminophen, tramadol, and duloxetine for the management of chronic musculoskeletal pain in otherwise healthy individuals.[41] Other nonpharmacological devices that can improve chronic musculo-skeletal pain conditions include the use of a cane, tibiofemoral knee brace, carpome-tacarpal joint orthosis, patellofemoral knee brace, or kinesiology taping.[41] These chronic musculoskeletal pain treatment recommendations are applicable to stroke survivors except for the use of oral NSAIDs and tramadol, which are not recommen-ded due to side effect profile.[31,43] **Fig. 2** outlines various treatment approaches to improve poststroke musculoskeletal pain, and the following section provides evidence-based management of poststroke shoulder pain.

Poststroke shoulder pain
Shoulder pain is a common complication after stroke. Zhang and colleagues conducted a systematic review and meta-analysis to investigate the prevalence of poststroke shoulder pain and found that among 10 cross-sectional studies, the pooled prevalence of poststroke shoulder pain was 33%.[45] The pathophysiology of poststroke shoulder pain is complex and multifactorial. Many causes of shoulder pain have been docu-mented—glenohumeral subluxation, glenohumeral joint arthritis, scapular dyskinesis, subacromial bursitis, shoulder impingement syndrome, rotator cuff injury, adhesive cap-sulitis, bicipital tendinopathy, myofascial pain, peripheral nerve entrapment, CRPS, cen-tral poststroke pain, central hypersensitivity, contracture, and spasticity.[5,45,46]

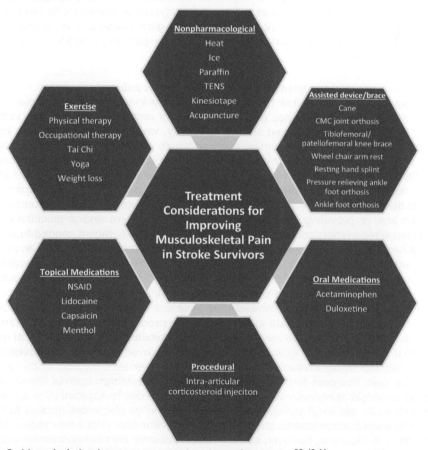

Fig. 2. Musculoskeletal treatment considerations after stroke.[38–42,44]

Identifying poststroke shoulder pain
Early detection of shoulder pain after stroke may lead to earlier intervention, improved pain control, and better functional outcomes. The positivity of 3 simple physical examination findings—pain with Neer's test, moderate-to-severe pain when shoulder is externally rotated and abducted with hand-behind-neck maneuver, and greater than 10° difference in passive external rotation when comparing range of motion of the hemiparetic shoulder to unaffected shoulder—is associated with a 98% probability of predicting early poststroke shoulder pain with a sensitivity of 96.7%.[47] Special tests may aid in the diagnosis of shoulder pathology; however, the sensitivity and specificity of these physical examination maneuvers is variable and conflicting throughout the literature. Positive Jobe test, full can test, drop arm test, Neer's test, or Hawkins/Kennedy impingement test may indicate supraspinatus pathology. Although positive lift off test, belly press test, or bear hug test may point toward subscapularis pathology. Infraspinatus injury can be associated with external rotation lag sign or Hornblower's sign. Positive speed's test or pain with palpation at the bicipital groove may suggest biceps tendon pathologic condition.[48] Other pertinent physical examination findings for poststroke shoulder pain include assessing active and passive range of motion at the glenohumeral joint since reduction in range of motion may indicate pain, spasticity, or adhesive capsulitis.[46] The degree of glenohumeral joint subluxation, which can be quantified by the number of fingerbreadths between the acromion and the humeral head is often evaluated during a shoulder physical examination; however, the association of shoulder subluxation causing hemiplegic shoulder pain is not known.[49] Diagnostic imaging used to further evaluate shoulder pathologic condition includes x-ray, ultrasound, and MRI.[50]

Nonpharmacological treatments of poststroke shoulder pain
The shoulder joint is a shallow ball-and-socket type with support from muscles and ligaments. This articulation has the widest range of motion among all joints in the body but at the cost of reduced structural stability, which makes the shoulder joint prone to injury. After stroke, hemiparesis can cause glenohumeral joint subluxation and shoulder instability, further placing the shoulder joint at risk for injury and pain. Guidelines for proper positioning of a hemiplegic arm during ADLs to prevent shoulder injury have not been well established and further research is needed. Avoiding movements that can exacerbate shoulder pain and instability—such as pulling on the hemiparetic arm or providing underarm assistance for transfers and ambulation—are reasonable recommendations.[51] Arm slings are not routinely recommended to position a hemiplegic extremity and have not been shown to improve glenohumeral joint subluxation, pain, or function.[52] The addition of a modified wheelchair arm support to a standard wheelchair can decrease the incidence of shoulder pain in stroke survivors and should be considered when writing a wheelchair prescription.[44]

Physical and occupational therapists are essential in the treatment plan of poststroke shoulder pain. Moderate intensity exercise programs with a focus on range of motion and shoulder stabilization are beneficial. Avoiding aggressive range of motion that inflicts pain and exercises that incorporate overhead pullies is advised.[53] Therapists can apply kinesiology taping to the shoulder as a method to decrease shoulder pain; however, further research is needed to establish optimal kinesiology taping protocols specifically for poststroke shoulder pain.[54] Application of surface neuromuscular electrical stimulation (NMES) delivered by electrodes applied to the skin surface of the hemiparetic shoulder within 6 months after stroke may reduce glenohumeral subluxation; however, surface NMES does not improve poststroke shoulder pain.[49,55] If shoulder pain continues despite preventative strategies, physical and occupational therapy, then additional pharmacologic or interventional modalities should be considered.

Pharmacologic and interventional treatments of poststroke shoulder pain

Presently, no controlled trials evaluating the effect of oral analgesics or oral spasticity medications on poststroke shoulder pain exist. **Fig. 2** illustrates various treatment modalities that can be trialed to improve musculoskeletal pain after stroke. Applying topical NSAIDs, lidocaine, or capsaicin to the skin of the hemiparetic shoulder may improve pain. Among simple oral analgesic medications, acetaminophen is advised over NSAIDs in stroke survivors when managing shoulder pain.[38,40,41]

If pain continues despite conservative treatments, then interventional procedures may be explored to improve pain and function. Subacromial corticosteroid injection is shown to be effective in improving poststroke shoulder pain, range of motion, and function in stroke survivors who have rotator cuff pathologic condition.[56] A suprascapular nerve block is another injection approach that can improve shoulder pain. The suprascapular nerve is a mixed nerve that provides motor innervation to the supraspinatus and infraspinatus along with sensory input to the acromioclavicular joint and glenohumeral joints.[57] Blocking the suprascapular nerve with a mixture of lidocaine and corticosteroid can be effective for treating poststroke shoulder pain.[58] If adhesive capsulitis is contributing to poststroke shoulder pain, clinicians may empirically treat with an intra-articular glenohumeral corticosteroid injection or perform an ultrasound-guided capsule hydrodilation, which uses a higher volume mixture of corticosteroid, saline, and anesthetic to distend the shoulder capsule.[59]

Neuromodulation through peripheral nerve stimulation of motor nerve fibers to elicit muscle contraction or sensory nerve fibers to create paresthesia is a promising intervention for the treatment of pain. Percutaneous peripheral nerve stimulation of the axillary nerve is an emerging treatment of chronic hemiplegic shoulder pain.[60] A randomized control trial concluded that a fine wire percutaneous electrode, inserted through the skin into the deltoid muscle, simulating the axillary nerve to cause contraction of the middle and posterior deltoid, 6 hours a day for 3 weeks duration, was safe and effective in decreasing shoulder pain after stroke.[61] A follow-up multisite case series evaluated the safety and efficacy of a fully implanted axillary peripheral nerve stimulator system for the treatment of poststroke shoulder pain and reported significant improvement in hemiplegic shoulder pain without any reported serious adverse events.[62]

Spasticity Pain After Stroke

Stroke survivors can develop spasticity as a complication from the upper motor neuron lesion of the stroke. Spasticity has been defined as a motor disorder characterized by velocity-dependent increase in muscle resistance to passive stretch, which is associated with hyperexcitable tendon jerks and stretch reflexes.[63,64] Spasticity can present as intermittent or sustained involuntary activation of muscles due to impaired sensorimotor control.[65] Muscle hypertonicity from spasticity can cause pain, and untreated spasticity can progress to other painful complications including joint contracture and skin break down.[66] Stroke survivors who have spasticity are more likely to have pain compared with those without spasticity.[67]

Poststroke spasticity treatment considerations

Current literature recognizes the benefits that spasticity treatments have on improving functional outcomes and quality of life; however, there is a paucity of research that specifically evaluates the effectiveness of spasticity treatment on pain out-comes.[64,66,68,69] Nonetheless, it is imperative that clinicians recognize and treat spasticity to prevent further complications that can cause additional pain.

When spasticity becomes a barrier in function or causes discomfort, treatment should be initiated. Conservative management begins with physical and occupational therapy, stretching, range of motion, casting, splint, and bracing.[66] **Table 1** outlines various pharmacologic treatment options for spasticity along with the associated mechanism of action and side effect profile. Common oral medications prescribed to decrease spasticity include baclofen, tizanidine, dantrolene, and benzodiazepines; however, the side effect profile limits use for many of these drugs.[64] Botulinum toxin type A and type B injections into spastic muscles are effective, for approximately 3 months, in decreasing pain from spasticity, preventing contracture, improving range of motion and hygiene.[70–74] Improvement in spasticity can be seen immediately after phenol and alcohol neurolysis and the duration of effect can last 3 to 9 months.[64] Intrathecal baclofen (ITB) is FDA approved for the management of severe spasticity of cerebral and spinal origin, and ITB therapy has shown improvement in pain and quality of life in stroke survivors who have severe spasticity.[75] Cryoneurotomy is an emerging therapy for the management of spasticity, which has been reported to be safe and efficacious. Similar to phenol, the improvement in spasticity after cryoneurotomy is immediate and longer lasting than botulinum toxin.[76,77] Additional research is needed to assess if cryoneurotomy improves spasticity-related pain.

Complex Region Pain Syndrome Type 1 After Stroke

CRPS Type 1 is a painful condition that can further impair function after stroke. The prevalence of poststroke CRPS varies between 9% and 50% depending on study methods.[81–84] Stroke survivors with severe motor impairment and glenohumeral joint subluxation are at greater risk for developing poststroke CRPS.[84] The pathophysiology of CRPS is not well defined and various mechanisms—autonomic nervous system dysfunction, somatic nervous system dysfunction, inflammation, local hypoxia, and psychological factors—may contribute to the painful syndrome.[85] In the fifth edition of the CRPS practical diagnostic and treatment guidelines, Harden and colleagues described CRPS as a syndrome characterized by regional pain (pain not in a specific nerve or dermatome distribution) that is disproportionate in time or degree to the usual course of trauma or lesion.[86] CRPS is further characterized by variable progression over time and commonly has a distal predominance of abnormal sensory, motor, sudomotor, vasomotor, or trophic findings. **Table 2** outlines the clinical diagnostic criteria for CRPS, which was accepted by the International Association for the Study of Pain.[86,87]

Treatment considerations for complex regional pain syndrome after stroke

The rarity and complexity of CRPS contributes to the lack of high-quality research, which adds to the challenge of treating patients with this disease. Given the multifactorial causes and clinical presentations of CRPS, there is not a single treatment that is effective for everyone, and some people may not find adequate pain relief with any of the treatment options. Expert consensus recommends a multidisciplinary treatment approach with a focus on functional restoration.[86] Members of the team include the patient, physician, psychologist, occupational, physical, recreational, and vocational rehabilitation therapists. According to Harden and colleagues, functional restoration emphasizes physical activity (reanimation), desensitization and normalization of sympathetic tone in the affected limb, and involves a steady progression from the most gentle, least invasive interventions, to the ideal of complete rehabilitation (such as

Table 1
Spasticity treatments after stroke[64,77–80]

Medication/Treatment	Mechanism of Action	Side Effects that May Limit Use in Stroke Survivors
Baclofen	Gamma-Aminobutyric Acid-B (GABA-B) receptor agonist	Weakness, drowsiness, withdrawal from abrupt discontinuation
Tizanidine	Alpha 2-adrenergic receptor agonist	Hepatotoxicity, hypotension
Dantrolene	Ryanodine receptor 1 antagonist, which blocks calcium release from sarcoplasmic reticulum in skeletal muscle	Weakness, drowsiness, hepatotoxicity
Benzodiazepines (diazepam/clonazepam)	GABA-A receptor agonist	Cognitive side effects, decrease attention, memory, drowsiness, withdrawal from abrupt discontinuation
Botulinum toxin A	Presynaptically blocks acetylcholine release into the neuromuscular junction by cleaving synaptosomal-associated protein-25	Weakness. Distant toxin spread causing difficulty with breathing and swallowing, which can be life threatening
Botulinum toxin B	Presynaptically blocks acetylcholine release into the neuromuscular junction by cleaving vesicle-associated membrane protein	Weakness. Distant toxin spread causing difficulty with breathing and swallowing, which can be life threatening
Phenol or alcohol	Protein denaturation resulting in nerve fiber destruction	Dysesthesia, swelling, weakness. Intravascular injection of phenol can cause hypotension, arrhythmia, respiratory depression, and death
Cryoneurotomy	Axonotmesis and nerve destruction by Wallerian degeneration	Dysesthesia

Table 2
Poststroke complex regional pain syndrome diagnosis and treatment[86–89]

CRPS Diagnostic Criteria	Poststroke CRPS Management
1. Continuing pain disproportionate to inciting event	Multidisciplinary team
2. Must report at least one symptom in 3 of 4 categories:	• Patient
• *Sensory:* hyperalgesia or allodynia	• Physician
• *Vasomotor:* temperature asymmetry, skin color changes, or skin color asymmetry	• Psychologist
• *Sudomotor/Edema:* edema, sweating changes or sweating asymmetry	• Physical, occupational, vocational, and recreational therapists
• *Motor/Trophic:* decreased range of motion, motor dysfunction (weakness, tremor, dystonia), or trophic changes (hair, nail, skin)	Nonpharmacological treatments
3. Must display at least 1 sign at time of evaluation in 2 or more categories:	• Physical therapy
• *Sensory:* hyperalgesia (to pinprick) or allodynia (to light touch and/or deep somatic pressure and/or joint movement)	• Occupational therapy
	• Mirror therapy
	• Graded motor imagery
	• Pain exposure
	• Aerobic exercise
• *Vasomotor:* temperature asymmetry or skin color asymmetry/change	Pharmacologic treatments
• *Sudomotor/Edema:* edema or sweating asymmetry/change	• Bisphosphonate
• *Motor/Trophic:* decreased range of motion, motor dysfunction (weakness, tremor, dystonia), or trophic changes (hair, nail, skin)	• Corticosteroid
4. No other diagnosis to explain the signs and symptoms	

return to work/studies) in all aspects of the patient's life.[86] **Table 2** illustrates treatment strategies for managing CRPS in stroke survivors.

In addition to conventional physical and occupation therapy, other conservative nonpharmacological therapies such as mirror therapy, motor imagery, pain exposure, and aerobic exercise maybe beneficial components to the comprehensive treatment plan for someone who has CRPS.[88] Studies report low-quality evidence that mirror therapy and graded motor imagery may improve motor function and decrease pain from CRPS.[88,89] Additionally, there is low-quality evidence that suggests pain exposure therapy and upper extremity aerobic exercise may improve CRPS pain.[88] It remains unclear if fluidotherapy, transcutaneous electrical nerve stimulation, acupuncture, ultrasound, manual lymphatic drainage, and laser therapy are effective treatments for CRPS.[88]

Various pharmacotherapies and interventions have been proposed to help treat patients with CRPS progress through the stages of functional restoration; however, the literature is sparse and lacking high-quality randomized controlled trials. Several studies report improvement in signs and symptoms of CRPS after oral corticosteroids in stroke survivors.[90–93] Clinicians are advised to assess risk and benefits before initiating oral corticosteroid treatment of CRPS in stroke survivors. Side effects of systemic corticosteroids include hyperglycemia, hypertension, and osteoporosis.[94]

Blood pressure and blood glucose monitoring is recommended if corticosteroids are initiated to treat poststroke CRPS since hypertension and diabetes are modifiable risk factors for stroke. Current literature supports the use of bisphosphonates for the treatment of CRPS, and bisphosphonates can be beneficial in stroke survivors who also have comorbid osteopenia or osteoporosis.[90,94–96] Clinicians may empirically prescribe calcitonin, tricyclic antidepressants, N-methyl-D-aspartate (NMDA) receptor antagonists, gabapentin, pregabalin, carbamazepine, opioids, clonidine, nifedipine, lidocaine patches, or topical capsaicin but the evidence that these treatments improve CRPS is uncertain.[86] Based on current literature, intravenous regional blocks with guanethidine, reserpine, droperidol, ketanserine, atropine, lidocaine, methylprednisolone, or ketorolac are not effective treatments for CRPS.[90] Peripheral sympathetic blocks and dorsal root ganglion neurostimulation show promise for some people who have refractory CRPS; however, larger scale clinical trials are necessary.[90]

Central Pain After Stroke

Central poststroke pain (CPSP) syndrome is a central neuropathic pain disorder that can be seen in people who had a stroke injuring any part of the somatosensory spinothalamocortical pathway.[97] The prevalence of CPSP has been reported between 2% and 31% and most commonly presents within the first year after stroke.[1,98,99] Infarcts in the lateral medulla and ventroposterior thalamus have a higher propensity for CPSP.[100] Stroke survivors may describe pain from CPSP as burning, squeezing, aching, pricking, freezing, lacerating, or shooting. **Table 3** illustrates a proposed guide for diagnosing CPSP since standardized criteria have not been established.[97] Further research to develop a universal diagnostic criterion for CPSP is highly recommended and imperative for the advancement of the understanding and treatment of CPSP.

Treatment considerations for central pain after stroke

CPSP can be a challenging pain syndrome to treat, and current literature is very limited. Studies evaluating efficacy of conservative therapies including physical therapy, occupational therapy, psychotherapy, exercise, desensitization on CPSP are needed. Higher quality studies are necessary to assess efficacy of nonpharmacological therapies — repetitive transcranial magnetic stimulation, transcranial direct current stimulation,

Table 3
Central poststroke pain diagnostic criteria and treatment considerations[1,99,100]

CPSP Diagnostic Criteria	CPSP Pharmacotherapies
CPSP mandatory diagnostic criteria	• Pamidronate
1. Pain within area of the body corresponding to the lesion of the central nervous system (CNS)	• Prednisone
	• Levetiracetam
2. History of stroke and onset of pain at or after stroke onset	• Lamotrigine
	• Etanercept
3. Confirmation of a CNS lesion by imaging or negative or positive sensory signs confined to area of body corresponding to the lesion	• Gabapentin
	• Pregabalin
4. Other causes for pain ruled out	• Duloxetine
CPSP supportive criteria	
1. No primary relation to movement, inflammation, or other local tissue damage	
2. Descriptors such as burning, painful cold, electric shocks, aching, pressing, stinging, and pins and needles	
3. Allodynia or dysesthesia to touch or cold	

acupuncture, and caloric vestibular stimulation—as potential treatments for CPSP.[101] First-line treatment of CPSP relies on pharmacotherapy, and there is no consensus on which medication is most efficacious. **Table 3** illustrates various medications that can be used to decrease CPSP. Meta-analyses report that pamidronate, prednisone, levetiracetam, lamotrigine, etanercept, gabapentin, pregabalin, and duloxetine can be effective for reducing CPSP.[99,100] The paucity of research on CPSP treatment highlights the opportunity for future scientific discovery in this domain.

SUMMARY

Stroke survivors commonly experience pain, which can prolong or reduce potential recovery. Headache, musculoskeletal pain, spasticity-related pain, CRPS, and CPSP are common in stroke survivors and rehabilitation specialists who treat this population should be aware of diagnoses and treatments that are available.

CLINICS CARE POINTS

- Poststroke pain is associated with decreased quality of life.[6]
- Pain can be a significant barrier to a stroke survivors' rehabilitation, and uncontrolled pain can prevent stroke patients from reaching maximal functional potential.
- Nonaspirin NSAID use after acute stroke is not advised—due to side effects of hypertension, edema, heart failure, gastritis, and the increased risk of myocardial infarction and stroke.[27,28,30,31]
- Beta blockers—propranolol, metoprolol, atenolol, and bisoprolol—and angiotensin receptor blocker, candesartan, are potential pharmacologic treatments that may be favorable to use after stroke to decrease blood pressure and headache; although, no specific studies have established treatment guidelines for headache after stroke.[23]
- Percutaneous peripheral nerve stimulation of the axillary nerve is an emerging treatment of chronic hemiplegic shoulder pain, which is safe and efficacious.[60–62]
- Cryoneurotomy is an emerging therapy for the management of spasticity, which has been reported to be safe and efficacious.[76,77]
- Multidisciplinary treatment approach is recommended when providing care to stroke survivors who have CRPS.[86]
- Pharmacotherapies that may benefit stroke survivors who have CPSP include pamidronate, prednisone, levetiracetam, lamotrigine, etanercept, gabapentin, pregabalin, and duloxetine; however, the care of stroke survivors would benefit from further studies that allow creation of comprehensive clinical guidelines for the treatment of CPSP.[99,100]

DISCLOSURE

J. Zakel does not have any commercial or financial conflicts of interest. R.D. Wilson receives grant support from the National Institutes of Health, United States. J. Chae is a consultant to SPR Therapeutics and owns equity in SPR Therapeutics.

REFERENCES

1. O'Donnell MJ, Diener HC, Sacco RL, et al. Chronic pain syndromes after ischemic stroke: PRoFESS trial. Stroke 2013;44(5):1238–43.

2. Appelros P. Prevalence and predictors of pain and fatigue after stroke: a population-based study. Int J Rehabil Res 2006;29(4):329–33.

3. Lundstrom E, Smits A, Terent A, et al. Risk factors for stroke-related pain 1 year after first-ever stroke. Eur J Neurol 2009;16(2):188–93.

4. Tang WK, Liang H, Mok V, et al. Is pain associated with suicidality in stroke? Arch Phys Med Rehabil 2013;94(5):863–6.

5. Harrison RA, Field TS. Post stroke pain: identification, assessment, and therapy. Cerebrovasc Dis 2015;39(3–4):190–201.

6. Paolucci S, Iosa M, Toni D, et al. Prevalence and Time Course of Post-Stroke Pain: A Multicenter Prospective Hospital-Based Study. Pain Med 2016;17(5): 924–30.

7. Hoang CL, Salle JY, Mandigout S, et al. Physical factors associated with fatigue after stroke: an exploratory study. Top Stroke Rehabil 2012;19(5):369–76.

8. Sackley C, Brittle N, Patel S, et al. The prevalence of joint contractures, pressure sores, painful shoulder, other pain, falls, and depression in the year after a severely disabling stroke. Stroke 2008;39(12):3329–34.

9. Morrison RS, Siu AL. A comparison of pain and its treatment in advanced dementia and cognitively intact patients with hip fracture. J Pain Symptom Manage 2000;19(4):240–8.

10. Bernabei R, Gambassi G, Lapane K, et al. Management of pain in elderly patients with cancer. SAGE Study Group. Systematic Assessment of Geriatric Drug Use via Epidemiology. JAMA 1998;279(23):1877–82.

11. Semla TP, Cohen D, Paveza G, et al. Drug use patterns of persons with Alzheimer's disease and related disorders living in the community. J Am Geriatr Soc 1993;41(4):408–13.

12. Scherder E, Oosterman J, Swaab D, et al. Recent developments in pain in dementia. BMJ 2005;330(7489):461–4.

13. Kehayia E, Korner-Bitensky N, Singer F, et al. Differences in pain medication use in stroke patients with aphasia and without aphasia. Stroke 1997;28(10): 1867–70.

14. Arsyawina P, Widiastuti Hesti Prawita, Hilda. The Validity of the Abbey Pain Scale for Assessing Pain in Stroke Patient. Journal Of Nursing Practice 2021;5(1): 162–7.

15. Lord B. Paramedic assessment of pain in the cognitively impaired adult patient. BMC Emerg Med 2009;9:20.

16. Abbey J, Piller N, De Bellis A, et al. The Abbey pain scale: a 1-minute numerical indicator for people with end-stage dementia. Int J Palliat Nurs 2004;10(1):6–13.

17. Nesbitt J, Moxham S, Ramadurai G, et al. Improving pain assessment and management in stroke patients. BMJ Qual Improv Rep 2015;4(1). https://doi.org/10.1136/bmjquality.u203375.w3105.

18. Brown D. Pain Assessment with Cognitively Impaired Older People in the Acute Hospital Setting. Rev Pain 2011;5(3):18–22.

19. Harriott AM, Karakaya F, Ayata C. Headache after ischemic stroke: A systematic review and meta-analysis. Neurology 2020;94(1):e75–86.

20. Lebedeva ER, Ushenin AV, Gurary NM, et al. Persistent headache after first-ever ischemic stroke: clinical characteristics and factors associated with its development. J Headache Pain 2022;23(1):103.

21. Tseng PT, Yang CP, Su KP, et al. The association between melatonin and episodic migraine: A pilot network meta-analysis of randomized controlled trials to compare the prophylactic effects with exogenous melatonin supplementation and pharmacotherapy. J Pineal Res 2020;69(2):e12663.

22. Halkes PH, van Gijn J, Kappelle LJ, et al. European/Australasian Stroke Prevention in Reversible Ischaemia Trial Study G. Risk indicators for development of headache during dipyridamole treatment after cerebral ischaemia of arterial origin. J Neurol Neurosurg Psychiatry 2009;80(4):437–9.

23. Kurth T, Diener HC. Migraine and stroke: perspectives for stroke physicians. Stroke 2012;43(12):3421–6.

24. Lindgren A, Husted S, Staaf G, et al. Dipyridamole and headache–a pilot study of initial dose titration. J Neurol Sci 2004;223(2):179–84.

25. Buring JE, Peto R, Hennekens CH. Low-dose aspirin for migraine prophylaxis. JAMA 1990;264(13):1711–3.

26. Wilmshurst PT, Nightingale S, Walsh KP, et al. Clopidogrel reduces migraine with aura after transcatheter closure of persistent foramen ovale and atrial septal defects. Heart 2005;91(9):1173–5.

27. Becker WJ, Findlay T, Moga C, et al. Guideline for primary care management of headache in adults. Can Fam Physician 2015;61(8):670–9.

28. Eigenbrodt AK, Ashina H, Khan S, et al. Diagnosis and management of migraine in ten steps. Nat Rev Neurol 2021;17(8):501–14.

29. Ailani J, Burch RC, Robbins MS, et al. The American Headache Society Consensus Statement: Update on integrating new migraine treatments into clinical practice. Headache 2021;61(7):1021–39.

30. Antman EM, Bennett JS, Daugherty A, et al. Use of nonsteroidal antiinflammatory drugs: an update for clinicians: a scientific statement from the American Heart Association. Circulation 2007;115(12):1634–42.

31. Meek IL, Van de Laar MA, E Vonkeman H. Non-Steroidal Anti-Inflammatory Drugs: An Overview of Cardiovascular Risks. Pharmaceuticals 2010;3(7): 2146–62.

32. Headache Classification Committee of the International Headache Society (IHS) The International Classification of Headache Disorders, 3rd edition. Cephalalgia 2018;38(1):1-211. doi.

33. Sommer BR, Fenn HH. Review of topiramate for the treatment of epilepsy in elderly patients. Clin Interv Aging 2010;5:89–99.

34. Ezhilarasan D, Mani U. Valproic acid induced liver injury: An insight into molecular toxicological mechanism. Environ Toxicol Pharmacol 2022;95:103967.

35. Lokk J, Delbari A. Management of depression in elderly stroke patients. Neuropsychiatr Dis Treat 2010;6:539–49.

36. Hettiarachchi C, Conaghan P, Tennant A, et al. Prevalence and impact of joint symptoms in people with stroke aged 55 years and over. J Rehabil Med 2011;43(3):197–203.

37. Nguyen-Oghalai TU, Ottenbacher KJ, Granger CV, et al. Impact of osteoarthritis on the rehabilitation of patients following a stroke. Arthritis Rheum 2005;53(3): 383–7.

38. Qaseem A, McLean RM, O'Gurek D, et al. Nonpharmacologic and Pharmacologic Management of Acute Pain From Non-Low Back, Musculoskeletal Injuries in Adults: A Clinical Guideline From the American College of Physicians and American Academy of Family Physicians. Ann Intern Med 2020;173(9):739–48.

39. Rannou F, Pelletier JP, Martel-Pelletier J. Efficacy and safety of topical NSAIDs in the management of osteoarthritis: Evidence from real-life setting trials and surveys. Semin Arthritis Rheum 2016;45(4 Suppl):S18–21.

40. Welsh TP, Yang AE, Makris UE. Musculoskeletal Pain in Older Adults: A Clinical Review. Med Clin North Am 2020;104(5):855–72.

41. Kolasinski SL, Neogi T, Hochberg MC, et al. 2019 American College of Rheumatology/Arthritis Foundation Guideline for the Management of Osteoarthritis of the Hand, Hip, and Knee. Arthritis Care Res 2020;72(2):149–62.

42. Babatunde OO, Jordan JL, Van der Windt DA, et al. Effective treatment options for musculoskeletal pain in primary care: A systematic overview of current evidence. PLoS One 2017;12(6):e0178621.

43. Scuteri D, Mantovani E, Tamburin S, et al. Opioids in Post-stroke Pain: A Systematic Review and Meta-Analysis. Front Pharmacol 2020;11:587050.

44. Pan R, Zhou M, Cai H, et al. A randomized controlled trial of a modified wheelchair arm-support to reduce shoulder pain in stroke patients. Clin Rehabil 2018; 32(1):37–47.

45. Zhang Q, Chen D, Shen Y, et al. Incidence and Prevalence of Poststroke Shoulder Pain Among Different Regions of the World: A Systematic Review and Meta-Analysis. Front Neurol 2021;12:724281.

46. Wilson RD, Chae J. Hemiplegic Shoulder Pain. Phys Med Rehabil Clin N Am 2015;26(4):641–55.

47. Rajaratnam BS, Venketasubramanian N, Kumar PV, et al. Predictability of simple clinical tests to identify shoulder pain after stroke. Arch Phys Med Rehabil 2007; 88(8):1016–21.

48. Jain NB, Luz J, Higgins LD, et al. The Diagnostic Accuracy of Special Tests for Rotator Cuff Tear: The ROW Cohort Study. Am J Phys Med Rehabil 2017;96(3): 176–83.

49. Iruthayarajah J., Iliescu A., Saikaley M., et al., Painful Hemiplegic Shoulder. In: Teasell R., editor. Evidence-based review of stroke rehabilitation. chap. Hemiplegic shoulder pain and complex regional pain syndrome. 2016:1-54. HEart and Stroke Foundation Canadian Partnership for Stroke Recovery; London, Ontario, Canada.

50. Dogun A, Karabay I, Hatipoglu C, et al. Ultrasound and magnetic resonance findings and correlation in hemiplegic patients with shoulder pain. Top Stroke Rehabil 2014;21(Suppl 1):S1–7.

51. Li Z, Alexander SA. Current evidence in the management of poststroke hemiplegic shoulder pain: a review. J Neurosci Nurs 2015;47(1):10–9.

52. van Bladel A, Lambrecht G, Oostra KM, et al. A randomized controlled trial on the immediate and long-term effects of arm slings on shoulder subluxation in stroke patients. Eur J Phys Rehabil Med 2017;53(3):400–9.

53. Kumar R, Metter EJ, Mehta AJ, et al. Shoulder pain in hemiplegia. The role of exercise. Am J Phys Med Rehabil 1990;69(4):205–8.

54. Wang Y, Li X, Sun C, et al. Effectiveness of kinesiology taping on the functions of upper limbs in patients with stroke: a meta-analysis of randomized trial. Neurol Sci 2022;43(7):4145–56.

55. Vafadar AK, Cote JN, Archambault PS. Effectiveness of functional electrical stimulation in improving clinical outcomes in the upper arm following stroke: a systematic review and meta-analysis. BioMed Res Int 2015;2015:729768.

56. Rah UW, Yoon SH, Moon DJ, et al. Subacromial corticosteroid injection on poststroke hemiplegic shoulder pain: a randomized, triple-blind, placebo-controlled trial. Arch Phys Med Rehabil 2012;93(6):949–56.

57. Basta M, Sanganeria T, Varacallo M. Anatomy, Shoulder and Upper Limb, Suprascapular Nerve. StatPearls; 2023.

58. Adey-Wakeling Z, Crotty M, Shanahan EM. Suprascapular nerve block for shoulder pain in the first year after stroke: a randomized controlled trial. Stroke 2013; 44(11):3136–41.

59. Elnady B, Rageh EM, Hussein MS, et al. In shoulder adhesive capsulitis, ultrasound-guided anterior hydrodilatation in rotator interval is more effective than posterior approach: a randomized controlled study. Clin Rheumatol 2020;39(12):3805–14.

60. Wilson RD, Kim CH. Percutaneous and Implanted Peripheral Nerve Stimulation for the Management of Pain: Current Evidence and Future Directions. Curr Phys Med Rehabil Rep 2020/03/01 2020;8(1):1–7.

61. Wilson RD, Gunzler DD, Bennett ME, et al. Peripheral nerve stimulation compared with usual care for pain relief of hemiplegic shoulder pain: a randomized controlled trial. Am J Phys Med Rehabil 2014;93(1):17–28.

62. Wilson RD, Bennett ME, Nguyen VQC, et al. Fully Implantable Peripheral Nerve Stimulation for Hemiplegic Shoulder Pain: A Multi-Site Case Series With Two-Year Follow-Up. Neuromodulation 2018;21(3):290–5.

63. Lance JW. Disordered muscle tone and movement. Clin Exp Neurol 1981;18: 27–35.

64. Francisco GE, Wissel J, Platz T, et al. Post-stroke spasticity. In: Platz T, editor. Clinical pathways in stroke rehabilitation: evidence-based clinical Practice recommendations. New York: Springer; 2021. p. 149–73.

65. Bhimani R, Anderson L. Clinical understanding of spasticity: implications for practice. Rehabil Res Pract 2014;2014:279175.

66. Treister AK, Hatch MN, Cramer SC, et al. Demystifying Poststroke Pain: From Etiology to Treatment. Pharm Manag PM R 2017;9(1):63–75.

67. Wissel J, Schelosky LD, Scott J, et al. Early development of spasticity following stroke: a prospective, observational trial. J Neurol 2010;257(7):1067–72.

68. Chang E, Ghosh N, Yanni D, et al. A Review of Spasticity Treatments: Pharmacological and Interventional Approaches. Crit Rev Phys Rehabil Med 2013; 25(1–2):11–22.

69. Nair KP, Marsden J. The management of spasticity in adults. BMJ 2014;349: g4737.

70. Jost WH, Hefter H, Reissig A, et al. Efficacy and safety of botulinum toxin type A (Dysport) for the treatment of post-stroke arm spasticity: results of the German-Austrian open-label post-marketing surveillance prospective study. J Neurol Sci 2014;337(1–2):86–90.

71. O'Brien CF. Treatment of spasticity with botulinum toxin. Clin J Pain 2002;18(6 Suppl):S182–90.

72. Shaw LC, Price CI, van Wijck FM, et al. Botulinum Toxin for the Upper Limb after Stroke (BoTULS) Trial: effect on impairment, activity limitation, and pain. Stroke 2011;42(5):1371–9.

73. Trompetto C, Marinelli L, Mori L, et al. Effectiveness of Botulinum Toxin on Pain in Stroke Patients Suffering from Upper Limb Spastic Dystonia. Toxins 5 2022; 14(1). https://doi.org/10.3390/toxins14010039.

74. Wu T, Fu Y, Song HX, et al. Effectiveness of Botulinum Toxin for Shoulder Pain Treatment: A Systematic Review and Meta-Analysis. Arch Phys Med Rehabil 2015;96(12):2214–20.

75. Creamer M, Cloud G, Kossmehl P, et al. Effect of Intrathecal Baclofen on Pain and Quality of Life in Poststroke Spasticity. Stroke 2018;49(9):2129–37.

76. Winston P, Mills PB, Reebye R, et al. Cryoneurotomy as a Percutaneous Mini-invasive Therapy for the Treatment of the Spastic Limb: Case Presentation, Review of the Literature, and Proposed Approach for Use. Arch Rehabil Res Clin Transl 2019;1(3–4):100030.

77. Rubenstein J, Harvey AW, Vincent D, et al. Cryoneurotomy to Reduce Spasticity and Improve Range of Motion in Spastic Flexed Elbow: A Visual Vignette. Am J Phys Med Rehabil 2021;100(5):e65.

78. Brashear A, Elovic E. Spasticity : diagnosis and management. New York: Demos Medical Pub.; 2011. p. 448, xv.

79. Krause T, Gerbershagen MU, Fiege M, et al. Dantrolene–a review of its pharmacology, therapeutic use and new developments. Anaesthesia 2004;59(4): 364–73.

80. Dressler D, Saberi FA, Barbosa ER. Botulinum toxin: mechanisms of action. Arq Neuropslquiatr 2005;63(1):180–5.

81. Do JG, Choi JH, Park CH, et al. Prevalence and Related Factors for Poststroke Complex Regional Pain Syndrome: A Retrospective Cross-Sectional Cohort Study. Arch Phys Med Rehabil 2022;103(2):274–81.

82. Van Ouwenaller C, Laplace PM, Chantraine A. Painful shoulder in hemiplegia. Arch Phys Med Rehabil 1986;67(1):23–6.

83. Kocabas H, Levendoglu F, Ozerbil OM, et al. Complex regional pain syndrome in stroke patients. Int J Rehabil Res 2007;30(1):33–8.

84. Gokkaya NK, Aras M, Yesiltepe E, et al. Reflex sympathetic dystrophy in hemiplegia. Int J Rehabil Res 2006;29(4):275–9.

85. de Mos M, Sturkenboom MC, Huygen FJ. Current understandings on complex regional pain syndrome. Pain Pract 2009;9(2):86–99.

86. Harden RN, McCabe CS, Goebel A, et al. Complex Regional Pain Syndrome: Practical Diagnostic and Treatment Guidelines, 5th edition. Pain Med. 2022;23(Suppl 1):S1-S53. doi.

87. Harden RN, Oaklander AL, Burton AW, et al. Complex regional pain syndrome: practical diagnostic and treatment guidelines, 4th edition. Pain Med. 2013;14(2):180-229. doi.

88. Shafiee E, MacDermid J, Packham T, et al. The Effectiveness of Rehabilitation Interventions on Pain and Disability for Complex Regional Pain Syndrome: A Systematic Review and Meta-analysis. Clin J Pain 2023;39(2):91–105.

89. Pervane Vural S, Nakipoglu Yuzer GF, Sezgin Ozcan D, et al. Effects of Mirror Therapy in Stroke Patients With Complex Regional Pain Syndrome Type 1: A Randomized Controlled Study. Arch Phys Med Rehabil 2016;97(4):575–81.

90. Duong S, Bravo D, Todd KJ, et al. Treatment of complex regional pain syndrome: an updated systematic review and narrative synthesis. Can J Anaesth 2018;65(6):658–84. Traitement du syndrome douloureux regional complexe : etude systematique actualisee et synthese narrative.

91. Braus DF, Krauss JK, Strobel J. The shoulder-hand syndrome after stroke: a prospective clinical trial. Ann Neurol 1994;36(5):728–33.

92. Kalita J, Vajpayee A, Misra UK. Comparison of prednisolone with piroxicam in complex regional pain syndrome following stroke: a randomized controlled trial. QJM 2006;99(2):89–95.

93. Kalita J, Misra U, Kumar A, et al. Long-term Prednisolone in Post-stroke Complex Regional Pain Syndrome. Pain Physician 2016;19(8):565–74.

94. Eun Young H, Hyeyun K, Sang Hee I. Pamidronate effect compared with a steroid on complex regional pain syndrome type I: Pilot randomised trial. Neth J Med 2016;74(1):30–5.

95. Varenna M, Adami S, Rossini M, et al. Treatment of complex regional pain syndrome type I with neridronate: a randomized, double-blind, placebo-controlled study. Rheumatology 2013;52(3):534–42.

96. Varenna M, Zucchi F, Ghiringhelli D, et al. Intravenous clodronate in the treatment of reflex sympathetic dystrophy syndrome. A randomized, double blind, placebo controlled study. J Rheumatol 2000;27(6):1477–83.

97. Klit H, Finnerup NB, Jensen TS. Central post-stroke pain: clinical characteristics, pathophysiology, and management. Lancet Neurol 2009;8(9):857–68.

98. Bo Z, Jian Y, Yan L, et al. Pharmacotherapies for Central Post-Stroke Pain: A Systematic Review and Network Meta-Analysis. Oxid Med Cell Longev 2022; 2022:3511385.

99. Liampas A, Velidakis N, Georgiou T, et al. Prevalence and Management Challenges in Central Post-Stroke Neuropathic Pain: A Systematic Review and Meta-analysis. Adv Ther 2020;37(7):3278–91.

100. Chen KY, Li RY. Efficacy and safety of different antidepressants and anticonvulsants in central poststroke pain: A network meta-analysis and systematic review. PLoS One 2022;17(10):e0276012.

101. Xu XM, Luo H, Rong BB, et al. Nonpharmacological therapies for central post-stroke pain: A systematic review. Medicine (Baltim) 2020;99(42):e22611.

Pathophysiology, Assessment, and Management of Post-Stroke Cognitive Impairment, Depression, and Fatigue

Abhishek Jaywant, PhD[a,b,c],*, Alexandra Keenan, BA[b]

KEYWORDS

- Cerebrovascular disease • Executive function • Memory • Mood disorder
- Behavior therapy

KEY POINTS

- Post-stroke cognitive impairment, depression, and fatigue are common, persistent, disabling, and require assessment and management to optimize recovery after stroke.
- Management of post-stroke cognitive impairment should include screening, comprehensive neuropsychological assessment, and referral for metacognitive strategy training with consideration for adjunctive computerized cognitive training.
- Management of post-stroke depression should include screening, diagnostic assessment, enhancement of social support, referral for cognitive-behavioral psychotherapy, and consideration of antidepressant medication.
- Management of post-stroke fatigue should include assessment and consideration of cognitive behavioral therapy and behavioral/environmental strategies; preliminary evidence suggests that modafinil may be beneficial.

INTRODUCTION

Cognitive impairment, depression, and fatigue are persistent and disabling sequelae of stroke.[1,2] This review summarizes current knowledge to aid in conceptualization, assessment, and management.

a Department of Psychiatry, Weill Cornell Medicine, 525 East 68th Street, New York, NY 10065, USA; b Department of Rehabilitation Medicine, Weill Cornell Medicine, 525 East 68th Street, New York, NY 10065, USA; c NewYork-Presbyterian Hospital/Weill Cornell Medical Center, 525 East 68th Street, New York, NY 10065, USA
* Corresponding author. 525 East 68th Street, Baker F-1232, New York, NY 10065
E-mail address: abj2006@med.cornell.edu

Phys Med Rehabil Clin N Am 35 (2024) 463–478
https://doi.org/10.1016/j.pmr.2023.06.028
1047-9651/24/© 2023 Elsevier Inc. All rights reserved.

POST-STROKE COGNITIVE IMPAIRMENT
Nature of the Problem

Approximately half of stroke survivors experience post-stroke cognitive impairment (PSCI).[3] Impairments are most common in executive functions, but also frequently occur in memory, spatial attention, and self-awareness.[3,4] There is some evidence that PSCI improves over 6 to 12 months post-stroke,[3,5] though the magnitude of change is likely small.[4] Deficits in language and spatial neglect are more associated with circumscribed lesions in left frontotemporal and right frontoparietal regions, respectively.[6] In contrast, impairment in higher order cognitive abilities such as executive functions arises from disconnection within and between an array of brain networks encompassing cortical and subcortical regions and the white matter pathways that connect them.[6,7] Indeed, measures of network disconnection are often stronger predictors of PSCI than lesion location or size.[6,8]

OBSERVATION/ASSESSMENT/EVALUATION
Screening

Screening should encompass clinician queries, collateral report, and use of objective screening assessments (**Fig. 1**). The Montreal Cognitive Assessment (MoCA)[9] demonstrates relatively strong diagnostic accuracy in identifying PSCI in acute and post-acute stages after stroke.[10,11] For remote assessment, there is a validated 22-point telephone version of the MoCA[12] that omits visually based items. The Brief Memory and Executive Test (BMET)[13] is an alternate screening measure that focuses on executive function and memory, includes multiple speed-dependent tasks, and correlates with everyday functioning and quality of life.[14]

The Oxford Cognitive Screen[15] is a freely available stroke-specific assessment that was developed to screen for impairment in a broad array of cognitive impairments including neglect, apraxia, reading/writing, in addition to attention, memory, and executive functions. It is more sensitive to impairment than the MoCA[16] and is less

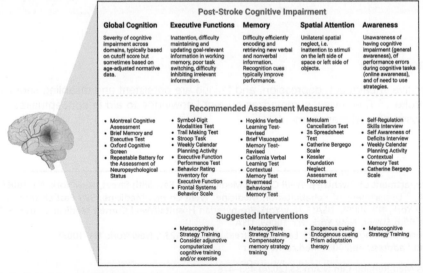

Fig. 1. Common manifestations of post-stroke cognitive impairment, recommended assessment measures, and suggested interventions. (Created with BioRender.)

impacted by aphasia.[15] It has been validated in stroke patients in multiple languages and in individuals with low income and low literacy.[17] A tablet-based version, the Oxford Cognitive Screen-Plus, is also available and has been validated.[18]

Neuropsychologic Assessment

Individuals who screen positive for cognitive impairment benefit from comprehensive neuropsychologic assessment. The National Institute of Neurologic Disorders and Stroke and the Canadian Stroke Network developed consensus guidelines for 30 minute and 60 minute neuropsychologic testing batteries to be used in stroke.[19] In acute inpatient stroke rehabilitation, a modified version of the consensus 30 minute battery that includes greater coverage of executive functions (ie, by adding the Trail Making Test and using the Symbol Digit Modalities Test) is sensitive to cognitive impairment and predicts functional outcomes after accounting for MoCA score.[20] Among specific neuropsychologic tests of the battery, the Symbol Digit Modalities Test is the most sensitive to impairment and had the strongest association with rehabilitation gain and independence in everyday activities at discharge.[20]

Neuropsychologic assessment should include testing for unilateral spatial neglect.[21] In viewer-centered neglect, the left side of space (relative to the observer) is failed to be attended to, whereas in stimulus-centered neglect, the left side of stimuli or objects are neglected regardless of where in space the stimulus is located. Cancellation tests such as the 3s Spreadsheet Test[22] are useful in assessing unilateral spatial neglect and differentiating between egocentric viewer-centered and allocentric stimulus-centered neglect.

Functional Cognitive Assessment

Functional cognitive assessments complement impairment-based neuropsychologic testing by measuring the ability to apply cognitive functions in contexts that closely mirror real-world activities. This provides useful information to guide rehabilitation. Examples that can be used in stroke include the Weekly Calendar Planning Activity,[23] the Multiple Errands Test,[24] and the Executive Functional Performance Test.[25] For unilateral spatial neglect, the Catherine Bergego Scale is a reliable and valid assessment that uses clinician observations to quantify the extent of neglect on everyday activities such as grooming, eating, looking to the left, and finding personal belongings.[26] The Kessler Foundation Neglect Assessment Process is a modification of the Catherine Bergego Scale that provides more detailed and specific administration and scoring instructions.[27]

Assessment of Awareness

Unawareness moderates the association between PSCI and limitations in everyday activities.[28,29] Individuals with PSCI and poor awareness of deficits are less likely to see the need to implement compensatory strategies and less likely to effectively use self-regulation and self-management strategies. Deficits can occur in general awareness and online awareness. General awareness or "metacognitive knowledge" refers to the individual's overall self-perception of their abilities that are not linked to a specific task or situation.[30] General awareness is typically assessed by interview questions that probe whether and to what extent the person has noticed cognitive difficulties in everyday life. The Self-Regulation of Skills Interview[31] can be used to assess awareness.

Deficits also occur in online awareness, which is the awareness of task difficulty, errors, and the need to use compensatory strategies during a cognitively based activity.[32] It can be operationalized and quantified by assessing the difference between estimated performance and actual performance on a task. It can also be assessed by observing whether the individual self-corrects errors during a task or spontaneously verbalizes challenges and/or uses compensatory strategies. The Weekly Calendar Planning Activity can be used to assess the difference between actual accuracy and an individual's perceived accuracy using a brief after-task interview.[33] Relative to age-matched adults, individuals with stroke demonstrate impaired online awareness on the Weekly Calendar Planning Activity as they less frequently self-recognize errors and more frequently overestimate their accuracy.[34]

Therapeutic Options

The American Congress of Rehabilitation Medicine (ACRM)'s Cognitive Rehabilitation Task Force[35] recommends the use of metacognitive strategy training for executive functions, which broadly speaking is the class of interventions with the most compelling evidence in stroke to date. Metacognitive interventions focus on increasing the individual's awareness of cognitive performance and errors, and to self-generate and implement strategies to manage cognitive errors. Metacognitive interventions incorporate goal setting, planning, executing the task/strategy, checking work for errors, and modifying strategies as needed. The evidence for transfer to everyday activities is mixed, and which patients are most likely to respond is still largely unknown.

For memory, compensatory strategy training has demonstrated efficacy.[36] Further, there is evidence for the benefit of assistive technology such as auditory or visual reminders, alarms, and organizational devices, though studies that evaluate these technologies are primarily drawn from the traumatic brain injury literature. There is preliminary evidence that use of a digital calendar smartphone application with mobile reminders may be efficacious.[37]

The above-mentioned interventions target the ability to self-manage and regulate cognitive performance. A related line of research focuses on restorative approaches to treating PSCI, primarily using computerized cognitive training. Current cognitive training paradigms demonstrate mixed evidence for efficacy and transfer to everyday activities. RehaCom is perhaps the most studied program in stroke, but evidence for transfer is mixed.[38–40] The ACRM Cognitive Rehabilitation Taskforce recommends against the standalone use of computerized cognitive training.[35] More research is needed to evaluate targeted and personalized training approaches, as it may be that only a subset of patients derive benefit from cognitive training. Combining computerized cognitive training with metacognitive strategy training is also an important area of future research.[41]

Among additional intervention approaches, use of cholinesterase inhibitors may be a helpful pharmacologic treatment for PSCI.[42] Exercise is also an emerging intervention that may promote neural restoration and rewiring. In a recent trial, individuals with stroke randomized to high intensity interval training demonstrated improvement on a neuropsychologic test of executive function that was sustained at 12 month follow-up.[43]

To date, intervention trials for unilateral spatial neglect have low-quality evidence, are underpowered, and show limited evidence for efficacy in improving functional abilities.[44] In this context, there is evidence for behavioral cueing. Cueing helps the individual to shift their attention to the neglected side. Cues can be both exogenous (highlighted letters/words in a line when reading) and endogenous (eg, therapist cues the individual to search for a specific letter/word or cues the individual to say to themselves "look to the left").[45] Multiple trials have studied prism adaptation therapy, with mixed findings in terms of improving everyday function suggesting that effects may be relatively small and temporary.[46]

POST-STROKE DEPRESSION
Nature of the Problem

Post-stroke depression (PSD) affects 30% of stroke survivors.[47] PSD arises in part from structural and functional changes to brain regions involved in experiencing and regulating emotions, including frontostriatal regions, limbic regions, and white matter pathways.[48,49] Concurrently with these biologic changes, stroke survivors must contend with a sudden loss of function, participation, life roles, and self-identity. In this context, negative thoughts and beliefs, loss of self-esteem, helplessness, and hopelessness can emerge.

OBSERVATION/ASSESSMENT/EVALUATION
Risk Factors

Individuals with pre-existing depression are at higher risk of PSD.[50] Another risk factor is the overall burden of small vessel disease, including white matter hyperintensities, silent lacunar infarcts, and microbleeds.[51,52] Greater stroke severity, functional disability, and cognitive impairment are also risk factors for PSD.[50]

Screening

Patient-reported screening assessments have shown relatively strong diagnostic accuracy, sensitivity, and specificity in identifying PSD[53,54] (Fig. 2, Table 1). Instruments such as the Hospital Anxiety and Depression Scale and the Montgomery Asberg Depression Rating Scale minimize the impact of somatic symptoms, which can overlap between stroke and depression, complicating diagnostic assessment. The 9-item Patient Health Questionnaire is also useful for screening given its free availability, its inclusion of questions asking about all 9 DSM-5 criteria of major depression, and its relatively strong diagnostic accuracy, though caution should be taken in diagnosing PSD in individuals where somatic items are predominantly endorsed. Turner and colleagues[55] provide cutoff points for various screening measures and associated sensitivity and specificity.

Clinical Interview

Clinician interview should focus on key symptoms and their frequency, intensity, and impact on everyday functioning. This enables the clinician to distinguish between PSD

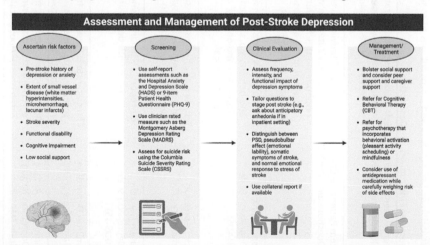

Fig. 2. Recommended approach to assessing and managing post-stroke depression. (Created with BioRender.)

Table 1
Description and advantages and disadvantages of common screening assessments for post-stroke depression

Assessment Instrument	Description	Advantages	Disadvantages
9-item Patient Health Questionnaire (PHQ-9)	Self-report. Respondent rates frequency of each of the 9 symptoms of major depression on a 0–4 scale.	Strong diagnostic accuracy, sensitivity, and specificity. Brief, easy to administer, and freely available.	Somatic items may overlap with physical symptoms of stroke. Anhedonia may be difficult for respondent to gauge during acute stroke hospitalization.
2-item Patient Health Questionnaire (PHQ-2)	Self-report. Abbreviated version of PHQ-9 that includes 2 items in which respondent rates frequency of depressed mood and loss of interest/pleasure on a 0–4 scale.	Very brief, easy to administer, and freely available.	Weaker sensitivity and specificity, and likely too crude to capture relevant clinical information to inform diagnosis. Anhedonia may be difficult for respondent to gauge during acute stroke hospitalization.
Hospital Anxiety and Depression Scale (HADS)	Self-report. 14 items assessing symptoms and behaviors associated with depression and anxiety, rated on a 0–4 Likert-type scale	Strong diagnostic accuracy, sensitivity, and specificity. Brief, easy to administer. Items specifically tailored to hospital setting and to minimize somatic confounds.	Can be used in acute and post-acute stages of stroke. For community dwelling respondents, relatively restricted range of symptoms and behaviors are queried.
Beck Depression Inventory (BDI)	Self-report. 21 items assessing cognitive, affective, and somatic symptoms of depression, rated on a 0–4 Likert-type scale.	Strong sensitivity at acute and post-acute stages, moderately comprehensive assessment of range of depression symptoms.	Risk of misclassification due to inclusion of somatic symptoms.
15-item Geriatric Depression Scale (GDS-15)	Self-report. 15 binary yes/no questions associated with depression.	Research evidence is more limited but does demonstrate strong sensitivity and specificity.	Yes/No responses to questions can result in information that lacks fine-grained conceptualization of key depression symptoms and treatment targets.
Hamilton Depression Rating Scale (HDRS)	Clinician-rated. Presence, frequency, and severity of depression symptoms are rated on a 0–4 point scale.	Strong sensitivity and specificity. Gold-standard outcome in depression clinical trials.	Requires training to administer with fidelity and reliability. Misdiagnosis may occur due to somatic items.
Montgomery Asberg Depression Rating Scale (MADRS)	Clinician-rated. Presence, frequency, and severity of depression symptoms are rated on a 0–7 point scale.	Strong sensitivity and specificity. Minimizes somatic items.	Requires training to administer with fidelity and reliability.

and normative levels of sadness and grief that can occur after a major medical illness such as a stroke. Individuals with PSD present with symptoms that are relatively frequent and not just brief periods of sadness or other fleeting emotional responses to situational stressors. As with other syndromes post-stroke, collateral reports from a caregiver or family member can be crucial in understanding the impact of a patient's symptoms on their behavior and everyday function. In extreme cases, the individual with stroke may minimize their symptoms whereas a caregiver may describe their observation of for example, frequent tearfulness, restricted activity participation, and persistent verbalization of self-critical thoughts.

Depression is a highly heterogeneous condition and after stroke, can present quite differently across individuals. Some individuals may not identify as feeling "depressed" per se, but instead report feeling blue, empty, or irritable. Depressed mood itself is not a necessary criterion for a diagnosis of depression and it is important to ask about loss of interest or pleasure in daily activities. There is evidence that PSD may cluster into 3 distinct subtypes characterized by depressed mood, anxious distress, and apathy.[56]

During the clinical interview, the clinician should take care to distinguish between PSD and pseudobulbar affect (also referred to as emotional lability). This emotional "overflow" can present as a mismatch between the individual's subjective, inner emotional experience and observable behavior. Thus, although tearfulness is associated with PSD, the clinician should not necessarily assume that tearfulness is a specific marker of depression and should always ask about subjective feeling states.

Clinician interviewing for depression can be especially challenging during the acute hospitalization and acute inpatient rehabilitation phase of recovery. Patients may have a difficult time answering a question about anhedonia because they have not had an opportunity to engage in typical activities while hospitalized. The clinician may wish to substitute questions about anticipatory interest/reward instead (eg, does the patient look forward to resuming their activities? Do they feel excited or enthusiastic or another positive emotion when imagining returning to a previously engaged activity?). Note that the transition from inpatient hospitalization to the community is a particularly vulnerable time for the emergence of PSD.[57] Individuals with more severe strokes and who are unmarried (possibly due to the lack of social support from a spouse) are especially vulnerable to depression during this time.[58]

Suicide Risk Assessment

Individuals with stroke have an elevated risk of suicide, particularly in the first year post-stroke.[59] Thus, suicide screening is recommended in individuals with PSD. The Columbia Suicide Severity Rating Scale is a validated, reliable, and freely available instrument with accompanying training that provides an easy-to-use stepped approach to assessing suicidal ideation, intent, plan, and behavior.[60] Individuals with stroke who endorse suicidal ideation should be referred promptly for treatment tailored to the severity of ideation.

THERAPEUTIC OPTIONS
Behavioral Interventions

Helping a patient to identify social supports and engaging in social activities may help in those at risk of PSD or who have mild depression symptoms.[61,62] Peer support interventions such as support groups are also a potentially helpful option for patients with PSD. A meta-analysis of peer support interventions for stroke survivors showed a positive benefit on depression symptoms and functional independence; however, the quality of evidence was rated as low to very low.[63] Providing support and education to caregivers may help to guard against worsening anxiety and depression symptoms in stroke survivors with mild mood disturbances.[64]

Among psychotherapies, cognitive behavioral therapy (CBT) helps the patient to reframe unhelpful thoughts and beliefs, and to decrease avoidance behaviors. CBT has demonstrated efficacy in PSD—both alone and in combination with antidepressant treatment[65] with gains maintained at 3 months.[66] CBT delivered via telemedicine has also shown efficacy in a pilot trial.[67] Behavioral activation is a form of CBT developed specifically for depression that focuses on increasing participation in meaningful, rewarding activities that promote pleasure and/or mastery. An intervention called "CALM" that helps patients with PSD to schedule and engage in pleasant activities has shown efficacy.[68] Relatedly, mindfulness-based interventions promote present moment awareness of thoughts, emotions, and experiences and are also associated with improvement in depression symptoms post-stroke, though effect sizes are small.[69]

Pharmacologic Interventions

Antidepressant medications (eg, selective serotonin reuptake inhibitors) are associated with greater response and remission rates than placebo, although the quality of the evidence was rated as low due to substantial heterogeneity across studies and risk of biases.[70] Prophylactic antidepressant use is associated with lower risk of incident depression and a reduction in depression symptom severity.[71] The risk of side effects—particularly bleeding risk, gastrointestinal side effects, and central nervous system side effects—has been the subject of some controversy. Villa and colleagues[50] reviewed this conflicting literature and summarized it as a slightly increased relative risk of hemorrhage, but a relatively low absolute risk. Other meta-analyses have found an increased risk of gastrointestinal side effects and central nervous system side effects.[70,72] Thus, initiation of antidepressant therapy should be weighed carefully with the possibility of side effects.

Anxiety

Approximately 29% of stroke survivors meeting criteria for an anxiety disorder during the first year after stroke.[73] Among stroke survivors, post-stroke anxiety is indeed associated with depression, as well as with cognitive and motor deficits, fatigue, and lack of social support.[74]

Screening measures may include the anxiety subscale of the Hospital Anxiety and Depression Scale or the 7-item Generalized Anxiety Disorder questionnaire. As with PSD, a careful assessment should distinguish between anxiety that is relatively normative given the psychosocial stress associated with a stroke versus anxiety that is distressing and functionally impairing. The clinician should ask about frequency, intensity, and duration of periods of anxiety. Also asked should be whether anxiety is perceived to be overwhelming and difficult to control. As with PSD, somatic/bodily symptoms of anxiety (muscle tension, sleep disruption, panic symptoms) can overlap with the physical symptoms of stroke. CBT is a gold-standard treatment for anxiety in the general population. In stroke, CBT shows a large effect size in treating post-stroke anxiety.[66] Remotely delivered CBT has shown benefit in reducing post-stroke anxiety for remotely delivered CBT compared with relaxation training.[67]

POST-STROKE FATIGUE
Nature of the Problem

Approximately 50% of stroke survivors experience post-stroke fatigue (PSF).[75] PSF can manifest as feelings of being tired and having lack of energy, exhaustion after physical/mental activity, and avoidance of physical or mental effort.[76] Depression, anxiety, sleep disturbances, diabetes mellitus, medical comorbidity, greater disability, and female sex are all associated with PSF.[77] In contrast, PSF is not associated with stroke type or severity, infarct volume, or brain atrophy indices.[78] The pathophysiology of PSF may include loss in structural and functional connectivity in prefrontal regions.[79]

Observation/Assessment/Evaluation

Clinicians should routinely assess for fatigue during clinical encounters (**Fig. 3**). **Fig. 3** displays assessment and management approaches. Useful patient-reported outcome measures are the Fatigue Severity Scale, Visual Analog Scale-Fatigue, and the Short Form-36 Vitality scale; however, these scales have limitations because they were not developed specifically for individuals with stroke, inadequately assess fatigue onset and duration, do not ask about coping strategies, and do not ask about fluctuations or diurnal variations in fatigue.[80] Thus, it is important for the clinician to ask how quickly after an activity fatigue begins, how long it tends to last (and relatedly how fast fatigue alleviates with rest, if at all), how the individual has tried to manage fatigue, and whether and how feelings of fatigue fluctuate during the day (diurnal variation). Clinicians should also ask about mental or cognitive fatigue, which can be supplemented by a patient-reported outcome measure, the Mental Fatigue Scale.

Therapeutic Options

There is limited evidence for the efficacy of interventions to manage PSF, though recent studies have shown promise of CBT, modafinil, and graded activity increases. CBT strategies include pacing activities with planned rest breaks, engaging in valued activities that are chosen and modified based on energy levels, scheduling high energy activities

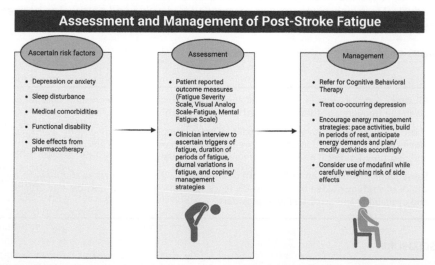

Fig. 3. Suggested approach to assessing and managing post-stroke fatigue. (Created with BioRender.)

for after a period of rest, preplanning rest prior to energy demanding activities, modifying the environment, and restructuring tasks to minimize physical effort, keeping a daily routine in which energy demands are anticipated and planned for, reframing unhelpful thoughts and beliefs about fatigue and rest, and optimizing diet, nutrition, and sleep.[76,81] A recent pilot study found that CBT was associated with reduced fatigue with gains maintained at 2-month follow-up, though the sample included only 15 participants and no active control condition.[81] Another study evaluated the combination of CBT and graded activity training in which participants engaged in treadmill walking and strength training starting at 40% of maximum heartrate/strength and progressing to 70% based on tolerance. A greater proportion of participants who received the combination of CBT and graded activity training experienced a clinically meaningful reduction in fatigue compared with those who received CBT alone.[82] There is emerging evidence that mindfulness may help improve mental fatigue.[83]

In a small study of 36 participants, modafinil—a pharmacologic agent that promotes arousal and wakefulness—was associated with improved fatigue relative to placebo.[84] Alleviation of fatigue in the modafinil group was associated with increased functional connectivity in the hippocampus and decreased connectivity in the somatosensory, parietal, and temporal cortex.[85] Another small study of 41 participants demonstrated that modafinil was associated with improved fatigue on one patient-reported outcome measure but not another.[86] Fluoxetine has not shown benefit for fatigue.[87]

SUMMARY AND FUTURE DIRECTIONS

Post-stroke cognitive impairment, depression, and fatigue emerge from complex pathophysiologic mechanisms. They are underrecognized and undertreated. Clinicians should routinely screen for the presence of cognitive impairment, depression, and fatigue at all stages post-stroke. Assessment should entail screening measures, patient-reported outcome measures, and clinician interviews. Both behavioral and pharmacologic interventions can help with management. Unfortunately, much of the literature on interventions is hampered by studies with small samples, inadequate control conditions, and a high risk of bias. Effect sizes of interventions tend to be small to medium at the group level, which may reflect the heterogeneity of stroke and variability of treatment benefits across individuals. More high-quality studies are needed to develop and personalize interventions that are optimally effective and tailored to the individual.

CLINICS CARE POINTS

- All stroke survivors should be screened for cognitive impairment, depression, and fatigue given the frequency of these neuropsychiatric complications.
- Those who screen positive should undergo more comprehensive diagnostic assessment, ideally using a combination of patient-reported outcome measures, clinician interview, and neuropsychological assessment if relevant and available.
- Subsequent treatment can include both pharmacologic and behavioral strategies with the choice of strategy guided by available evidence, careful weighing of possible side effects, and availability and accessability of providers.

DISCLOSURE

The authors have no conflicts to declare. A. Jaywant receives salary support from the National Institute of Mental Health, United States grant K23MH129849.

REFERENCES

1. Laakso HM, Hietanen M, Melkas S, et al. Executive function subdomains are associated with post-stroke functional outcome and permanent institutionalization. Eur J Neurol 2019;26(3):546–52.

2. Kapoor A, Lanctot KL, Bayley M, et al. Screening for Post-Stroke Depression and Cognitive Impairment at Baseline Predicts Long-Term Patient-Centered Outcomes After Stroke. J Geriatr Psychiatr Neurol 2019;32(1):40–8.

3. Turunen KEA, Laari SPK, Kauranen TV, et al. Domain-specific cognitive recovery after first-ever stroke: A 2-year follow-up. J Int Neuropsychol Soc 2018;24(2):117–27.

4. Ebaid D, Bird LJ, McCambridge LJE, et al. Mood and Cognitive Trajectories Over the First Year after Mild Ischemic Stroke. J Stroke Cerebrovasc Dis 2022;31(4):106323.

5. Lo JW, Crawford JD, Desmond DW, et al. Long-Term Cognitive Decline After Stroke: An Individual Participant Data Meta-Analysis. Stroke 2022;53(4):1318–27.

6. Siegel JS, Ramsey LE, Snyder AZ, et al. Disruptions of network connectivity predict impairment in multiple behavioral domains after stroke. Proc Natl Acad Sci USA 2016;113(30):E4367–76.

7. Lim JS, Lee JJ, Woo CW. Post-Stroke Cognitive Impairment: Pathophysiological Insights into Brain Disconnectome from Advanced Neuroimaging Analysis Techniques. J Stroke 2021;23(3):297–311.

8. Kuceyeski A, Navi BB, Kamel H, et al. Structural Connectome Disruption at Baseline Predicts 6-Months Post-Stroke Outcome. Hum Brain Mapp 2016;37:2587–601.

9. Nasreddine Z, Phillips N, Bédirian V, et al. The Montreal Cognitive Assessment, MoCA: a brief screening tool for mild cognitive impairment. J Am Geriatr Soc 2005;53(4):695–9.

10. Jaywant A, Toglia J, Gunning FM, et al. The diagnostic accuracy of the Montreal Cognitive Assessment in inpatient stroke rehabilitation. Neuropsychol Rehabil 2017;29(8):1163–76.

11. Pendlebury ST, Mariz J, Bull L, et al. MoCA, ACE-R, and MMSE versus the National Institute of Neurological Disorders and Stroke-Canadian Stroke Network vascular cognitive impairment harmonization standards neuropsychological battery after TIA and stroke. Stroke 2012;43(2):464–9.

12. Zietemann V, Kopczak A, Müller C, et al. Validation of the Telephone Interview of Cognitive Status and Telephone Montreal Cognitive Assessment Against Detailed Cognitive Testing and Clinical Diagnosis of Mild Cognitive Impairment After Stroke. Stroke 2017;48(11):2952–7.

13. Brookes RL, Hollocks MJ, Khan U, et al. The Brief Memory and Executive Test (BMET) for detecting vascular cognitive impairment in small vessel disease: A validation study. BMC Med 2015;13(1):1–8.

14. Hollocks MJ, Brookes R, Morris RG, et al. Associations between the Brief Memory and Executive Test (BMET), Activities of Daily Living, and Quality of Life in Patients with Cerebral Small Vessel Disease. J Int Neuropsychol Soc 2016;22(5):561–9.

15. Demeyere N, Riddoch MJ, Slavkova ED, et al. The Oxford Cognitive Screen (OCS): Validation of a stroke-specific short cognitive screening tool. Psychol Assess 2015;27(3):883–94.

16. Webb SS, Hobden G, Roberts R, et al. Validation of the UK English Oxford cognitive screen-plus in sub-acute and chronic stroke survivors. Eur Stroke J 2015; 7(4):476–86.

17. Humphreys GW, Duta MD, Montana L, et al. Cognitive Function in Low-Income and Low-Literacy Settings: Validation of the Tablet-Based Oxford Cognitive Screen in the Health and Aging in Africa: A Longitudinal Study of an INDEPTH Community in South Africa (HAALSI). GERONB 2017;72(1):38–50.

18. Demeyere N, Haupt M, Webb SS, et al. Introducing the tablet-based Oxford Cognitive Screen-Plus (OCS-Plus) as an assessment tool for subtle cognitive impairments. Sci Rep 2021;11(1):8000.

19. Hachinski V, Iadecola C, Petersen RC, et al. National Institute of Neurological Disorders and Stroke-Canadian Stroke Network vascular cognitive impairment harmonization standards. Stroke 2006;37(9):2220–41.

20. Jaywant A, Toglia J, Gunning FM, et al. The clinical utility of a 30-minute neuropsychological assessment battery in inpatient stroke rehabilitation. J Neurol Sci 2018;390(April):54–62.

21. Durfee AZ, Hillis AE. Unilateral Spatial Neglect Recovery Poststroke. Stroke 2023; 54(1):10–9.

22. Chen P, Toglia J. The 3s Spreadsheet Test version 2 for assessing egocentric viewer-centered and allocentric stimulus-centered spatial neglect. Appl Neuropsychol: Adult 2022;29(6):1369–79.

23. Toglia J. Weekly calendar planning activity (WCPA): a performance test of executive function. North Bethesda, MD: AOTA Press; 2015.

24. Clark AJ, Anderson ND, Nalder E, et al. Reliability and construct validity of a revised Baycrest Multiple Errands Test. Neuropsychol Rehabil 2017;27(5): 667–84.

25. Baum CM, Connor LT, Morrison T, et al. Reliability, validity, and clinical utility of the Executive Function Performance Test: A measure of executive function in a sample of people With stroke. Am J Occup Ther 2008;62(4):446–55.

26. Azouvi P, Olivier S, de Montety G, et al. Behavioral assessment of unilateral neglect: Study of the psychometric properties of the Catherine Bergego Scale. Arch Phys Med Rehabil 2003;84(1):51–7.

27. Chen P, Chen CC, Hreha K, et al. Kessler Foundation Neglect Assessment Process Uniquely Measures Spatial Neglect During Activities of Daily Living. Arch Phys Med Rehabil 2015;96(5):869–76.e1.

28. Ownsworth T, Clare L. The association between awareness deficits and rehabilitation outcome following acquired brain injury. Clin Psychol Rev 2006;26(6): 783–95.

29. Villalobos D, Caperos JM, A Bilbao, et al. Self-awareness moderates the association between executive dysfunction and functional independence after acquired brain injury. Arch Clin Neuropsychol 2020;35(7):1059–68.

30. Toglia J. The Dynamic Interactional Model and the Multicontext Approach. In: Katz N, Toglia J, editors. Cogn. Occup. Across lifesp. model. Interv. Occup. Ther. North Bethesda, MD: American Occupational Therapy Association; 2018. p. 355–85.

31. Ownsworth TL, Mcfarland K, Young RM. Development and standardization of the Self-Regulation Skills Interview (SRSI): A new clinical assessment tool for acquired brain injury. Clin Neuropsychol 2000;14(1):76–92.

32. Toglia J, Foster ER. The multicontext approach to cognitive rehabilitation: a metacognitive strategy intervention to optimize functional cognition. Columbus, OH: Gatekeeper Press; 2021.

33. Arora C, Frantz C, Toglia J. Awareness of performance on a functional cognitive performance based assessment across the adult lifespan. Front Psychol 2021; 12(753016). https://doi.org/10.3389/fpsyg.2021.753016.

34. Jaywant A, Arora C, Lussier A, et al. Impaired performance on a cognitively-based instrumental activities of daily living task, the 10-Item Weekly Calendar Planning Activity, in individuals with stroke undergoing acute inpatient rehabilitation. Front Neurol 2021;12(July). https://doi.org/10.3389/fneur.2021.704775.

35. Cicerone KD, Goldin Y, Ganci K, et al. Evidence-Based Cognitive Rehabilitation: Systematic Review of the Literature From 2009 Through 2014. Arch Phys Med Rehabil 2019;100(8):1515–33.

36. Miller LA, Radford K. Testing the effectiveness of group-based memory rehabilitation in chronic stroke patients. Neuropsychol Rehabil 2014;24(5):721–37.

37. Andreassen M, Danielsson H, Hemmingsson H, et al. An interactive digital calendar with mobile phone reminders (RemindMe) for people with cognitive impairment: A pilot randomized controlled trial. Scand J Occup Ther 2022;29(4): 270–81.

38. Nie P, Liu F, Lin S, et al. The effects of computer-assisted cognitive rehabilitation on cognitive impairment after stroke: A systematic review and meta-analysis. J Clin Nurs 2022;31(9–10):1136–48.

39. Veisi-Pirkoohi S, Hassani-Abharian P, Kazemi R, et al. Efficacy of RehaCom cognitive rehabilitation software in activities of daily living, attention and response control in chronic stroke patients. J Clin Neurosci 2020;71:101–7.

40. Yoo C, Yong MH, Chung J, et al. Effect of computerized cognitive rehabilitation program on cognitive function and activities of living in stroke patients. J Phys Ther Sci 2015;27:2487–9.

41. Jaywant A, Mautner L, Waldman R, et al. Feasibility and Acceptability of a Remotely Delivered Executive Function Intervention That Combines Computerized Cognitive Training and Metacognitive Strategy Training in Chronic Stroke. IJERPH 2023;20(9):5714.

42. Kim JO, Lee SJ, Pyo JS. Effect of acetylcholinesterase inhibitors on post-stroke cognitive impairment and vascular dementia: A meta-analysis. In: Ginsberg SD, editor. PLoS One 2020;15(2):e0227820.

43. Gjellesvik TI, Becker F, Tjønna AE, et al. Effects of High-Intensity Interval Training After Stroke (The HIIT Stroke Study) on Physical and Cognitive Function: A Multicenter Randomized Controlled Trial. Arch Phys Med Rehabil 2021;102(9): 1683–91.

44. Longley V, Hazelton C, Heal C, et al. Interventions for Spatial Neglect After Stroke or Nonprogressive Brain Injury: A Cochrane Systematic Review. Stroke 2021; 52(9). https://doi.org/10.1161/STROKEAHA.121.036590.

45. Turgut N, Möller L, Dengler K, et al. Adaptive Cueing Treatment of Neglect in Stroke Patients Leads to Improvements in Activities of Daily Living: A Randomized Controlled, Crossover Trial. Neurorehabil Neural Repair 2018;32(11):988–98.

46. Li J, Li L, Yang Y, et al. Effects of Prism Adaptation for Unilateral Spatial Neglect After Stroke: A Systematic Review and Meta-Analysis. Am J Phys Med Rehabil 2021;100(6):584–91.

47. Towfighi A, Ovbiagele B, El Husseini N, et al. Poststroke Depression: A scientific statement for healthcare professionals from the American Heart Association/ American Stroke Association. Stroke 2016;47:1–15.

48. Shen XY, Fan ZX, Wang L, et al. Altered white matter microstructure in patients with post-stroke depression detected by diffusion kurtosis imaging. Neurol Sci 2019;40:2097–103.

49. Jaywant A, DelPonte L, Kanellopoulos D, et al. The Structural and Functional Neuroanatomy of Post-Stroke Depression and Executive Dysfunction: A Review of Neuroimaging Findings and Implications for Treatment. J Geriatr Psychiatry Neurol 2022;35(1):3–11.

50. Villa RF, Ferrari F, Moretti A. Post-stroke depression: Mechanisms and pharmacological treatment. Pharmacology & Therapeutics 2018;184:131–44.

51. Zhang X, Tang Y, Xie Y, et al. Total magnetic resonance imaging burden of cerebral small-vessel disease is associated with post-stroke depression in patients with acute lacunar stroke. Eur J Neurol 2017;24(2):374–80.

52. Zhang F, Ping Y, Jin X, et al. White matter hyperintensities and post-stroke depression: A systematic review and meta-analysis. J Affect Disord 2023;320: 370–80.

53. Meader N, Moe-Byrne T, Llewellyn A, et al. Screening for poststroke major depression: a meta-analysis of diagnostic validity studies. J Neurol Neurosurg Psychiatr 2014;85(2):198–206.

54. Kang HJ, Stewart R, Kim JM, et al. Comparative validity of depression assessment scales for screening poststroke depression. J Affect Disord 2013; 147(1–3):186–91.

55. Turner A, Hambridge J, White J, et al. Depression Screening in Stroke: A Comparison of Alternative Measures With the Structured Diagnostic Interview for the Diagnostic and Statistical Manual of Mental Disorders, Fourth Edition (Major Depressive Episode) as Criterion Standard. Stroke 2012;43(4):1000–5.

56. Kanellopoulos D, Wilkins V, Avari J, et al. Dimensions of Poststroke Depression and Neuropsychological Deficits in Older Adults. Am J Geriatr Psychiatr 2020; 28(7):764–71.

57. Fournier LE, Beauchamp JES, Zhang X, et al. Assessment of the Progression of Poststroke Depression in Ischemic Stroke Patients Using the Patient Health Questionnaire-9. J Stroke Cerebrovasc Dis 2020;29(4):104561.

58. Strong B, Fritz MC, Dong L, et al. Changes in PHQ-9 depression scores in acute stroke patients shortly after returning home. In: Gall S, editor. PLoS One 2021; 16(11):e0259806.

59. Vyas MV, Wang JZ, Gao MM, et al. Association Between Stroke and Subsequent Risk of Suicide: A Systematic Review and Meta-Analysis. Stroke 2021;52(4): 1460–4.

60. Posner K, Brown GK, Stanley B, et al. The Columbia–Suicide Severity Rating Scale: Initial Validity and Internal Consistency Findings From Three Multisite Studies With Adolescents and Adults. Aust J Pharm 2011;168(12):1266–77.

61. Lin FH, Yih DN, Shih FM, et al. Effect of social support and health education on depression scale scores of chronic stroke patients. Medicine 2019;98(44): e17667.

62. Volz M, Möbus J, Letsch C, et al. The influence of early depressive symptoms, social support and decreasing self-efficacy on depression 6 months post-stroke. J Affect Disord 2016;206:252–5.

63. Wan X, Chau JPC, Mou H, et al. Effects of peer support interventions on physical and psychosocial outcomes among stroke survivors: A systematic review and meta-analysis. Int J Nurs Stud 2021;121:104001.

64. Kang K, Li S. A WeChat-based caregiver education program improves satisfaction of stroke patients and caregivers, also alleviates poststroke cognitive impairment and depression: A randomized, controlled study. Medicine 2022;101(27): e29603.

65. Wang SB, Wang YY, Zhang QE, et al. Cognitive behavioral therapy for post-stroke depression: A meta-analysis. J Affect Disord 2018;235(March):589–96.
66. Ahrens J, Shao R, Blackport D, et al. Cognitive -behavioral therapy for managing depressive and anxiety symptoms after stroke: a systematic review and meta-analysis. Top Stroke Rehabil 2023;30(4):368–83.
67. Chun HYY, Carson AJ, Tsanas A, et al. Telemedicine Cognitive Behavioral Therapy for Anxiety After Stroke: Proof-of-Concept Randomized Controlled Trial. Stroke 2020;51(8):2297–306.
68. Thomas SA, Walker MF, Macniven JA, et al. Communication and Low Mood (CALM): a randomized controlled trial of behavioural therapy for stroke patients with aphasia. Clin Rehabil 2012;27(5):398–408.
69. Tao S, Geng Y, Li M, et al. Effectiveness of mindfulness-based stress reduction and mindfulness-based cognitive therapy on depression in poststroke patients- A systematic review and meta-analysis of randomized controlled trials. J Psychosom Res 2022;163:111071.
70. Allida S, Cox KL, Hsieh CF, et al. Pharmacological, psychological, and non-invasive brain stimulation interventions for treating depression after stroke. Cochrane database of systematic reviews 2020. https://doi.org/10.1002/14651858. CD003437.pub4. Published online January 28.
71. Cao JX, Liu L, Sun YT, et al. Escitalopram improves neural functional prognosis and endothelial dysfunction in patients with acute cerebral infarction. RNN 2020;38(5):385–93.
72. Kalbouneh HM, Toubasi AA, Albustanji FH, et al. Safety and Efficacy of SSRIs in Improving Poststroke Recovery: A Systematic Review and Meta-Analysis. JAHA 2022;11(13):e025868.
73. Rafsten L, Danielsson A, Sunnerhagen K. Anxiety after stroke: A systematic review and meta-analysis. J Rehabil Med 2018;50(9):769–78.
74. Sanner Beauchamp JE, Casameni Montiel T, Cai C, et al. A Retrospective Study to Identify Novel Factors Associated with Post-stroke Anxiety. J Stroke Cerebrovasc Dis 2020;29(2):104582.
75. Cumming TB, Packer M, Kramer SF, et al. The prevalence of fatigue after stroke: A systematic review and meta-analysis. Int J Stroke 2016;11(9):968–77.
76. Lanctôt KL, Lindsay MP, Smith EE, et al. Canadian Stroke Best Practice Recommendations: Mood, Cognition and Fatigue following Stroke, 6th edition update 2019. Int J Stroke 2020;15(6):668–88.
77. Zhang S, Cheng S, Zhang Z, et al. Related risk factors associated with post-stroke fatigue: a systematic review and meta-analysis. Neurol Sci 2021;42(4):1463–71.
78. Cotter G, Salah Khlif M, Bird L, et al. Post-stroke fatigue is associated with resting state posterior hypoactivity and prefrontal hyperactivity. Int J Stroke 2022;17(8): 906–13.
79. Schaechter JD, Kim M, Hightower BG, et al. Disruptions in Structural and Functional Connectivity Relate to Poststroke Fatigue. Brain Connect 2023;13(1):15–27.
80. Skogestad IJ, Kirkevold M, Indredavik B, et al. Lack of content overlap and essential dimensions – A review of measures used for post-stroke fatigue. J Psychosom Res 2019;124:109759.
81. Nguyen S, Wong D, McKay A, et al. Cognitive behavioural therapy for post-stroke fatigue and sleep disturbance: a pilot randomised controlled trial with blind assessment. Neuropsychol Rehabil 2019;29(5):723–38.
82. Zedlitz AMEE, Rietveld TCM, Geurts AC, et al. Cognitive and Graded Activity Training Can Alleviate Persistent Fatigue After Stroke: A Randomized, Controlled Trial. Stroke 2012;43(4):1046–51.

83. Johansson B, Bjuhr H, Rönnbäck L. Mindfulness-based stress reduction (MBSR) improves long-term mental fatigue after stroke or traumatic brain injury. Brain Inj 2012;26(13–14):1621–8.
84. Bivard A, Lillicrap T, Krishnamurthy V, et al. MIDAS (Modafinil in Debilitating Fatigue After Stroke): A Randomized, Double-Blind, Placebo-Controlled, Cross-Over Trial. Stroke 2017;48(5):1293–8.
85. Visser MM, Goodin P, Parsons MW, et al. Modafinil treatment modulates functional connectivity in stroke survivors with severe fatigue. Sci Rep 2019;9(1):9660.
86. Poulsen MB, Damgaard B, Zerahn B, et al. Modafinil May Alleviate Poststroke Fatigue: A Randomized, Placebo-Controlled, Double-Blinded Trial. Stroke 2015; 46(12):3470–7.
87. Hankey GJ, Hackett ML, Almeida OP, et al. Twelve-Month Outcomes of the AF-FINITY Trial of Fluoxetine for Functional Recovery After Acute Stroke: AFFINITY Trial Steering Committee on Behalf of the AFFINITY Trial Collaboration. Stroke 2021;52(8):2502–9.

Moving?

Make sure your subscription moves with you!

To notify us of your new address, find your **Clinics Account Number** (located on your mailing label above your name), and contact customer service at:

Email: journalscustomerservice-usa@elsevier.com

800-654-2452 (subscribers in the U.S. & Canada)
314-447-8871 (subscribers outside of the U.S. & Canada)

Fax number: 314-447-8029

Elsevier Health Sciences Division
Subscription Customer Service
3251 Riverport Lane
Maryland Heights, MO 63043

Printed and bound by CPI Group (UK) Ltd, Croydon, CR0 4YY

03/10/2024

01040471-0007